The Early Intervention Teaming Handbook

The Early Intervention Teaming Handbook
The Primary Service Provider Approach

Second Edition

by

M'Lisa L. Shelden, PT, Ph.D.
Department of Physical Therapy
Wichita State University
Wichita, Kansas

and

Dathan D. Rush, Ed.D., CCC-SLP
Family, Infant and Preschool Program
J. Iverson Riddle Developmental Center
Morganton, North Carolina

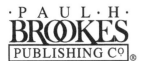
·P·A·U·L·H·
BROOKES
PUBLISHING Co ®

Baltimore • London • Sydney

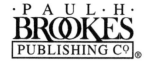

Paul H. Brookes Publishing Co.
Post Office Box 10624
Baltimore, Maryland 21285-0624
USA

www.brookespublishing.com

Typeset by Progressive Publishing Services, York, Pennsylvania.
Manufactured in the United States of America by Vicks, Yorkville, New York.

The individuals described in this book are composites or real people whose situations are masked and are based on the authors' experiences. In all instances, names and identifying details have been changed to protect confidentiality.

Library of Congress Cataloging-in-Publication Data

Names: Shelden, M'Lisa L., author. | Rush, Dathan D., author.
Title: The early intervention teaming handbook: the primary service
  provider approach / M'Lisa L. Shelden and Dathan D. Rush.
Description: Second edition. | Baltimore, Maryland: Paul H. Brookes
  Publishing Co., [2022] | Includes bibliographical references and index.
Identifiers: LCCN 2021038374 (print) | LCCN 2021038375 (ebook) |
  ISBN 9781681255002 (paperback) | ISBN 9781681255019 (epub) |
  ISBN 9781681255026 (pdf)
Subjects: LCSH: Children with disabilities—Education (Early
  childhood)—Handbooks, manuals, etc. | Early childhood special
  education—Handbooks, manuals
Classification: LCC LC4019.3.S54 2022 (print) | LCC LC4019.3 (ebook) |
  DDC 371.9—dc23
LC record available at https://lccn.loc.gov/2021038374
LC ebook record available at https://lccn.loc.gov/2021038375

British Library Cataloguing in Publication data are available from the British Library.

2026   2025   2024   2023   2022

10   9   8   7   6   5   4   3   2   1

Contents

About the Downloads

Purchasers of this book may download, print, and/or photocopy blank forms for professional and educational use.

To access the materials that come with this book:

1. Go to the Brookes Download Hub: http://downloads.brookespublishing.com

2. Register to create an account (or log in with an existing account)

3. Filter or search for the book title *The Early Intervention Teaming Handbook: The Primary Service Provider Approach, Second Edition*

About the Authors

M'Lisa L. Shelden, PT, Ph.D., Department of Physical Therapy, Wichita State University, Kansas

Dr. Shelden has a doctoral degree in special education from the University of Oklahoma. She also has a bachelor's degree in physical therapy from the University of Oklahoma Health Sciences Center and a master's degree in early childhood special education from the University of Oklahoma. Dr. Shelden currently serves as the Chair and Program Director of the Department of Physical Therapy in the College of Health Professions at Wichita State University in Wichita, Kansas. She and Dr. Rush provide ongoing technical assistance to statewide early intervention programs to implement evidence-based early intervention practices in natural settings. Dr. Shelden has over 30 years of experience as a physical therapist and special educator. In addition, Dr. Shelden received a 2000 National Institute on Disabilities and Rehabilitation Research Mary E. Switzer Merit Fellowship. She is a graduate fellow of ZERO TO THREE: National Center for Infants, Toddlers, and Families. Dr. Shelden has coauthored several articles related to early intervention teamwork, writing individualized family service plans (IFSPs), coaching, and supporting young children with disabilities and their families in natural learning environments. She has also written a chapter related to physical therapy personnel preparation and service delivery and coauthored a book titled *Physical Therapy Under IDEA* (McEwen, Arnold, Jones, & Shelden; American Physical Therapy Association, Section on Pediatrics, 2000). Dr. Shelden coauthored *The Early Childhood Coaching Handbook, Second Edition* (Rush; Paul H. Brookes Publishing Co., 2020) as well as a chapter on using a primary coach approach to teaming in *Working with Families of Young Children with Special Needs* (McWilliam; Guilford Press, 2010). Dr. Shelden has made numerous presentations nationally on the topics related to IFSP development and implementation, transition, inclusion, evaluation and assessment, coaching, primary service provider approach to teaming, and natural learning environment practices.

Dathan D. Rush, Ed.D., CCC-SLP, Family, Infant and Preschool Program, J. Iverson Riddle Developmental Center, Morganton, North Carolina

Dr. Rush, has a doctoral degree in child and family studies from Nova Southeastern University, Fort Lauderdale, Florida, and a master's degree in speech-language pathology from Oklahoma State University. Dr. Rush is currently Director/Researcher at the Family, Infant and Preschool Program in Morganton, North Carolina. He provides ongoing technical assistance to statewide early intervention programs to implement evidence-based early intervention practices in natural settings. Dr. Rush previously served as Clinical Assistant Professor at the University of Oklahoma Health Sciences Center, teaching early childhood intervention in the graduate program. He has more than 30 years of experience as a practitioner and early intervention program director and has managed a number of training contracts with various state agencies and organizations. He is a former editorial board member of Infants and Young Children and has published articles in the areas of coaching families in early intervention, in-service training, and teaming in early intervention. He is a past president and former executive council member of the Oklahoma Speech-Language-Hearing Association.

Dr. Rush has presented numerous workshops nationally on topics related to writing and implementing IFSPs, team building, using a primary service provider approach to teaming, coaching, and supporting young children with disabilities and their families in natural learning environments. Dr. Rush has also coauthored *The Early Childhood Coaching Handbook, Second Edition* (Shelden; Paul H. Brookes Publishing Co., 2020) as well as a chapter on using a primary coach approach to teaming in *Working with Families of Young Children with Special Needs* (McWilliam; Guilford Press, 2010).

Foreword

The *Early Intervention Teaming Handbook* sits on the shelves in many early intervention programs across the United States. Professionals have been drawn to the promise of guidance about teaming, with a certain knowledge that our business as usual might or might not contribute to teamwork (Bailey, McWilliam, & Winton, 1992). In community-based programs, where we endorse inter-agency collaboration—and where the fee-for-service, vendor model might prevail—we sometimes have plans with so-called teams of people from different agencies, including private vendors, on the individualized plan. Do these professionals talk to each other? Do they have access to each other's notes? Do they see families at similar frequencies?

Shelden and Rush, in this new edition, bring clarity to how services should be provided to build the capacity of parents and child care teachers, to have professionals working together, to streamline supports to children and families, and to promote relationships between caregivers and their early intervention (Birth to 3) professionals.

THE NEW CONTEXT

Since the first edition of this landmark book, I am astonished at two diametrically opposed phenomena: how much has changed and how little has changed. The field of early intervention seems aware of the importance of a primary service provider (PSP) approach: It shows up in the now-classic "Agreed-Upon Mission and Key Principles for Providing Early Intervention in Natural Environments" (Workgroup on Principles and Practices in the Natural Environment, 2008) and in the *DEC Recommended Practices* for teaming (Division for Early Childhood, 2014). Yet, across the country, we still see redundant, duplicative, confusing service pages on individualized family service plans. Shelden and Rush and others among us have beaten the bushes, raising awareness about the futility of three problems in service delivery related to the PSP approach. First, multidisciplinary service delivery tends to focus on a discipline-specific visit, with the professional addressing one area of development. Unfortunately, a corollary problem is that this area of development might not even be related to the child's *functioning* in everyday routines. Second, multidisciplinary service delivery tends not to include teamwork. Each person does his or her own thing and does not consult with others. Third, multidisciplinary service delivery misleads caregivers into thinking that young children learn during their early intervention sessions rather than between sessions. This second edition reiterates the need for the PSP approach and updates the rationale and resources available to help practitioners, administrators, and professional-development providers.

FIDELITY

Since the first edition, the term fidelity is tossed around as though it were an end in itself: "We need to do this to fidelity." *Fidelity* means faithfulness, so the question is faithful to what? As Dunst et al. (2013) have explained, fidelity is to procedures as planned or as intended by the purveyor. We therefore need a measure of this fidelity, such as performance checklists (Boavida, Akers, McWilliam, & Jung, 2015; Casey & McWilliam, 2011; Dunst, 2017). Shelden and Rush provide four checklists, for 1) preparing for a team-based approach, 2) using a primary service provider, 3) coordinating joint visits, and 4) conducting team meetings. I have long maintained that checklists serve three purposes: 1) to describe a practice, 2) to serve as a platform for feedback during training (coaching), and 3) to collect data on fidelity to a model. Shelden and Rush are clearly concerned with helping the field distinguish between claimants to implementing a practice (e.g., "Yeah, sure, I use the PSP approach") and practitioners who can document with checklists or other data that they are using the practice "to fidelity."

THREATS, TRUTH, TEAMING

These three Ts are intertwined. Among the threats to the PSP approach are a reluctance of some professionals to embrace the four foundational components described here: role expectation, role gap, role overlap, and role assistance. Delving into these interdependent components, described herein, will help understand the perceived threats. The myths about the PSP approach persist, and Shelden and Rush (2001) have spent 20 years differentiating between the myths and the truths about providing early intervention in natural environments, including the primary coach/service provider approach.

One of the persistent myths (maybe all myths, by definition, are persistent) is that the PSP is one person, from one discipline, obviously, working with the family. This is the maverick or sole service provider approach, which is emphatically what is not described in this book. The book is, after all, a *Teaming Handbook*. When I was a young early interventionist in Johnston County, North Carolina, our little team of three contracted with an occupational therapist, a physical therapist, and a speech-language pathologist, who would separately venture into the wilds of Johnston County, while we whisked them around from one family to another, sapping their knowledge and strategies. Between their joint visits (see the chapter in this book on joint visits), we supported the family in carrying out strategies. This was the best professional development I ever received: It was straight from experts in different fields, applied to children and families I really cared about, and these experts ensured that families and I had a good grasp on what to do and why. Shelden and Rush continue to re-envision the early intervention team, from a bunch of signatures on the service page to a functioning, collaborative team.

This second edition provides the field with the rationale for the PSP approach, descriptions of how the approach works, and tools to put the approach into practice and to teach it to others.

Robin A. McWilliam, Ph.D.
The University of Alabama

REFERENCES

Bailey, D. B., McWilliam, P. J., & Winton, P. J. (1992). Building family-centered practices in early intervention: A team-based model for change. *Infants and young children, 5,* 73–82.

Boavida, T., Akers, K., McWilliam, R. A., & Jung, L. A. (2015). Rasch analysis of the Routines-Based Interview Implementation Checklist. *Infants & Young Children, 28,* 237–247. doi:10.1097/IYC.0000000000000041

Casey, A. M., & McWilliam, R. A. (2011). The impact of checklist-based training on teachers' use of the zone defense schedule. *Journal of Applied Behavior Analysis, 44,* 397–401.

Division for Early Childhood. (2014). *DEC recommended practices in early intervention/early childhood special education.* Retrieved from http://www.dec-sped.org/recommendedpractices

Dunst, C. J. (2017). Procedures for developing evidence-Informed performance checklists for improving early childhood intervention practices. *Journal of Education and Learning, 6,* 1–13.

Dunst, C. J., Trivette, C. M., & Raab, M. (2013). An implementation science framework for conceptualizing and operationalizing fidelity in early childhood intervention studies. *Journal of Early Intervention, 35,* 85–101.

Shelden, M. L., & Rush, D. D. (2001). The ten myths about providing early intervention services in natural environments. *Infants & Young Children, 14,* 1–13.

Workgroup on Principles and Practices in the Natural Environment, O. T. C. o. P. e. P. C. S. (2008). *Agreed upon mission and key principles for providing early intervention services in natural environments.* Retrieved from http://www.ectacenter.org/~pdfs/topics/families/Finalmissionandprinciples3_11_08.pdf

Preface

In 1985, M'Lisa L. Shelden was working as a physical therapist at a residential facility in Oklahoma, where many of the residents were deemed (by school personnel) unable to attend the segregated school on the campus. Because of this, physical therapy sessions became the big event of their day. With the work of Lou Brown, Michael Giangreco, and others in her head, M'Lisa began to visualize a different approach for physical therapy. With support from the administration (Jerry Poyner, Superintendent), the notion of what the life of residents could be began to shift, and the therapies became the strategy for supporting participation in real-life activities; a means to an end . . . not the end. For some of the residents, this meant leaving the facility for jobs or new lives in their home communities. For others, this opened the door to attending school, increasing independence in self-care, and planning for life beyond the residential facility. Instead of physical therapy sessions focusing on attainment of developmental skills, the strategies employed often involved the use of assistive technology to support access, participation, and independence. The intrusion of the therapy supports into the lives of the residents became one of the major challenges in implementing this approach. The number of times each day or week that classes, mealtimes, or leisure time was interrupted by the different therapies actually became problematic. The shift to supporting the residents in their daily activities was the impetus for M'Lisa to return to graduate school to learn more about educational support for young children, especially those with severe challenges. She was on a mission to learn more about teaming approaches, more specifically transdisciplinary teaming. During her master's degree program and continuing into her doctoral studies, M'Lisa focused on learning about inclusion and teaming approaches that supported families, teachers, and children with severe disabilities.

In 1990, M'Lisa joined the faculty at the University of Oklahoma Health Sciences Center. One of her primary roles was to support the newly formed statewide SoonerStart early intervention program in hiring therapists and implementing recommended practices. The SoonerStart program had made the decision to implement a transdisciplinary teaming approach. M'Lisa and Dathan D. Rush first met this same year. Dathan was newly recruited to serve on an early intervention team as a speech-language pathologist, and M'Lisa joined the same team to serve as a physical therapist and learn more about teaming in early intervention. As many of you know, the Dathan and M'Lisa journey began here. We were very fortunate to have true visionary leadership at the time in early intervention in Oklahoma. Specifically, Marileigh Dougherty, Department of Health; Cathy Perri, Department of Education; Cyd Roberts, Department of Health and Human Services; and Ann Taylor, State Interagency Coordinating Council Chair, who provided the space, trust, and fortitude to support the program and the two of us as we developed in our roles as technical assistance providers and Dathan when he joined the leadership team at the Department of Health as the assistant director and training coordinator for the statewide early intervention program. We often share with early intervention providers that we have been doing this a long time. This most often refers to using a primary service provider (PSP) approach to teaming. After more than 25 years of practicing, we like to believe we have made every mistake possible related to using this approach, and we cannot be convinced that we have not heard every reason (excuse) why the approach should not be implemented.

One year at a Division for Early Childhood conference, M'Lisa attended a presentation by Robin McWilliam and Don Bailey that included a discussion on the difficulties of studying transdisciplinary teaming. They remarked on the challenges of quantifying teaming and capturing all of the ways that effective team members support one another. This presentation and additional work by Robin and others (Geneva Woodruff, Mary McGonigel, Michael Giangreco, and Corrine Garland) helped us in our desire to continue to explore what teaming using a PSP approach should look like when well implemented. In the early years, we had the opportunity in Oklahoma, Nebraska, and Georgia to help teams with members that were 1) very interested in learning about teaming using a PSP, 2) scared to death about implementing a PSP approach to teaming, and 3) repulsed by every aspect of the approach. We both agree that although we might have a favorite group, we learned immensely from all team members whom we had the opportunity to support.

Of course, over the years, the constraints and challenges in early intervention have increased in number and complexity. Two issues surface as the most frustrating for us. The first issue is the complication of billing for services that further drives the notion of a service-based approach to intervention that is outdated and not considered best practice in early intervention. The second issue is the role expectation of practitioners working in early intervention. We discuss this at length in this text, but the idea is that early intervention is redefining what it takes to be an effective practitioner. To be skilled solely in one's discipline or technical craft is not enough. All early intervention practitioners must understand typical child development (beyond their own discipline), parent and parenting support, and maintain up-to-date knowledge in evidence-based practices in order to be helpful to parents and child care providers. For example, to serve as a helpful PSP in early intervention, M'Lisa cannot be defined as simply the motor expert, and expectations of Dathan must extend beyond that of understanding communication development. When a PSP approach to teaming is implemented with fidelity to the evidence-based characteristics, safety nets and accountability strategies are in place to help ensure that all children and families receive equitable, high-quality supports and services that are responsive to family-identified priorities that make a meaningful difference in the lives of children enrolled in the program.

In 2002, we joined the team at the Family, Infant and Preschool Program in Morganton, North Carolina. With the support of Carl Dunst, Melinda Raab, and other team members, we worked diligently to identify evidence-based characteristics, implementation conditions, and logistical recommendations to clearly define a PSP approach to teaming. Our journey has been challenging and rewarding. We have learned so much from the teams we have worked with and applaud their courage and tenacity needed to move practices forward in a world where often the right thing to do is never the easy thing to do.

Our intent with the second edition of this book is to provide a resource to help states, programs, teams, and individual practitioners work through the process of implementing a PSP approach to teaming. We have included practical tools to support implementation and hope that *The Early Intervention Teaming Handbook* will serve as a companion to *The Early Childhood Coaching Handbook* to assist you in your work with children and their families. We have added new tools to support team meeting facilitators in their very important (and difficult) role. Also new to this revision are resources to support program administrators, team meeting facilitators, and professional development providers. The new PSP Teaming Scenario Matrix includes the topic, characteristics of the child, team members involved, chapter, and page number. The purpose of this matrix is to help the reader easily find scenarios of interest. Because the topic of PSP approach to teaming continues to generate many questions, we have developed a table of Commonly Asked Questions listing the topic, chapter, and page numbers where the answers can be found.

We continue to imagine a day in the (not-so-distant) future when we are remembering back to the old days of IFSPs that contained service delivery statements identifying multiple providers responsible for outcomes that are based on child deficits. We muse about the day when early intervention providers everywhere say to one another, "Remember when we all made separate visits to see the child and family?' "Can you believe we used to do that?" "How did that ever make sense to us?" The exciting fact that keeps us hopeful is that one does not need to travel far or look very hard to find teams of providers that will share this type of information now. Early intervention teams across the country are forming, changing, and perfecting their practices based on current evidence. If you are skeptical of using a PSP approach to teaming, then we challenge you to read on with your mind open to the possibilities. If you want to learn more, then we have worked hard to provide you with new ideas, information, and tools that you can use immediately to support you in your work. Finally, if you are a change leader—a PSP who can never go back to working without a team—then we congratulate you on your hard work and challenge you to keep an open mind as we continue learning about our practices to ensure the best possible experience for every child and family enrolled in early intervention.

Acknowledgments

The authors would like to acknowledge and thank Laura Hansen, PT, M.S., and Vito DiBona, M.S., for their contributions to the studies included in Chapter 2.

To the early intervention teams and their leaders from across the country with whom we have worked who demonstrated courage, tenacity, and perseverance in helping to shift the paradigm of how families and practitioners can work together on behalf of infants and young children

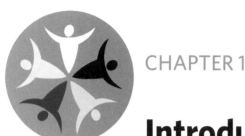

CHAPTER 1

Introduction to a Primary Service Provider Approach to Teaming

The audience was already a bit unsettled: 200 early intervention providers in tiered stadium-type seating ready to fight for their professional identities and ethics. It was 1990, and the group was gathered to learn more about primary service provider (PSP) teaming, a transdisciplinary model of service delivery in early intervention set to be implemented statewide. Participants were members of existing teams that included psychologists, social workers, child development specialists, speech-language pathologists (SLPs), and newly added members from occupational therapy and physical therapy. Many resented that the state was trying to cram another program with more regulations and requirements down their throats. Moreover, the state was attempting to dictate how they were to provide their services. This was crossing a line, and providers were not willing to sit by passively and be told how to practice their chosen professions.

Sandwiched in the crowd was a speech-language pathology supervisor tapped to work in the new Part H early intervention program. He seated himself with a group of SLP supervisors and other members of his team. They had been anticipating this event for weeks and were not supportive of this misguided new model. The implications of transdisciplinary teaming were unsettling: "If I'd wanted to be a physical therapist, I would have gone to physical therapy school." "How am I expected to teach someone everything I learned about communication intervention in graduate school?" "I don't want to be held liable if someone does something wrong and a child is injured." "Well, I'm an SLP, I'm not about to do stretching exercises with a child." "I'm just not going to do it!"

Like a gladiator thrown to the lions in ancient Rome, the program director entered the room. She approached the microphone and made a few brief remarks about the federal regulations in IDEA Part H, requirements for teaming, and best practice in transdisciplinary service delivery. This, she told the crowd, would be the first of several meetings to help providers learn how to use the PSP model.

Silence.

The director then introduced the speaker—a physical therapy faculty member from a large state-funded university. Wearing her signature mismatched earrings and red Converse high-tops, she approached the podium seemingly unaware of the intense feelings surrounding her. She went through her presentation, trying to make her case for a transdisciplinary model of service delivery in early intervention. As she reviewed the other models of service delivery, some providers recognized that they had been using a variation of multidisciplinary service delivery already—they met weekly to report about children on their caseload but typically did not receive feedback, information, or support from other team members. Outside of the team meeting, each service provider worked independently on separate treatment plans.

After the morning break, the audience members could contain their angst no longer. In fact, most were unable or unwilling to listen to what the speaker had said prior to this time because they had such intense preconceived notions about what she was going to say that conflicted with their personal values and beliefs about how they should work with young children. The first words out of the speaker's mouth once everyone was settled back in their seats were, "Does anyone have any questions about what I have shared so far?" Hands shot up across the auditorium. Some people, unable to precede their words with a raised hand, yelled out their questions and concerns.

"What research do you have that says this is what we should be doing?"

"Why is this so much better than what we already do?"

"If a child has severe disabilities, then don't more therapists naturally have to be involved?"

"Maybe this can work for children with mild disabilities, but I can't imagine how it would work for children with multiple and severe disabilities or children with autism."

"Yeah, maybe if the child only has speech issues and the speech-language pathologist is the primary provider, then it might work."

"What are the liability issues of having a speech-language pathologist do occupational therapy?"

"What if a parent wants all of the therapists involved, wouldn't we be violating family-centered practices if we tell them they have to pick just one?"

"This sounds unethical and against my practice act. What do the professional organizations have to say about all of this?"

"One specific service delivery model isn't the best option for every family. Why can't teams decide which service delivery model to use? After all, we are professionals!"

"This sounds like watered-down service to me. Is the state trying to save money or something?"

"Yeah, it makes me think you believe that just anybody can come in and provide services to the children. Are you trying to minimize the need for specialized therapists?"

Many of the questions were followed by applause from the audience. One by one, the speaker addressed each of the questions and concerns as she continued through the presentation and showed a videotape of assessment and intervention using a transdisciplinary model.

At the end of the day, one of the SLPs turned to her supervisor and asked, "What do you think about all of this?"

"I'm not sure. She made some interesting points. I've been concerned about all of the people coming and going from the families' homes. It seems like such a disruption in their lives. I didn't hear her say that the physical therapist would be doing speech and the speech-language pathologist would be doing occupational therapy. I heard that we need to work more closely together on the goals for the child and family, and we need to change what we do when we are with the family in their home or community. From what she said, it sounds like other team members can go with the primary person if there are questions. I mean, it wouldn't make sense for them to need to go every time, but . . ."

"I hear what you're saying, but I think it's going to be a huge change for all of us."

"I don't disagree with that. I think I need to read the handouts more carefully and look up some of these reference articles that she gave us. You know, people can get research to back up just about any position they want to promote. I need to read some of this for myself. If I need to rethink how I have been practicing or if I can even improve my practices a little bit to have better results for children and families, then I'm willing to do that. I don't quite understand why the federal government, the state, and some of the researchers in these articles would be promoting this if it was such a bad thing to do."

"I don't know either."

"Maybe they're paying her big bucks to do this."

They looked at each other simultaneously and said, "Not!"

"With the hostility in this room, I'd say she earned whatever she got."

"I'd say so."

The speech-language services supervisor struggled with the questions and what the physical therapist (PT) had shared during the presentation. He searched to find any available written information about the practices in order to help him better understand the rationale and research. If this type of teaming model really was the way in which early intervention should be provided to infants, toddlers, and their families, then he wished for a comprehensive resource that would explain how to operationalize these practices, beginning with a synthesis of the available research followed by how to prepare a program for this type of team-based approach to procedures for how to operationalize these practices in real early intervention programs.

The speech-language services supervisor's journey to understanding a PSP approach to teaming in early intervention began in 1990. He served on a team with the PT who provided the initial statewide training on a primary provider approach. Together, they have continued to work together to better understand how to use evidence-based practices in early childhood intervention to support the growth and development of young children and families via a PSP (e.g., primary provider, primary coach, team lead, lead provider, team liaison, key worker) as well as support other early intervention team members in using these practices. So far, their journey has taken them from the homes of families with whom they have individually worked to most every state in the country and abroad as they continue to define, refine, and examine the effectiveness of a primary provider teaming model. Many viewpoints, perceptions, and misperceptions exist about using a PSP in early intervention, as experienced by the SLP in this partnership.

The purpose of this text is to provide a common definition, characteristics of the practice, and implementation strategies for using a PSP approach to teaming within the context of evidence-based practices in early childhood intervention. This information is based on research in how people learn, early childhood intervention, family-centered helpgiving, and team-based supports as operationalized through the authors' more than 30 years of experience in the fields of physical therapy, speech-language pathology, early childhood special education (ECSE), and early intervention as well as the experiences of early intervention teams using these practices across the United States and beyond.

A BRIEF OVERVIEW OF COMMON TEAMING MODELS

Using teams comprised of individuals with a variety of expertise and knowledge in the field of early childhood intervention has been a consistent component of education legislation (Individuals with Disabilities Education Act Amendments [IDEA] of 1997 [PL 105-17]), recommended practice documents (Division for Early Childhood, 2014), and theoretical and research literature over the last 40 years (Antoniadis & Videlock, 1991; Briggs, 1997; Dunst et al., 2007; King et al., 2009; Nash, 1990; Nash, 2008; Sloper et al., 2006; Woodruff & McGonigel, 1988). Bell (2007) stated that a survey of U.S. organizations indicated that more than 48% use teams of some sort. Acknowledging the large amount of work contributed by teams in the workplace is commonplace in business and industry (West, 2012) as well as in education (Malone & Gallagher, 2010; Silverman et al., 2010) and health care contexts (Nandiwada & Dang-Vu, 2010; Weller et al., 2014).

Historically, several different teaming models for providing early childhood services have been suggested in the literature. The multidisciplinary, interdisciplinary, and transdisciplinary team approaches are three models of team interaction that have been readily discussed. The approaches differ based on the level of team interaction, parental involvement, the assessment process, and intervention methods (Fewell, 1983; Haynes, 1976; Kingsley & Mailloux, 2013; Peterson, 1987; Woodruff & McGonigel, 1988).

A *multidisciplinary approach* to teaming was initially defined as a group of professionals who work independently and interact minimally with each other (McGonigel et al., 1994; Woodruff & McGonigel, 1988). Each member of the team performed a separate evaluation and wrote an individual report, including discipline-specific goals. Each practitioner then performed intervention at separate times and focused on the remediation of the weaknesses noted during the evaluation (McGonigel et al., 1994; Rush & Shelden, 1996). When a multidisciplinary team functioned in this manner, team members viewed the child based on identified deficits from their own discipline's perspective and children received discipline-specific interventions that may have resulted in overlaps and gaps in services (Giangreco, 1986; Orelove & Sobsey, 1996).

Interdisciplinary teams traditionally had more interaction among the team members on an ongoing basis. Each team member continued to perform a discipline-specific evaluation and write discipline-specific goals. The team met to discuss the results of each evaluation and develop an intervention plan (McGonigel et al., 1994; Woodruff & McGonigel, 1988). Team members provided intervention services at different times and discussion among team members occurred primarily at team meetings (Fewell, 1983; Peterson, 1987; Rush & Shelden, 1996). The primary purpose of team meetings in an interdisciplinary approach was for each discipline to report on child status.

Several authors described transdisciplinary services as a team of professionals who work in a collaborative fashion (Garland et al., 1989; Haynes, 1976; McGonigel et al., 1994; York et al., 1990). The professionals share the responsibilities of evaluating, planning, and implementing early intervention services for infants and toddlers. Families are integral members of the team, and practitioners value the family's involvement in all aspects of early intervention. One person is chosen as the PSP for a child and family in a transdisciplinary approach. Other team members provide support to this individual through consultation regarding strategies to specifically include during interventions with the child and family. This approach decreases the number of professionals with whom the family is in contact on a regular basis (McGonigel et al., 1994; Woodruff & McGonigel, 1988).

Members of a transdisciplinary team must first develop competence in their own skill areas and then expand their knowledge by learning to observe development and provide intervention in areas outside their own discipline. As a practitioner's skills improve, team members engage in role release of intervention strategies from their disciplines to the other team member so the PSP has the necessary skills to work with the child and family (Briggs, 1997; Woodruff & McGonigel, 1988; York et al., 1990).

The stages of transdisciplinary team development involve six steps (Haynes, 1976; Woodruff & McGonigel, 1988). Role extension is the first step and refers to professional development activities including, but not limited to, self-study, workshops, conferences, and university coursework intended to deepen one's knowledge in his or her own discipline (e.g., a PT attending a course on lower extremity splinting for infants and toddlers with low muscle tone). Role enrichment is the second step and involves individual team members developing an understanding of the terminology and core practices of the other disciplines on the team. This can happen through conversations at team meetings, journal club review and discussion, and sharing information via a resource library. Role expansion is the third step and occurs based on individual team members' acquisition of enough information to make informed observations and program decisions outside of their own disciplines. Role exchange is the fourth step of transdisciplinary team development and occurs when team members have adequate knowledge of the theories, methods, and procedures from other disciplines to incorporate them into their own intervention process while working alongside or with the other team member. For example, role exchange occurs when an SLP is implementing newly acquired positioning techniques during a joint visit with the team's PT. Role release is the fifth step and occurs when a team member is fully functioning in the role of PSP and implements intervention methods typically associated with another discipline with accountability to the team member from the associated discipline. Role support is the sixth step and occurs when the PSP needs support of a specific discipline because intervention strategies are complex, new, or require the direct involvement of a particular discipline. For example, a child needs to learn how to use a walker and is currently being supported by an occupational therapist (OT) as the PSP. The PT would provide support to the child, OT, and family by teaching the child how to safely and successfully use the walker.

Three fundamental differences exist between transdisciplinary teams and the other commonly referenced models of team interaction. First, one team member is chosen as the PSP in a transdisciplinary team and has consistent interaction with the child and family (McGonigel et al., 1994; Woodruff & McGonigel, 1988). Second, members of the transdisciplinary team must collaborate to meet the needs of a child and family (Garland et al., 1989; McGonigel et al., 1994; Rush & Shelden, 1996; Woodruff & McGonigel, 1988). Third, transdisciplinary team members must commit to teaching, working, and learning across disciplinary boundaries (McGonigel et al.,1994; Woodruff & McGonigel, 1988).

AGREED-ON TEAMING APPROACH IN EARLY INTERVENTION

Using a PSP is most commonly associated with a transdisciplinary model of team development in which one member of the team is chosen to work directly with the child. Role release, or teaching the skills traditionally associated with one discipline to another team member who functions in direct service capacities with the child, is a distinguishing feature of transdisciplinary teamwork (Woodruff & McGonigel, 1988). The need for a teaming approach using a PSP is based on the fact that focusing on services and multiple disciplines implementing decontextualized, child-focused, and deficit-based interventions has not proven optimally effective (Boyer & Thompson, 2014; Campbell & Halbert, 2002; Dunst, Bruder, et al., 2001; Dunst et al., 2007; Dunst, Trivette, et al., 2001; Garcia-Grau et al., 2019; Hughes-Scholes et al., 2015; McWilliam, 2000). A PSP can be used effectively with young children and their families (American Occupational Therapy Association [AOTA], 2019; American Physical Therapy Association Academy of Pediatric Physical Therapy, 2013; American Physical Therapy Association Section on Pediatrics, 2010; American Speech-Language-Hearing Association [ASHA], 2008a, b; Division for Early Childhood, 2014; Pilkington, 2006; Vanderhoff, 2004; Workgroup on Principles and Practices in Natural Environments, 2007b).

The AOTA web site (http://www.aota.org) includes a document on transdisciplinary teaming, which discusses the role of the OT and use of a primary interventionist for supporting young children and their families in natural learning environments (Pilkington, 2006). More specifically, the document details information about how the OT serving as a coach and working as a transdisciplinary team member exemplifies several key principles of occupational therapy practice. Pilkington also referred to the importance of the OT going into the home "bare-handed (i.e., no toy bag) bringing the practitioner's therapeutic use of self to all team and family interactions, coaching and guiding rather than directing and doing" (p. 12).

The Academy of Pediatric Physical Therapy of the American Physical Therapy Association web site (http://www.pediatricapta.org) contains two resources: 1) a question and answer document containing facts specifically about a PSP teaming approach and 2) a fact sheet on team-based approaches used by PTs. Transdisciplinary teaming and use of a PSP is specifically cited as a "recommended practice in early intervention settings" (Section on Pediatrics of the American Physical Therapy Association, 2013, p. 2). The fact sheet stated the following:

> Role release and delegation of intervention strategies can be both ethical and legal and exist within the scope of physical therapy practice. The American Physical Therapy Association's Guide to Physical Therapist Practice provides instruction for coordinating, communicating, and documenting patient/client-related interventions. In other words, PTs may teach others activities or intervention strategies. (p. 2)

In 2008, ASHA put forth three documents regarding the roles and responsibilities of SLPs in early intervention. The documents include a position statement, guidelines, and a technical report. Each of the documents indicates that the SLP may practice within a transdisciplinary model and serve as the primary provider "based on the needs of the child, relationships already developed with the family, and special expertise" (ASHA, 2008b, p. 16) of the practitioner. Due to the emphasis on team interaction, members of transdisciplinary "teams benefit from joint professional development and can enhance each other's knowledge and skills as well as through role extension and role release for specific children and families" (ASHA, 2008b, p. 4). More recently, ASHA added an early intervention practice portal to their web site (https://www.asha.org/practice-portal/professional-issues/early-intervention/) that includes a description of the use of a PSP.

The Division for Early Childhood of the Council for Exceptional Children recommended practices document states that practitioners and families collaborate with each other to identify one practitioner from the team to serve as the PSP between the family and other team members based on child and family priorities and needs (Division for Early Childhood, 2014). The document further states that using multiple providers is not recommended. Rotating multiple practitioners in and out of a family's life on a regular basis has been found to negatively affect family functioning (Dunst et al., 2007; Greco & Sloper, 2004; Law et al., 1998; Sloper, 2004). Furthermore, using a PSP minimizes any negative consequences of having multiple and/or changing practitioners (Bell et al., 2009; Dunst et al., 2007; Law et al., 1998; Shelden & Rush, 2010; Sloper, 2004; Sloper et al., 2006).

Prior to 2007, the National Early Childhood Technical Assistance Center (NECTAC) formed the Workgroup on Principles and Practices in Natural Environments to develop agreed-on practices for supporting infants and toddlers with disabilities and their families. Specifically, the workgroup was charged with reaching consensus on the mission, key principles, and practices for providing early intervention in natural environments. The workgroup was comprised of individuals representing multiple perspectives, including state-level policy makers, Part C coordinators, faculty from institutions of higher education, ECSE researchers, early intervention practitioners, and parents, as well as state and national training and technical assistance providers representing all of the key disciplines involved in early intervention (i.e., ECSE, occupational therapy, physical therapy, psychology, service coordination, speech-language pathology). The workgroup created three documents:

1. *Agreed Upon Mission and Key Principles for Providing Early Intervention Services in Natural Environments* (http://www.nectac.org/~pdfs/topics/families/Finalmissionandprinciples3_11_08.pdf)

2. *Seven Key Principles: Looks Like/Doesn't Look Like* (https://ectacenter.org/~pdfs/topics/families/Principles_LooksLike_DoesntLookLike3_11_08.pdf)

3. *Agreed Upon Practices for Providing Early Intervention Services in Natural Environments* (https://ectacenter.org/~pdfs/topics/families/AgreedUponPractices_FinalDraft2_01_08.pdf)

Table 1.1 summarizes the mission and seven key principles developed by the workgroup. Principle 6 states, "The family's priorities, needs, and interests are addressed most appropriately by a primary provider who represents and receives team and community support" (Workgroup on Principles and Practices in Natural Environments, 2007b, p. 7). Principle 6 also delineates concepts that support using a primary provider, such as formalized communication mechanisms, opportunities for joint visits, and shared responsibility for achievement of individualized family service plan (IFSP) outcomes.

Haynes (1976) first introduced a transdisciplinary model of teaming into the literature. The original intent of this teaming model was to provide efficient patient-focused services to remediate deficits in a variety of locations. This approach was originally adopted by many early intervention teams in the late 1980s as a recommended practice in early intervention. In this text, we put forth a refinement of the transdisciplinary approach to teaming and the use of a PSP as it applies to Part C early intervention. In our experience, if teams are not using a multidisciplinary or interdisciplinary approach, then they refer to their teaming model as a PSP approach. In fact, we attempted to change the nomenclature and identify a new name for a teaming approach that used a PSP coaching interaction style and focused on supporting family members and teachers to promote child learning through everyday, interest-based opportunities. We began using the term *primary*

Table 1.1.   Agreed upon mission and key principles for providing early intervention services in natural environments

Mission
IDEA Part C early intervention builds upon and provides supports and resources to assist family members and care givers to enhance children's learning and development through everyday learning opportunities.

Key principles
Infants and toddlers learn best through everyday experiences and interactions with familiar people in familiar contexts.
All families, with the necessary supports and resources, can enhance their children's learning and development.
The primary role of a service provider in early intervention is to work with and support family members and care givers in children's lives.
The early intervention process, from initial contacts through transition, must be dynamic and individualized to reflect the child's and family members' preferences, learning styles, and cultural beliefs.
IFSP outcomes must be functional and based on children's and families' needs and family-identified priorities.
The family's priorities, needs, and interests are addressed most appropriately by a primary provider who represents and receives team and community support.
Interventions with young children and family members must be based on explicit principles, validated practices, best available research, and relevant laws and regulations.

From Workgroup on Principles and Practices in Natural Environments. (2007b, November). *Agreed upon mission and key principles for providing services in natural environments.* Available at http://www.nectac.org/topics/families/families.asp; reprinted by permission.

Key: IDEA, The Individuals with Disabilities Education Act Amendments of 1997 (PL 105-17); IFSP, individualized family service plan.

coach approach to teaming (Shelden & Rush, 2007, 2010) because commonly used definitions of the transdisciplinary model of team interaction lacked the essential elements of a focus on the adults in the child's life instead of a sole focus on practitioner–child interventions, as well as how to interact with and support the adults in a way to promote confidence and competence in using everyday life activities as the venue for learning, growth, and development. In yielding to the terminology most commonly used in early intervention, this text intends to provide a common definition for the field, practice characteristics, and detailed information on how to operationalize this teaming approach. Regardless of the terminology used, the field of early childhood intervention has moved beyond the use of a pure transdisciplinary model of team interaction.

Woodruff and McGonigel (1988) provided a table that compared the elements of practice of multidisciplinary, interdisciplinary, and transdisciplinary models of team interaction. They compared how teams conduct assessment, develop and implement the service plan, communicate with one another, involve parents, participate in staff development, and guide philosophy. We offer an additional comparison of a PSP approach to teaming in Table 1.2. More specifically, a PSP approach to teaming differs from a transdisciplinary service delivery model in that the PSP is not asked to engage in role release and take on the role of practitioners from other disciplines involving specific techniques targeted at skill development. Rather, the PSP becomes an expert on a family's and child's activity settings, routines, and interests in order to promote parent mediation of child participation in everyday activities. For example, for a child who is having difficulty walking on their own and has an IFSP outcome targeting playing with their twin brother and/or sister in the backyard, many team members across all disciplines would be equipped to support the parents in promoting the child's interest and success of playing with their brother and/or sister. If, however, the child needed foot splints to support their success in this interest-based activity setting, then the PT (PSP or not) would be responsible for either constructing or assisting the family in acquiring the needed assistive technology.

In a PSP approach to teaming in early intervention, the PSP acts as the principle program resource and point of contact among other program staff, the family, and other care providers (i.e., the team). The PSP mediates the family's and other care providers' skills and knowledge in relation to a range of needed or desired resources (i.e., child learning, child development, parenting supports). A PSP approach to teaming is characterized by the team members' use of coaching practices to build the capacity of parents, other primary care providers, and professional colleagues to improve existing abilities, develop new skills, and gain a deeper understanding of how to promote

Table 1.2. Models of team interaction

	Multidisciplinary	Interdisciplinary	Transdisciplinary	Primary service provider (PSP)
Assessment	Team members conduct separate assessments.	Team members conduct separate assessments.	Team members and family conduct joint assessment.	Fewest number of service providers needed participate in the assessment based on improving the child's participation across activity settings and learning opportunities.
Parent participation	Parents meet with team members individually.	Parents meet with entire team or a representative of the team.	Parents are full, active members of the team.	Parents and other care providers are equal team members.
Service plan development	Team members develop separate, discipline-specific plans.	Team members develop separate, discipline-specific plans but share them with each other.	Team members and family develop joint plan based on family priorities, needs, and resources.	Outcomes/goals are developed based on improving the child's participation across activity settings and learning opportunities.
Service plan responsibility	Team members are responsible for their discipline-specific plan.	Team members share information with each other about their part of the plan.	Team members are jointly responsible and accountable for how the PSP implements the plan.	Team members are jointly responsible and accountable for how the PSP implements the plan.
Service plan implementation	Team members implement their discipline-specific plans.	Team members implement their portion of the plan and incorporate other sections where possible.	A PSP implements the plan with the family.	Team members provide coaching to the PSP to effectively implement the plan across activity settings and care providers.
Lines of communication	Informal	Occasional case-specific staffing	Regular team meetings to exchange information, knowledge, and skills among team members	Ongoing interaction among team members for reflecting and sharing information occurs beyond scheduled meetings.
Guiding philosophy	Team members recognize the importance of information from other disciplines.	Team members are willing to share and be responsible for providing services as part of the comprehensive service plan.	Team members commit to teach, learn, and work across traditional discipline lines to implement a joint service plan.	Service and care providers engage in learning and coaching to develop the necessary expertise to improve the child's participation across activity settings and learning opportunities.
Staff development	Independent and discipline specific	Independent within and outside of own discipline	A critical component of team meetings for learning across discipline boundaries and for team building	Team members implement an annual team development plan to identify any gaps in skills and knowledge and improve expertise across disciplines.

From *Early intervention team approaches: The transdisciplinary model* by G. Woodruff & M.J. McGonigel (1988) (p. 166) in J.B. Jordon, J.J. Gallagher, P.L. Huntinger, & M.B. Karnes (Eds.), *Early Childhood Special Education: Birth to Three.* Copyright 1988 by The Council for Exceptional Children. Reprinted with permission.

child learning and development within the context of interest-based, everyday learning opportunities (Dunst, Bruder, et al., 2001; Rush & Shelden, 2005; Shelden & Rush, 2007, 2010). Using a PSP approach to teaming does not equate to only one practitioner supporting a child and family nor does it imply any prescription for frequency and intensity of service provision. In this approach, the child and family have access to any and all team members as needed via joint visits with the PSP and team meetings. Determining frequency and intensity is an IFSP team decision based on many factors rather than the perception that frequency and intensity equals the amount of service provision delivered by one member of a multidisciplinary or interdisciplinary team (e.g., 1 hour per week).

Whereas Woodruff and McGonigel (1988) described the six linear phases of transdisciplinary team development, the process in a PSP approach to teaming is based on four foundational interdependent components:

1. Role expectation

2. Role gap

3. Role overlap

4. Role assistance

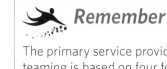

Remember

The primary service provider approach to teaming is based on four foundational interdependent components: 1) role expectation, 2) role gap, 3) role overlap, and 4) role assistance.

These components refer to individual team member involvement when using a PSP approach as opposed to the discipline represented by each person.

Role expectation refers to three minimal areas of competency when practicing in Part C and using a PSP approach to teaming. The first expectation is that each team member will be an evidence-based practitioner, which includes knowing the evidence to support practice in his or her own discipline, early intervention (Part C federal regulations and the mission and key principles for providing early intervention in natural environments), and early childhood development (beyond the areas of development typically associated with a particular discipline). The second expectation is that every team member is competent in providing parent and parenting support. *Parent support* is defined as assisting families related to identification, use, and evaluation of needed resources such as transportation, housing, crisis intervention, and medical services. *Parenting support* involves evidence-based information, techniques, strategies, and approaches that assist parents in meeting identified needs related to topics such as toileting, supporting positive behavior, helping a child sleep through the night in his or her own bed, and/or expanding a child's repertoire of foods. Finally, the third expectation is that all team members know how to mediate parents' and care providers' abilities to support child learning and development by using evidence-based adult learning and interaction methods (e.g., coaching) (Rush & Shelden, 2020). The Role Expectation Checklists (see Appendix 1A) may be used by practitioners to conduct self-assessments of current knowledge and skills related to preparedness for working on teams providing Part C services using a PSP approach to teaming. The Role Expectation Checklists—Administrator's Guide (see Appendix 1B) can be used by team leaders and supervisors to help structure an interview for a new staff member or contract provider, conduct orientation, and identify professional development needs of team members.

Role gap occurs when the PSP or another team member realizes that the primary provider does not have all of the needed knowledge and skills to adequately support a child's learning or implement necessary parent/parenting supports. This may occur at the time in which the PSP is being selected or while serving as the PSP for a particular child and family. Individual practitioners may opt out of serving as the primary provider when role gap occurs as the PSP is being selected, or the individual practitioner and team may determine that role gap will be bridged through role assistance from other team members. Role gap may also occur while a practitioner is serving as the primary provider. This might occur when a child makes substantial progress in a particular developmental area or

Remember

Role expectation includes three minimal areas of competency. Each team member will be

1. An evidence-based practitioner

2. Competent in providing parenting and parent support

3. Able to mediate parents' and care providers' abilities to support child learning and development

Remember

Role gap occurs when the primary service provider does not have all of the needed knowledge and skills to adequately support a child's learning or implement necessary parent/parenting supports.

Remember

Role overlap occurs when multiple team members feel confident and competent to fill the role of the primary service provider for a particular child and family.

Remember

Role assistance is

- The ongoing support provided by the team or a specific team member to the primary service provider

- Focused learning opportunities for the team at large and individual team members to fill an identified role gap

when a parent encounters a new or unexpected situation requiring knowledge and expertise beyond the primary provider's training and experience. The team has two options to consider when the primary provider is in this circumstance. First, other team members provide role assistance to the primary provider, which could occur during a team meeting, joint visit, colleague-to-colleague coaching opportunity, or formalized training event. Second, replace the PSP with another team member. Changing the PSP is the option of last resort (see Chapter 5). Due to the relationship-based nature of early intervention, this option should be considered only when role assistance is inadequate because of the significance, urgency, or seriousness of the situation. Another role gap that a team may experience is when the entire team is lacking an area of expertise or knowledge (e.g., assistive technology alternatives for a child with hearing impairment or vision loss). In these limited instances, the team must identify an external resource to support the PSP, child, and family. This can be achieved through contractual arrangements or by tapping another early intervention team member within the program or region with the needed expertise. The team's long-term development plan should include formalized training opportunities for an individual team member or entire team to obtain the necessary information to fill the role gap.

Role overlap is when multiple team members feel confident and competent to fill the role of the PSP for a particular child and family. Role overlap maximizes flexibility and efficiency for teams in selecting the PSP. For example, when identifying the most likely primary provider for an infant with Down syndrome whose mother is challenged by feeding him, many team members would have the knowledge, skills, and expertise necessary to support this child and family with role assistance from other team members as needed. When role overlap occurs, role assistance would most likely take the form of colleague-to-colleague coaching opportunities, conversations during team meetings, and joint visits with the family. Role overlap occurs more frequently as team members work together for longer periods of time. This occurs not necessarily because team members are releasing or exchanging intervention techniques or strategies, but due to collective experience implementing evidence-based practices in early intervention and shared conversations at team meetings, observations during joint visits, and supporting one another over time.

Role assistance is 1) the ongoing direct support provided by the team or a specific team member to the PSP and 2) focused learning opportunities for the team at large and individual team members filling an identified role gap. Role assistance is provided through regular team meetings, joint visits between the PSP and another team member, colleague-to-colleague coaching conversations, and coursework, training, and other professional development activities. Role assistance should be provided when any team member identifies that additional support is needed. Role assistance is required if an evidence-based intervention is perceived to be too complicated, new, or beyond the scope of practice of the PSP. This is not to say that a joint visit is required any time a PSP feels uncomfortable or challenged. Role assistance, however, should be prompt and could be in the form of a one-to-one or small-group conversation, a joint visit, coaching during a team meeting, or additional in-depth training for an identified role gap situation. See Chapter 6 for more information about joint visits.

A PSP approach to teaming differs from a transdisciplinary or other approach in which one practitioner serves as the liaison

Transdisciplinary team development process	≠	PSP approach to teaming process

Role extension refers to professional development activities including, but not limited to, self-study, workshops, conferences, and university coursework intended to deepen one's knowledge in his or her own discipline.
Role enrichment involves individual team members developing an understanding of the terminology and core practices of the other disciplines on the team.
Role expansion occurs based on individual team members' acquisition of enough information to make informed observations and program decisions outside of their own disciplines.
	→	Role expectation refers to three minimal areas of competency when practicing Part C and using a PSP approach to teaming.
		1. Evidence-based practices
		  • Own discipline-specific evidence-based practice
		  • Early intervention regulations/mission and key principles
		  • Early childhood evidence-based practices including typical development across all developmental domains and the roles and basic practices of other disciplines working in early intervention
		2. Parent support
		3. Adult interaction/adult learning

Role exchange occurs when team members have adequate knowledge of the theories, methods, and procedures from other disciplines to incorporate them into their own intervention process while working alongside or directly with the other team member.	⊘	Role gap is the circumstance in which the PSP or another team member realizes that the primary provider does not have the needed knowledge and skills to adequately support a child's learning or implement necessary parent/parenting supports.
Role release occurs when a team member is fully functioning in the role of PSP and implements intervention methods typically associated with another discipline with accountability to the team member from the associated discipline.	⊘	Role overlap is the situation in which multiple team members feel confident and competent to fill the role of the PSP for a particular child and family.
Role support occurs when the PSP needs support of a specific discipline because intervention strategies are complex, new, or require the direct involvement of a particular discipline.	→	Role assistance is 1) the ongoing direct support provided by the team or a specific team member to the PSP and 2) focused learning opportunities for the team at large and individual team members to fill an identified role gap.

Figure 1.1. Comparison of the transdisciplinary team development process and the primary service provider (PSP) approach to teaming process. (*Source:* Woodruff & McGonigel, 1988.)

between the family and other team members (Woodruff & McGonigel, 1988) by an explicit focus on the multiple individuals (i.e., parents/care providers, children) in the environment, the content of intervention (i.e., natural learning environment practices—everyday activity settings, child interests, parent responsiveness), the type of interactions (i.e., coaching practices), and the interconnectedness of all team members (i.e., PSP approach to teaming) regarding their role in promoting parent-mediated child learning and development. Figure 1.1 illustrates the similarities and differences of the four components of a PSP approach to teaming and the six stages of transdisciplinary team development. Role expectation includes the stages of transdisciplinary team development referred to as *role extension, role enrichment,* and *role expansion.* Role expectation in the PSP approach to teaming includes Stages 1–3 of the transdisciplinary teaming process and refers to the minimum expectation that all early interventionists have a mastery of evidence-based practices in early childhood across developmental domains and a detailed understanding of the roles and basic practices of other disciplines working in early intervention. The PSP approach to teaming does not involve or include role exchange or role release to implement deficit-based and skill-focused intervention methods typically associated with another discipline. Instead, practitioners using a PSP approach to teaming identify role gap and role overlap situations and recognize the need for role assistance (i.e., discipline-specific expertise), which is known as *role support* in the transdisciplinary teaming process.

EVIDENCE-BASED DEFINITION OF A PRIMARY SERVICE PROVIDER APPROACH TO TEAMING

In light of information and resource documents from AOTA, American Physical Therapy Association, ASHA, Division for Early Childhood, and the Workgroup on Principles and Practices in Natural Environments and as required by Part C, early childhood practitioners are faced with the task of reconceptualizing their roles with families of children with disabilities from independent, child-focused interventionists to members of family-centered teams using a PSP. An interdependent team of highly qualified practitioners is more likely to support families in a manner that will build their capacity to confidently and competently promote their children's growth and development.

A PSP approach to teaming is implemented when an early intervention program is identified as a formal resource for early childhood intervention and family support, and the program employs or contracts with practitioners with diverse knowledge and experiences to support the child's parents and other primary care providers. Using a PSP approach to teaming is not intended to limit a family's access to a range of supports and services, but instead to expand support for families of children with disabilities. The PSP is the lead program resource and point of contact among other program staff, the family, and other care providers (i.e., the team). The PSP mediates the family's and other care providers' skills and knowledge in relation to a range of priorities and needed or desired resources. The operational definition of a PSP approach to teaming is

> An established team consisting of multiple disciplines that meets regularly and selects one member as the primary service provider who receives coaching and support from other team members, and uses coaching as an interaction style with parents and other care providers to support and strengthen their confidence and competence in promoting child learning and development and obtaining desired supports and resources in natural learning environments. (Shelden & Rush, 2010, p. 176)

 Remember

A geographically based team is a group of early intervention practitioners minimally consisting of an early childhood educator or special educator, occupational therapist, physical therapist, speech-language pathologist, and service coordinator(s) responsible for all referrals to an early intervention program within a predetermined area defined by zip code or other geographical boundary.

The operational definition of a PSP approach to teaming is the requirement of a geographically based team consisting of individuals representing multiple disciplines, in which one member is selected as the PSP, receives support from other team members and provides support to the parents and other care providers using coaching and natural learning environment practices to strengthen parenting competence and confidence. A geographically based team is a group of early intervention practitioners consisting minimally of an early childhood educator or special educator, OT, PT, SLP, and service coordinator(s) responsible for all referrals to an early intervention program within a predetermined area defined by zip code or other geographical boundary. A specific child's IFSP team is composed of members from the geographically based team.

PRIMARY SERVICE PROVIDER APPROACH WITHIN THE CONTEXT OF RECOMMENDED EARLY CHILDHOOD PRACTICES

Although a PSP approach to teaming may be used in isolation as part of early intervention under Part C, the law requires that services be provided in natural learning environments and the intervention focuses on supporting parents and other care providers in confidently and competently promoting child learning and development. This text focuses on using a PSP approach as one of three key components of an evidence-based approach to early intervention. The other two components are implementing natural learning environment practices or, more specifically, using child interests and everyday activity settings as the contexts for learning, and coaching as the strategy for building the capacity of the important adults in the child's life (see Figure 1.2). Enhanced capacity of parents and other care providers in early intervention includes both global child and family outcomes. Desired child outcomes include supporting child learning, promoting positive social relationships, and providing opportunities for children to learn and use appropriate behaviors to meet their needs. Family outcomes in early intervention involve assisting parents in understanding their children's strengths and needs, knowing their rights and how to advocate effectively, helping their children learn and develop, ensuring availability of family support systems, and gaining access to desired resources in their community.

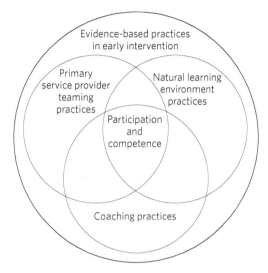

Figure 1.2. Evidence-based practices in early intervention.

Natural Learning Environment Practices

Under Part C, the content of the intervention must be evidence based and provided in the natural learning environments of eligible infants and toddlers (Workgroup on Principles and Practices in Natural Environments, 2007b). Natural learning environments are the locations where children would be if they did not have disabilities. Natural learning environment practices support parents of children with disabilities and other care providers in understanding the critical role of everyday activity settings and child interests as the foundation for children's learning opportunities (Campbell & Sawyer, 2007; Chiarello, 2017; Dunn et al., 2012; Dunst, Hamby, et al., 2000; Dunst, Trivette, et al., 2001; Graham et al., 2009; Hughes-Scholes et al., 2015; Humphrey & Wakeford, 2008; Hwang et al., 2013; Keilty & Galvin, 2006; Kellegrew, 2000; Kramer et al., 2018; Lim et al., 2016; McWilliam, 2000; Spagnola & Fiese, 2007). Activity settings include, but are certainly not limited to, taking a walk, eating a snack, going down a slide at the park, feeding the cat, making dinner, riding in a car, watering the garden, and fishing with Grandpa. Using these practices also supports parents and other care providers in recognizing and using child interests to capitalize on the number and variety of learning opportunities that naturally occur in the lives of all young children. *Interest-based learning* is defined as children's engagement in activities and with people and objects they find interesting, fun, exciting, and enjoyable (Dunst, Herter, et al., 2000; Raab, 2005). For example, when children are involved with objects (a favorite spoon) or people (brother or sister) that they find interesting, research shows that they will be more motivated to pay attention longer, resulting in positive benefits related to child learning (Dunst, Herter, et al., 2000; Raab, 2005).

Most practitioners are trained to determine a child's delays in skill development and either directly attempt to remediate the deficits through practitioner–child interventions and/or teach parents strategies to work on delayed or absent skills within a daily routine or activity setting. For example, if a child lacks head control, then a practitioner might recommend more opportunities for tummy time throughout the day and teach the parent ways to help the child tolerate being on the stomach for longer periods of time or encourage the child to push up on extended arms. Conversely, a practitioner who understands that child participation in activity settings is part of early childhood intervention will spend time with the parent observing and identifying the child's interests and existing opportunities for expression during which the child has an inherent opportunity to learn and practice new skills. For example, a practitioner learns that a child loves to lie on Daddy's stomach while he watches his favorite sports teams on television (i.e., activity setting/child interest). The practitioner encourages the father to continue this activity, discussing all the valuable learning opportunities the child experiences by participating in this interest-based activity setting on a regular basis (i.e., every evening and multiple opportunities on the weekends). If the father is interested and willing, then the practitioner also discusses ways to involve the child further in the activity. The father realizes that another one of his daughter's favorite activities is when they blow raspberries or she tries to imitate exaggerated mouth movements that he makes. While she is on his stomach when he is watching the game, he blows raspberries and makes silly faces to engage her more or extend the amount of time she is happy in this position. This is an example of a simple, interest-based, responsive strategy the father could easily use to maintain the child's engagement in a fun and interesting activity that would not only lead to improved head control but also promote the child's social, cognitive, and communication skill development while spending quality time with her daddy in a naturally and frequently occurring context. Evidence-based strategies and techniques are taught by early intervention team members as parent-mediated tools for supporting child participation in interest-based everyday activity settings.

Coaching Families

Early intervention practitioners should use a capacity-building approach with families of infants and toddlers with disabilities in order to support parent competence and confidence for promoting child learning within the context of natural learning opportunities (Trivette & Dunst, 2007). Capacity building is a process that assists parents in recognizing and taking advantage of everyday activities and situations that have development-enhancing qualities to increase children's learning (Dunst et al., 2010, 2014; Mangin, 2014; Rush & Shelden, 2020, Stormont & Reinke, 2012). Practitioners must adopt a method of parent engagement that is consistent with how people learn in order for parents to benefit from early intervention practitioners' use of a capacity-building approach to increase parenting skills and abilities (Donovan et al., 1999).

As previously mentioned, coaching is one style of interaction identified as a practice for building the capacity of parents, care providers, and colleagues in early intervention (AOTA, 2010; ASHA, 2008a; Hanft et al., 2004; Rush & Shelden, 2020; Trivette et al., 2009; Workgroup on Principles and Practices in Natural Environments, 2007b). Coaching does not mean just telling another person what to do; it is a process that starts with what the other person already knows and does and supports that person according to his or her needs and priorities. Coaching is an interactive process of reflection, sharing information, and action on the part of the coach and coachee used to provide support and encouragement, refine existing practices, develop new skills, and promote continuous self-assessment and learning. Coaching involves asking questions; jointly thinking about what works, does not work, and why; trying new ideas with the child; modeling with the child for the parent; sharing information; and jointly planning next steps (Hanft et al., 2004; Rush & Shelden, 2020). A coaching interaction style is as hands on by the PSP as necessary, but it also ensures that what the practitioner is doing and discussing with the parent is meaningful and functional within the context of everyday life and promotes the parents' ability to support child learning and development during the times when the practitioner is not present.

Operational Definition of Coaching Practices

The definition of coaching developed and used by the authors focuses on the operationalization of the relationship between coaching practices and the intended consequences, as well as the processes used to produce the observed changes, and is based on a comprehensive review of research on coaching practices. *Coaching* may be defined as

> An adult learning strategy in which the coach promotes the learner's ability to reflect on his or her actions as a means to determine the effectiveness of an action or practice and develop a plan for refinement and use of the action in immediate and future situations. (Rush & Shelden, 2005, p. 3; Rush & Shelden, 2020)

Following is a brief example of how a practitioner would engage a grandparent in a coaching interaction. Consider a situation in which a grandmother tells a practitioner that she would like for her granddaughter to sit in her highchair during mealtime. The practitioner asks what they have currently been doing during mealtime and how well it has worked. The practitioner and grandmother then brainstorm some ideas, building on what the grandmother has tried, and plan to meet during lunchtime on the next visit. The grandmother places the child in the highchair in the kitchen. The child begins to fuss and cry and reaches out her arms toward the grandmother. The practitioner asks her why she thinks the child might be crying. The grandmother believes that the child is angry about being in the highchair because she prefers to sit on her grandmother's lap during meals. The practitioner then asks what ideas the grandmother might have to help the child be happier in the highchair. The grandmother says she is not sure and also states, "I think I hold her too much. I really think she's ready to sit in the highchair by herself." The practitioner affirms the grandmother and then asks, "How can we use what you already know about your granddaughter's interests to help her be more content in the highchair?" The grandmother shares that she likes to play with a set of plastic measuring spoons and she sometimes gives them to her when she's cooking. Then the practitioner asks, "Can we try that right now?" The grandmother gives the child the measuring spoons and she calms down immediately. The grandmother states, "I should have thought of this before, but I don't usually give her a toy when she needs to eat." The practitioner affirms the grandmother's concerns about the measuring spoons and asks, "What other ideas do you have?" The grandmother responds with handing the child her favorite spoon and cup and says to the practitioner, "What about just giving her these?" The practitioner agrees that the spoon and cup seem to be working well. The grandmother then states, "Before we know it, she'll be feeding herself." Following the meal, the practitioner and grandmother develop a plan that includes ways for the grandmother to use the child's interests at every meal in ways that will not be distracting to the mealtime routine.

Coaching Characteristics

The characteristics of a particular practice inform a practitioner of what to do to achieve the desired effect. A review of coaching research by the authors suggests that coaching has five practice characteristics that lead to intended outcomes: 1) joint planning, 2) observation, 3) action/practice, 4) reflection, and 5) feedback (Rush & Shelden, 2020).

Joint Planning

Joint planning ensures the parent's active participation in using new knowledge and skills between coaching sessions. The two-part joint plan occurs during all coaching conversations, which typically involve discussing what the parent agrees to do between coaching interactions to use the information discussed or skills that were practiced (Part 1) and planning for the activity setting that will be used as the context for intervention during the next visit (Part 2). For example, as a result of a coaching interaction between a parent and practitioner and a child's love of playing in water, the two-part plan involves the parent's decision to purchase an inexpensive plastic wading pool, fill it up, and play with her toddler in the backyard between visits (Part 1). The next visit will occur in the afternoon when they are playing in the wading pool (Part 2).

Observation

Observation typically occurs with the practitioner directly viewing an action on the part of the parent, which then provides an opportunity for later reflection and discussion (e.g., a practitioner observes a parent moving the child from playing with a favorite toy to the bedroom for a nap). Observation may also involve modeling by the practitioner for the parent. When the practitioner models for the parent, the practitioner discusses what the parent is going to do with the child and asks the parent to make specific observations while the modeling occurs. The practitioner builds on what the parent is already doing and demonstrates additional strategies. Following the model, the practitioner prompts reflection by the parent regarding how the parent's actions match intent, are similar to or different from what the parent typically does, and are consistent with what research informs about child learning and what the parent wants or is willing to try based on the practitioner's modeling (e.g., following further discussion, the practitioner demonstrates preparing the child for the transition from play to naptime by talking about what will happen and offering the child a choice of what favorite snuggly the child would like to take to bed).

Action/Practice

Actions are events or experiences that are planned or spontaneous, occur in the context of a real-life activity, and might take place when the coach is or is not present. The characteristic of action provides opportunities for the family member or care provider to use the information discussed during the coaching interaction. This type of active participation is a key characteristic of effective helpgiving and is an essential component for building the capacity of the person being coached. For example, the parent offers the child a choice of milk or water during snack time and waits for the child to attempt to verbally respond.

Reflection

Reflection occurs during the visit and follows an observation or action, providing the parent an opportunity to analyze current strategies and refine knowledge and skills. The practitioner may ask the parent to describe what did or did not work during observation or action as part of the visit or between visits, followed by generating alternatives and actions for continually improving his or her knowledge and skills.

Feedback

Feedback occurs after the parent has the opportunity to reflect on their observations, actions, or opportunity to practice new skills. Feedback includes statements by the practitioner that affirm the parent's reflections (e.g., "I know what you mean") or add information to deepen the parent's understanding of the topic. It also includes jointly developing new ideas and actions. The coach provides feedback by sharing information based on current research from his or her discipline-specific training, professional experience, and input from other team members. Sharing additional information about typical 2-year-old behavior following the parent's reflection on what they have tried and found to be either successful or unsuccessful around helping their child share favorite toys with a cousin is an example of informative feedback.

PURPOSE OF A PRIMARY SERVICE PROVIDER APPROACH TO TEAMING

The fundamental purpose of using a PSP approach to teaming is to enable families to establish and maintain an ongoing working relationship with a lead team member with needed expertise, who then becomes an expert on the whole child and family rather than promoting an isolated focus on developmental domains and deficits by each practitioner. The intent of this approach is to promote positive child and family outcomes and minimize any negative consequences of having multiple and/or changing practitioners involved in the family's life. Families are faced with varying degrees of consistency of approaches, information, and interaction styles when multiple practitioners are involved (Bell et al., 2009; Dunst et al., 2007; Law et al., 1998; Shelden & Rush, 2010; Sloper, 2004; Sloper et al., 2006). These circumstances can potentially lead to confusion or conflict, leaving the parent to decide what to do and whom to trust and believe.

BENEFITS OF A PRIMARY SERVICE PROVIDER APPROACH TO TEAMING

The relationship among the practitioner, family members, and other care providers is a significant benefit of a team approach that uses a primary provider. The important adults in the life of the eligible child can focus on developing trust, respect, and open communication with one key person instead of having to experience this process with multiple people who have different interaction styles, levels of expertise, and knowledge about the child and family.

Efficiently using family and program resources is another important benefit of a PSP approach to teaming. Using a primary provider allows for increased coordination of supports and services instead of a more fragmented approach to addressing child and family priorities. For example, in a more fragmented approach, a family could potentially be introduced to three or four practitioners with separate meeting times and reasons for visiting. The parent must then remember who does what (e.g., SLP to work on talking, PT to work on rolling), on what day and time (e.g., Tuesday at 4:00 p.m. for OT, Wednesday at 9:00 a.m. for SLP), the expectations for involvement during the visit (e.g., observer, active participant), the homework to be completed between visits (e.g., practice giving choices, pull-to-stand exercises), what needs to be available for the practitioner or whether to bring toys and materials, practitioner preference for sibling involvement, and how the environment should be set up and maintained while the practitioner is present (e.g., television on or off).

Decreasing both gaps and overlaps in supports and services is also a benefit when using a PSP. Because the child cannot be divided neatly into developmental domains and/or discrete areas of focus by a particular discipline, using multiple practitioners inherently invites redundancy across practitioners to address particular skills. For example, an OT may be working on feeding during visits, while during separate sessions an SLP also addresses a child's oral-motor abilities as they relate to managing foods. In addition, gaps can occur when multiple providers are involved because of a lack of communication and belief by one practitioner that another practitioner is addressing a particular issue.

Consider a situation in which an early childhood special educator and a PT are both involved with a family providing ongoing services at separate times. The child may need specialized equipment to be able to play with toys or interact more independently with the environment. Each believes the other practitioner will address the assistive technology needs of the child and family, but ultimately neither addresses the need or at best an unnecessary delay occurs in providing access to the technology. Multiple practitioners working with a particular family may all recognize signs of maternal depression, but because this issue does not fall clearly within the scope of practice of the disciplines involved, each makes the assumption that someone else will be responsible for addressing the issue either through referral or assisting the parent in gaining access to supports.

In contrast, a primary provider is responsible for focusing on the entire child within the context of the family and community. The focus of the primary provider is on parent promotion of child participation within and across family routines and activities rather than an emphasis on practitioner–child interventions to remediate deficits within a particular domain by a specific discipline. For example, in the previous scenario in which multiple providers failed to address the issue of maternal depression, a primary provider would recognize the parent's possible depression and its direct impact on the parent's ability to promote child participation during everyday activity settings. Thus, the primary provider would need to engage the parent in a conversation about the necessary supports and resources the parent could access.

Due to the complexity of working with families from a wide variety of diverse backgrounds, identifying one lead provider from the team diminishes the potential of violating a family's values, beliefs, rituals, and traditions. The advantage of a primary provider is that the provider can focus on the time necessary to embrace the uniqueness of the family situation and respectfully engage in conversations to better understand the family preferences.

ORGANIZATION OF THIS BOOK

This text is intended to be a working guide for how to operationalize a PSP approach to teaming in early intervention and, therefore, features learning tools to assist the reader in applying the content to everyday practice. The content is applicable to practitioners working in early intervention, parents, program administers, policy makers, technical assistance providers, and higher education faculty and students interested in learning more about teaming. Case studies and scenarios are provided to illustrate and provide examples for how PSP teaming practices are implemented in early intervention. The PSP Teaming Scenario Matrix (located directly after the References) provides a comprehensive list of all scenarios in the text (see p. 223). This matrix details the location of the scenario within the book, the topic of the scenario, and the specific disciplines involved. Readers are provided with opportunities to reflect, remember, and take action throughout the text. Reflection opportunities include thinking about current or future practices and applying or using the information learned to build on one's current knowledge and skills. Remember notations contain brief summations of critical points to assist readers in retaining key concepts. Take action opportunities challenge readers and include ideas for how to put information into action by applying what is being learned to a real-life context. A list of commonly asked questions about the PSP approach to teaming and the location of the answers in the text is provided at the end of this text (directly following the PSP Teaming Scenario Matrix on p. 225).

TERMINOLOGY USED IN THIS BOOK

This book contains terminology that may be familiar to the reader or may be defined by different readers in different ways. The authors have provided definitions of some of the terms used throughout the text to ensure a common understanding.

Blended service coordination: A model in which an early intervention practitioner also operates as a service coordinator (e.g., an OT serves as the team's OT and also provides service coordination).

Caregivers or care providers: Individuals other than parents who care for and are important in the child's life, including grandparents, aunts, uncles, family friends, baby sitters, and nannies.

Child care providers: Individuals who work in child care centers or family child care homes.

Dedicated service coordination: A separate individual operates as the service coordinator and solely provides this service to the family.

Geographically based team: Practitioners that provide services and supports to children and families within an identified geographic area of the region served by the program, such as a county, specific zip code area, or school district.

IDEA Part C: The federal legislation that provides regulations for how states provide early intervention services to eligible children from birth to age 3.

Individualized family service plan: The process used to develop and provide appropriate early intervention services for families to increase their capacity to care for their infants and toddlers with disabilities. Family members and service providers work together as a team through the IFSP process. The team plans, implements, and evaluates services tailored to fit the family's unique concerns, priorities, and resources. The IFSP is the vehicle through which effective early intervention is implemented in accordance with federal legislation (Part C).

Interdisciplinary team: Interdisciplinary teams have more interaction among team members than multidisciplinary teams. Each professional continues to perform a discipline-specific assessment and write discipline-specific goals. The team meets to discuss the results of each assessment and develop an intervention plan (McGonigel et al., 1994; Woodruff & McGonigel, 1988). Team members provide intervention services during different appointment times, with discussion among team members occurring primarily at team meetings (Fewell, 1983; Peterson, 1987; Rush & Shelden, 1996).

Joint visit: A visit in which a secondary service provider (SSP) accompanies the PSP in order to coach and support when a question or issue is identified by the PSP, family members, other care providers, or other team members. The joint visit may also be referred to as a *consultative visit, consultation,* or *covisit,* depending on the program or fiscal ramifications.

Multidisciplinary team: Professionals working independently of each other and interacting minimally with other team members (McGonigel et al., 1994; Woodruff & McGonigel, 1988). Each member of the team performs a separate evaluation and writes an individual report, including discipline-specific goals. Intervention is then performed by each service provider at separate times and focuses on the remediation of the weaknesses noted during the evaluation (McGonigel et al., 1994; Rush & Shelden, 1996).

Parents: Individuals who are directly responsible for the care of their biological, adopted, or foster child.

Practitioner: Staff members or contract providers working in an early intervention program. Practitioners may include, but are not limited to, audiologists, behavior specialists, early childhood educators, early childhood special educators, nurses, nutritionists, OTs, PTs, psychologists, service coordinators, social workers, SLPs, and vision and hearing specialists.

Primary service provider: The one team member selected to serve as the liaison between the family and other team members. This is the person who sees and interacts with a family most often and is responsible for becoming an expert on individual family priorities, activity settings, routines, and unique characteristics. The PSP assists family members and other care providers in promoting child participation within and across everyday activity settings, addressing parenting issues, and ensuring the family's access to needed and desired resources. Any core team member may be the PSP, with the exception of the service coordinator in systems that use a dedicated service coordinator. The person selected to be the PSP is the member of the team who is the best possible long-term match for a child and family.

Secondary service provider: A team member who uses coaching to support the PSP, parents, and other care providers directly related to the IFSP outcomes. This support may occur within the context of a team meeting, during a joint visit, or as part of a conversation between meetings and scheduled visits.

Service coordinator: The member of the team responsible for coordinating necessary evaluations and assessments, facilitating the initial IFSP meeting and subsequent reviews, assisting the family in receiving the services and supports described on the IFSP, and ensuring their rights and procedural safeguards.

Teachers: Individuals who teach in infant/toddler classrooms.

Team: A geographically based team designed to support children enrolled in early intervention and their families. Teams are not formed around individual children, but they consist of representatives from a variety of disciplines that are assigned to provide supports within a given catchment area, geographic region, or zip code. A core team must minimally include an early childhood educator or early childhood special educator, one OT, one PT, and one SLP for approximately every 100–125 children enrolled in Part C. The team must also include a service coordinator who is one of the core team members and also serves as a service coordinator or a dedicated service coordinator, depending on the state's guidelines for service coordination (e.g., approximately three service coordinators for every 100–125 children enrolled in the program).

Team facilitator: A member of the geographically based team who is responsible for conducting all team meetings.

Team meeting: A regularly scheduled (most often, weekly) formal opportunity for colleague-to-colleague coaching and support necessary to build the capacity of parents and care providers to promote child participation and parenting supports across home, community, and early childhood program settings.

Transdisciplinary team: Professionals who work in a collaborative fashion (Garland et al., 1989; Haynes, 1976; McGonigel et al., 1994; York et al., 1990) and share the responsibilities of evaluating, planning, and implementing services. Families are integral members of the team, and other team members value the family's involvement in all aspects of intervention. One person is chosen as the PSP for a child and family. Other team members provide support to this individual through consultation regarding activities to include during interventions with the child and family.

CONCLUSION

The purpose of this text is to define a PSP approach to teaming as one component of a three-part approach for providing evidence-based early intervention practices. This three-part approach also includes using natural learning environment practices as the context for intervention and coaching as the style of interaction with the important adults in the child's life. Using a PSP is a key principle identified by the Workgroup on Principles and Practices in Natural Environments of the NECTAC and is recognized by ASHA, AOTA, the Section on Pediatrics of the American Physical Therapy Association, and the Division for Early Childhood of the Council for Exceptional Children as an appropriate teaming approach in early intervention. The federal regulations for Part C clearly delineate the involvement of teams comprised of individuals from multiple disciplines in the design and delivery of early intervention supports and services. Furthermore, evidence, practical experience, and common sense inform us that having one primary liaison from the team to the family is an effective means of providing supports. This text is designed to assist the reader in operationalizing the research-based characteristics of the practices in early intervention contexts.

This text is intended to provide detailed information in such a way that practitioners and program leaders can consider how their current practices align with the approach described. The information is provided in a manner that could support a program in implementing the characteristics of this practice as well as serve as a resource for family members interested in learning more about the use of a primary provider. This text is also put forth as a resource for higher education faculty to use within and across disciplinary and departmental boundaries in order to prepare graduates to serve on teams in early intervention.

Role Expectation Checklists

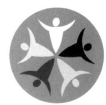

Practitioner's name: _____ Date: _____

	Knowledge and skills are characterized by the following:	Yes	No	Examples/notes/plan
Evidence-based practices	Practitioner can ensure that the practices he or she uses from his or her own discipline are evidence based.	Y	N	
	Practitioner has an understanding of Part C of the Individuals with Disabilities Education Act Amendments (IDEA) of 1997 (PL 105-17).	Y	N	
	Practitioner has reviewed the mission and key principles for providing early intervention services in natural environments.	Y	N	
	Practitioner implements practices in accordance with the mission and key principles.	Y	N	
	Practitioner demonstrates knowledge of typical child development across the five domains (adaptive, cognitive, communication, physical, and social-emotional).	Y	N	
	Practitioner demonstrates the ability to assess child functioning across the three global child outcomes (positive social-emotional skills, acquisition and use of knowledge and skills, and use of appropriate behaviors to meet his or her needs).	Y	N	

	Knowledge and skills are characterized by the following:	Yes	No	Examples/notes/plan
Parent support	Practitioner supports family members in identifying, gaining access to, and evaluating informal and formal resources needed to assist them in meeting their desired outcomes (e.g., employment, housing, medical/dental care, transportation).	Y	N	
	Practitioner implements evidence-based parenting support practices to assist family members and other care providers to achieve their desired outcomes (e.g., toileting, helping the child sleep through the night in his or her own bed, providing positive behavior support, eliminating the use of a pacifier, teaching basic nutrition).	Y	N	

	Knowledge and skills are characterized by the following:	Yes	No	Examples/notes/plan
Adult interaction/ adult learning	Practitioner uses methods and strategies when working with the adults in young children's lives that are likely to strengthen individual or family capacity to accomplish the family's desired outcomes.	Y	N	
	Practitioner recognizes and builds on what the family and other care providers already know and are doing related to child learning and parent support.	Y	N	
	Practitioners demonstrate respect for individual adult learning styles, preferred interaction methods, and cultural influences.	Y	N	

Role Expectation Checklists—Administrator's Guide

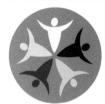

Practitioner's name: _____   Date: _____

	Knowledge and skills are characterized by the following:	Examples/notes/plan
Evidence-based practices	*Indicator* Practitioner can ensure that the practices he or she uses from his or her own discipline are evidence based. *Administrator probe questions* • What research does the practitioner have to support the practices that he or she uses? • How is the research relevant to children from birth to 3 years of age? • How does the research consider the importance of parents/caregivers and everyday contexts? • How does the practitioner vary his or her treatment methods or strategies with children/families based on current research and the child/family needs, activity settings, and so forth?	
	Indicator Practitioner has an understanding of Part C of the Individuals with Disabilities Education Act Amendments (IDEA) of 1997 (PL 105-17). *Administrator probe questions* • How recently has the practitioner reviewed IDEA Part C regulations and/or state policies and procedures for early intervention? • What were the topics discussed when the administrator, team leader, or supervisor had a conversation with the practitioner about how IDEA Part C regulations and state policies and procedures for early intervention are implemented in the program? • How does the practitioner demonstrate understanding of IDEA Part C? • How does this compare with the practitioner's prior work experiences?	
	Indicator Practitioner has reviewed the mission and key principles for providing early intervention services in natural environments. *Administrator probe questions* • How recently has the practitioner reviewed the mission and key principles? • What were the topics discussed when the administrator, team leader, or supervisor had a conversation with the practitioner about how the mission and key principles are applied in the program? • What is the practitioner's current level of understanding and agreement with the mission and key principles? • How does this compare with the practitioner's prior work experiences?	*(continued)*

	Knowledge and skills are characterized by the following:	Examples/notes/plan
Evidence-based practices	*Indicator* Practitioner implements practices in accordance with the mission and key principles. *Administrator probe questions* • How does the practitioner demonstrate practices in accordance with the mission and key principles? • What does the practitioner do when conflicted about implementing practices in accordance with the mission and key principles?	
	Indicator Practitioner demonstrates knowledge of typical child development across the five domains (adaptive, cognitive, communication, physical, and social-emotional). *Administrator probe questions* • How does the practitioner demonstrate knowledge of typical child development across the five domains? • Does the practitioner competently and confidently provide supports to families within the context of everyday activities regarding topics outside of their own area of expertise?	
	Indicator Practitioner demonstrates the ability to assess child functioning across the three global child outcomes (positive social-emotional skills, acquisition and use of knowledge and skills, and use of appropriate behaviors to meet his or her needs). *Administrator probe questions* • What is the practitioner's knowledge of the three global outcome areas and how the global outcomes are used? • How does the practitioner collect and share information related to the three global outcome areas?	

	Knowledge and skills are characterized by the following:	Examples/notes/plan
Parent support	*Indicator* Practitioner supports family members in identifying, gaining access to, and evaluating informal and formal resources needed to assist them in meeting their desired outcomes (e.g., employment, housing, medical/dental care, transportation). *Administrator probe questions* • What is the practitioner's knowledge about resource-based practices? • What is the practitioner's knowledge of formal and informal community resources? • How does the practitioner build the family's capacity to identify, gain access to, and evaluate resources rather than giving or procuring needed resources for family?	

(continued)

	Knowledge and skills are characterized by the following:	Examples/notes/plan
Parent support	*Indicator* Practitioner implements evidence-based parenting support practices to assist family members and other care providers to achieve their desired outcomes (e.g., toileting, helping the child sleep through the night in his or her own bed, providing positive behavior supports, eliminating the use of a pacifier, teaching basic nutrition). *Administrator probe questions* • What basic evidence-based knowledge does the practitioner have regarding typical parenting needs for support? • What evidence does the practitioner use for parenting supports? • How does the practitioner implement evidence-based parenting support practices?	

	Knowledge and skills are characterized by the following:	Examples/notes/plan
Adult interaction/adult learning	*Indicator* Practitioner uses methods and strategies when working with the adults in young children's lives that are likely to strengthen individual or family capacity to accomplish the family's desired outcomes. *Administrator probe questions* • What experience does the practitioner have using adult learning methods to support the adults in the child's life rather than only focusing on working directly with the child? • What methods and strategies does the practitioner use to build parent capacity to achieve his or her desired outcomes? • What is the evidence to support the methods and strategies the practitioner uses?	
	Indicator Practitioner recognizes and builds on what the family and other care providers already know and are doing related to child learning and parent support. *Administrator probe questions* • How does the practitioner obtain information about what family and care providers already know? • How does the practitioner use this information to guide the supports he or she provides?	
	Indicator Practitioners demonstrate respect for individual adult learning styles, preferred interaction methods, and cultural influences. *Administrator probe questions* • How does the practitioner gather information about the adult's learning style, preferred interaction methods, and cultural influences? • How does the practitioner use information about adult preferences within the context of interactions?	

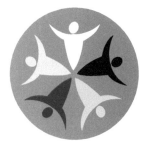

CHAPTER 2

Research Foundations of a Primary Service Provider Approach to Teaming

The information in Chapter 1 describes the requirement of teams under Part C early intervention. The chapter also acknowledges the use of a PSP as an accepted teaming approach by the professional associations representing the disciplines most closely aligned with early intervention (ECSE, occupational therapy, physical therapy, and speech-language pathology). Furthermore, the guidance documents provided by NECTAC stipulate the use of a PSP approach to teaming as one of the seven key principles for implementing early intervention in natural environments. To further support and substantiate using a PSP as specified in the key principles, we have identified three fundamental areas of research that define the characteristics and implementation conditions of PSP teaming practices: 1) a defined team, 2) a PSP as the team liaison to the family, and 3) team support for the PSP. This chapter describes the research, defines the characteristics, and identifies the implementation conditions required for effective use of this teaming approach.

Acknowledging the large amount of work contributed by teams in the workplace is commonplace in business and industry (West, 2012), as well as in education (Malone & Gallagher, 2010; Silverman et al., 2010) and health care contexts (Nandiwada & Dang-Vu, 2010; Weller et al., 2014).

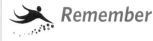

> ## Remember
>
> The three fundamental areas of research that define the characteristics and implementation conditions of primary service provider (PSP) teaming practices are
>
> 1. Using a defined team
>
> 2. Selecting a PSP as the team liaison to the family
>
> 3. Providing team support for the PSP

A DEFINED TEAM

Using teams to accomplish objectives that could not be accomplished otherwise is prevalent (West et al., 2004) in business and industry (West, 2012), education (Malone & Gallagher, 2010; Silverman et al., 2010), early childhood (Boyer & Thompson, 2014; Brito & Lindsay, 2016; Hong & Reynolds-Keefer, 2013; King et al., 2009; Moeller et al., 2013), and health care contexts (Nandiwada & Dang-Vu, 2010; Weller et al., 2014). Research indicates that teamwork in health care has also been reported to benefit health care workers (e.g., lower stress, higher retention rates, increased innovation by team members, increased job satisfaction) and recipients of services (e.g., lower mortality rates in hospitals, higher quality of care, improved cost-effectiveness) (West, 2012).

Characteristics of Effective Teams

The literature on effective teams contains many studies that describe positive outcomes for teams that use the following task and structure factors. Consider how these task and structure factors apply to early childhood intervention teaming contexts.

Team task(s) should allow members to use a variety of skills, result in meaningful work, and have significant consequences for other people (Bell, 2007; Borrill et al., 2001). Effective early intervention teams allow their members to use disciplinary expertise as well as other specialized knowledge and skills based on experience and other individual characteristics. As an example, a team member is identified to support a child and family because she has specialized knowledge about a diagnosis or condition. In addition to this specialized knowledge, the practitioner also happens to have personal experience of using public transportation. The family needing support also lives in the city and needs to gain access to public transportation to run errands. The team member is allowed and encouraged to support the family using all that she knows, not only her discipline-specific expertise. Team members' ability to successfully support a broader range of families and family circumstances is enhanced when they use the professional and personal knowledge and experience of individual team members.

 Remember

Using a defined team is a fundamental area of research supporting the use of a primary service provider approach to teaming.

The importance of a team's task is a critical component regarding inherent motivation of the team, the commitment the team members have to accomplishing the task, and the development of a collective team identity in terms of successfully completing a job. Motivation, commitment, satisfaction, and sense of responsibility are inherent to the task given to teams in the fields of health care and education. For example early intervention teams are charged with and fully responsible for assisting family members and care providers in developing the confidence and competence individually needed (despite any and all challenges) to support the growth and development of the children in their care (IDEA 2004).

The number of team members should be appropriate for the task (Bell, 2007; Larsson, 2000). The team should include enough members with the necessary specialized expertise to accomplish the assigned tasks (Bell, 2007). Although the meta-analysis of the teaming literature identifies no optimal number of team members, teams with unnecessary members are not as productive as teams with the membership limited to those required to perform the task (Bell, 2007). Early intervention programs are required by federal law to have a multidisciplinary team of practitioners available to families of children with disabilities (IDEA 2004). The team must have sufficient team members with necessary knowledge and skills to meet the needs of eligible children and their families for a designated catchment area.

Teams should have some degree of self-managing abilities because team self-management is related to enhanced team performance (Bell, 2007; Borrill et al., 2001; De Drue & West, 2001; Erez et al., 2002, West, 2012). Assigning a team leader (or facilitator) is essential in early intervention programs. Using a team decision-making process whenever possible, however, is a critical factor in team innovation (i.e., pursuit, assimilation, and implementation of new ideas). A team leader who has skills in group facilitation will most likely result in a team that has short decision times, self-implemented accountability strategies, and enhanced flexibility and efficiency. Teams with self-management do not need a multitude of supervisory or middle management positions. For example, an early intervention team that self-manages decisions related to the date, time, and length of team meetings will have enhanced participation and efficiency.

Characteristics of Effective Team Members

Effective teams consist of individuals who are agreeable, are conscientious, have high general mental ability, are competent in their area of expertise, are highly open to experience and mental stability, like teamwork, and have been with the organization long enough to be socialized or acculturated to the written and unwritten rules or norms (Bell, 2007). Being an agreeable team member is identified as an important characteristic of practitioners working together in early childhood. The term *agreeable* when used to describe effective team members is synonymous with being flexible, courteous, trusting, and respectful. Historically, the term *respectful* or the phrase "demonstrating mutual respect" is pervasive in teaming literature (Bell, 2007; DeGangi et al., 1994; Dinnebeil et al., 1996, 1999; Dunst & Trivette, 2009; Dunst et al., 1994; Harrison et al., 1990; Lowenthal, 1992; O'Connor, 1995; Park & Turnbull, 2003; Soodak & Erwin, 2000). Agreeableness should not be confused with serving as a rubber stamp for other team members' ideas and recommendations. Team members will disagree; however, effective teams are able to reach consensus and move forward in supporting the team's decision.

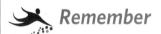

Remember

Effective team members

- Are agreeable
- Are conscientious
- Have high general mental ability
- Are competent in their area of expertise
- Are highly open to experience and mental stability
- Like teamwork
- Have been with the organization long enough to be socialized

Conscientious team members are described as reliable, responsible, punctual, and organized. Studies in early childhood intervention have repeatedly recognized this characteristic as a critical trait for practitioners (Bell, 2004; DeGangi et al., 1994; Dinnebeil et al., 1999; Dunst et al., 1994; Lowenthal, 1992; O'Connor, 1995; Park & Turnbull, 2003; Soodak & Erwin, 2000). For example, being prepared, organized, and mindful of the topics to be discussed at a home visit or team meeting is a clear way of demonstrating conscientious behavior so that scheduled conversations and visits do not exceed the planned time and do not negatively affect the timeliness of subsequent visits or meetings.

Teams are more effective when the individual members have high general mental ability; in other words, the team is comprised of smart people (Bell, 2007). The team is only as strong as the weakest team member. Team members must be able to think on their feet, make quick and effective decisions, and possess knowledge and skills beyond the content expected of a particular discipline. For example, an SLP working in early intervention is expected to contribute knowledge and expertise related to communication development. The SLP must also understand global child development from many perspectives when working on a team in early intervention in order to learn from and support other team members and caregivers. Team members who are viewed as lacking the knowledge or skills needed to complement the collective knowledge of the team can become marginalized and not sought out as a resource by other team members, potentially limiting the effectiveness of the team.

The characteristic of team member competence in their area of expertise is referenced across a number of studies (Bell, 2007; Boyer & Thompson, 2014; DeGangi et al., 1994; Dinnebeil et al., 1996, 1999; Dunst & Trivette, 2009; Dunst et al., 1994; Harrison et al., 1990; King et al., 2009; Lowenthal, 1992; O'Connor, 1995; Park & Turnbull, 2003; Soodak & Erwin, 2000). Early intervention teams using a PSP approach must consist of members representing a variety of disciplines because they have specialized training and often licensing or credentialing in a particular area of expertise or knowledge. Using practitioners who have recently graduated from preservice training programs is consistent with this characteristic. New graduates may lack experience, but they bring a fresh perspective, new energy, and the most up-to-date practices based on current research. An increased accountability for practitioner competence related to evidence-based practice has been emphasized in recent years not only to ensure the highest probability of achievement of desired outcomes but also as a consumer protection factor. Families enroll in early childhood programs and partner with practitioners because they trust and presume that needed or desired experiences and knowledge are available. They believe that the team members have expertise, knowledge, experience, and/or skills that will enhance their success in supporting the young children in their care. Competence and knowledge of early childhood development, family support, and adult learning are critical components for practitioners from every discipline associated with the field. Monitoring of required competencies is necessary at every level by individual practitioners, programs, agencies, and oversight systems to ensure that parents have not misplaced their trust or made false presumptions about the type and quality of support that is available.

The characteristics of openness to experience and mental stability of each team member are critical when supporting families and other team members in early intervention. A team member who is open to experience might be described as imaginative, objective, adaptable, innovative, and open minded. Openness to viewing new experiences as learning opportunities is specifically identified as an effective characteristic of team members. Factors related to openness and mental or emotional stability were reported across a number of early studies examining effective practitioner–parent interactions (DeGangi et al., 1994; Dinnebeil et al., 1996; Dunst & Trivette, 2009; Dunst et al., 1994; Lowenthal, 1992; O'Connor, 1995; Park & Turnbull, 2003; Soodak & Erwin, 2000).

Although the characteristic of "likes teamwork" may seem like an obvious statement, not every practitioner does. Working in isolation is often perceived to be faster, less stressful, and easier to some practitioners. Teamwork requires considering the perspectives of other team members, acknowledging different learning styles, building and maintaining relationships, and recognizing that an independent practitioner does not have all of the knowledge and skills necessary to appropriately support any child and family. Liking and respecting teamwork means that the individual practitioner believes the team's knowledge is always better than any one team member working alone.

Effective team members are socialized to the organization's culture. Every team has its own way of being and doing. The amount of time a team member spends in a particular environment or setting determines how they practice. For example, if a practitioner spends most of their time in a hospital setting and contracts a few hours each week with an early intervention program, then their dominant culture will most likely be the hospital. The early intervention team will need to make time to assist this individual in becoming acculturated and socialized to early intervention practices and team functioning. This culture may be disrupted whenever a member joins or leaves the team. The remaining members must ensure that the team is not swayed to the incoming member's culture or allow the team's culture to disintegrate or depart with the exiting team member.

The amount of time committed to the team and the longevity of team membership are particularly important when considering using consistent teams for children and their families in early intervention. This is especially true for those states using broker-type systems and vendors from a multitude of agencies in which providers contract for an hour here or there in addition to their real job (Dunst & Bruder, 2006; Sloper et al., 2006). Team members should be assigned to a consistent team so they can readily identify who is on their team. The system must be able to support these teams to minimize turnover, maximize involvement time, and promote long-term membership. Socialization and acculturation to the team and the use of research-based practices is more likely when team members do not rotate or change frequently. This socialization-acculturation effect is one of the most positive benefits of implementing a PSP approach to teaming (Bell, 2007; Borrill et al., 2001; West, 2012). The approach adds an inherent check and balance among team members, a heightened sense of responsibility, and programmatic accountability regarding the overall quality of supports and services for all families enrolled in the program.

PRIMARY SERVICE PROVIDER AS TEAM LIAISON TO FAMILY

Selecting one team member to serve as the liaison to the family and child is the second area of research that defines the characteristics and implementation conditions of PSP teaming practices. The need for a teaming approach using a PSP is based on the fact that focusing on services and multiple disciplines implementing decontextualized, child-focused, and deficit-based interventions has proven ineffective (Campbell & Halbert, 2002; Dunst et al., 2014; Dunst, Trivette, et al., 2001; Garcia-Grau et al., 2019; Hughes-Scholes et al., 2015; McWilliam, 2000; Shonkoff et al., 1992). Rotating multiple practitioners in and out of a family's life on a regular basis has been found to negatively affect family functioning (Dunst et al., 2007; Garcia-Grau et al., 2019; Greco & Sloper, 2004; Law et al., 1998; Shonkoff et al., 1992; Sloper, 2004).

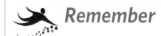

Remember

Selecting one team member to serve as the liaison to the family and child is another important area of research that defines the characteristics and implementation conditions of primary service provider teaming practices.

The results of a longitudinal investigation of 190 infants and their families after receiving 1 year of early intervention services indicate that those families receiving their services from a single provider compared with families receiving services from multiple providers reported less parenting stress (Shonkoff et al., 1992). In addition, the developmental outcomes for the infants of the families receiving services from a single provider were better than the infants who were receiving multidisciplinary services. These results persisted when the study controlled for the severity of disability of the child, the age of the child, and when both factors were controlled simultaneously. The only benefit actualized for the families of the children receiving services from multiple providers was an increase in the size of the mother's social support network. No differences were noted, however, in the mothers' reports of the helpfulness of their social support networks.

In a study of a statewide early intervention program in the northeastern United States, 250 parents completed surveys and follow-up parent and family outcome measures (Dunst et al., 2007). This study examined the level of family-centered practices received and resulting benefits for the children and families. Results indicated the more services that a family received, the less satisfied they were with early intervention, the less family centered the respondents rated the program, and the more negative the effects on personal and family well-being. The families reporting receipt of services that were not family centered also reported less child progress. Dunst et al. summarized that this study provides evidence that how early intervention is provided matters a great deal and that more service is not better in terms of outcomes for children and families.

Sloper and Turner (1992) reviewed the literature and summarized that families with multiple providers experienced increased parental stress, unmet needs, and confusion. More specifically, parents without a single provider reported a general lack of coordination of services resulting in increased stress related to parenting a child with disabilities. Surprisingly, having multiple providers resulted in unmet needs for a significant number of families, and most of the families had children with severe disabilities. This seems contrary to the commonly held belief that the needs of a child with severe disabilities cannot possibly be met by a PSP. In several studies reviewed, parents of children with disabilities reported confusion when multiple providers were involved on a regular basis. This confusion resulted from conflicting information and recommendations regarding intervention and resources. Parents were also confused about which practitioner to contact regarding specific questions or supports needed. For example, it might be clear to the professionals working with the family who addresses what issues, but parents reported ongoing struggles with role definitions when multiple providers were involved.

In the absence of a comparative study of teaming approaches in early intervention, we conducted a pilot study to compare the rate of achievement of IFSP outcomes, child outcomes, and service costs for children served by two geographically based early intervention teams using a PSP approach with those services provided to a matched cohort of children by multiple independent practitioners in the same catchment area. In this study, a *geographically based team* is defined as a group of practitioners consisting of an early childhood special educator, OT, PT, SLP, and service coordinator(s) responsible for all referrals within a predetermined area. The intervention 1) focused on promoting parent-mediated child learning in everyday activities (Dunst et al., 2006), 2) used coaching as the interaction style with parents (Rush & Shelden, 2020), and 3) used a PSP approach to teaming (Shelden & Rush, 2010).

The results from the study indicated that the children in the experimental group received fewer service hours, including team meeting time, than the control group that had no team meeting time; however, IFSP outcomes were met more often by children in the experimental group. No differences were noted between the groups for child developmental outcome data. Early intervention services and supports provided by the program using the PSP approach were less expensive than those services provided outside of this model. Practitioners in the experimental group not only met all federal requirements for Part C, but they also exceeded time frames for reviewing IFSP documents. Finally, fewer practitioners were involved in the lives of families, resulting in less disruption to family life. This pilot study of the use of geographically based early intervention teams using a PSP demonstrates promising data regarding efficient use of resources for early intervention programs. See Appendix 2A for the complete study.

TEAM SUPPORT FOR THE PRIMARY SERVICE PROVIDER

The support given by other team members to the PSP is the third area of research that defines the characteristics and implementation conditions of PSP teaming practices. This section describes the formal mechanism for team planning and sharing information as well as efficiently structuring the team meeting based on available research and a case study of one early intervention team.

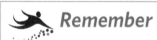

Remember

The support given by other team members to the primary service provider (PSP) is the third area of research that defines the characteristics and implementation conditions of PSP teaming practices.

The literature indicates that teams should have a common planning time, which is critical for effective team functioning (Borrill et al., 2001; Boyer & Thompson, 2014; West, 2012). This regularly scheduled shared meeting provides team members with a predictable time for discussion, idea generation, questioning, and analytical thinking; contributes to the acculturation and socialization of the team identity; and allows for the development of a heightened sense of accountability and commitment to complete the task.

In order to determine how to most effectively and efficiently conduct team meetings when using a PSP approach to teaming, we conducted a study to identify the characteristics of meetings to address three basic research questions:

1. Is the current team meeting structure providing the supports needed by team members?

2. What are the characteristics of an effective team meeting when using a PSP approach to teaming?

3. Would specific guidelines for presenting information and providing coaching in the team meeting be seen as useful to meeting participants?

The results of the study indicated that using a meeting facilitator, clearly defining roles of the facilitator and other meeting participants, and adopting a prepublished agenda led to meeting participants reporting that the team meeting better met their needs and accomplished the meeting purpose to provide and receive support related to working with families and gaining access to needed resources to ensure families are receiving comprehensive care. The team participating in this study met weekly and adhered to the characteristics of the PSP approach to teaming, including using an identified team of individuals from multiple disciplines, with one team member serving as PSP to the care provider(s) and the PSP receiving coaching from other team members through ongoing planned and spontaneous interactions. The complete study is located in Appendix 2B.

CHARACTERISTICS OF A PRIMARY SERVICE PROVIDER APPROACH TO TEAMING

In light of the literature previously discussed and adhering to the evidence-based approach for documenting characteristics of specific practices described by Dunst et al. (2002), the following list depicts the characteristics of a PSP approach to teaming. All of the characteristics must be adhered to by all team members in order to identify the practices as a PSP approach to teaming and ensure achievement of optimal benefits for young children and their families.

- A geographically based team of individuals from multiple disciplines having expertise in child development, family support, and coaching is assigned to each family in a program.

- One team member serves as PSP to the child and care provider(s).

- The PSP receives coaching from other team members through ongoing planned and spontaneous interactions.

Implementation Conditions

In addition to the three characteristics of a PSP approach to teaming, five implementation conditions are critical to putting the approach into practice. First, all therapists and educators on the team must be available to serve as a PSP. The flexibility of the entire team is compromised when only selected members or disciplines from the team serve in the role of PSP. Due to the nature of teamwork and the mandates of Part C (e.g., time lines, steps in the process), all team members must share the responsibility of serving as a PSP to equalize duties and maximize the quality of supports to children and families. In addition, ensuring that all members' roles and responsibilities are equal alleviates the tendency for hierarchical relationships to develop among team members.

Attendance by all members at regularly scheduled team meetings for the purpose of colleague-to-colleague coaching is another critical implementation condition. Coaching topics at team meetings are varied and include specific information for supporting team members in their role as a PSP to the families in the program. The process that a team uses to select a PSP is the third implementation condition. The PSP is selected according to four factors: 1) parent/family, 2) child, 3) environmental, and 4) practitioner. See Chapter 5 for more information for selecting the most likely PSP.

Joint visits are an essential condition of the PSP approach to teaming and give team members the opportunity to support one another and the child's care providers in a timely and effective manner. Joint visits by other team members must occur with the PSP at the same place and time whenever possible. When a joint visit occurs and the other team member is supporting the PSP, the relationship between the PSP and family is not disrupted or negatively affected. In addition, the opportunity for sharing information between the PSP and the other team member provides learning opportunities for the PSP, builds trust and respect among team members, and affords the caregivers prioritized and focused opportunities to interact with other team members. The PSP can assist the family in applying the information in an ongoing and contextualized manner with the support of the accompanying team member.

The last implementation condition is that the PSP for a family should change as infrequently as possible. One of the purposes of having a PSP is for the family to establish and maintain an ongoing working relationship with a single team member to minimize any negative consequences of having multiple and or changing practitioners. As a result, the PSP rarely changes. The PSP does not change when IFSP outcomes change, when primary learners change, or when the PSP may need specific supports from other team members. The PSP should change if the family does not

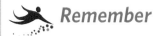 **Remember**

Five implementation conditions must be present when implementing a primary service provider (PSP) approach to teaming:

1. All therapists and educators on the team must be available to serve as a PSP.

2. All members attend regular team meetings for the purpose of colleague-to-colleague coaching.

3. The team uses a process to select a PSP according to four factors: 1) parent/family, 2) child, 3) environmental, and 4) practitioner.

4. Joint visits are required as a role assistance strategy to give team members the opportunity to support one another and the child's care providers in a timely and effective manner.

5. The PSP for a family should change as infrequently as possible.

like the manner or style of the PSP, the family specifically requests a change, or the PSP continually needs another team member on joint visits because of their lack of knowledge and skill.

Checklists for Implementing a Primary Service Provider Approach to Teaming

We developed a set of four checklists using the characteristics and implementation conditions of the PSP approach in order to assist teams in implementing a PSP approach to teaming (see Figure 2.1 and Appendix 2C). The indicators were based on a review of relevant research and were revised following feedback from practitioners and other professionals considered proficient in the use of the practices. Each indicator is worded to reflect different aspects of four practice areas of a PSP approach to teaming. The four sets of indicators include the following elements of a PSP approach to teaming:

1. *Preparing for a team-based approach.* This checklist includes practice indicators for establishing geographically based teams.

2. *Using a PSP.* This checklist includes indicators for selecting a PSP for a specific child and family as well as documenting the presence of coaching by the PSP with family members, care providers, and other team members.

3. *Coordinating joint visits.* This checklist includes indicators for implementing joint visits between the PSP and other team members with the family or other care providers.

4. *Conducting team meetings.* This checklist includes indicators for conducting effective team meetings based on the study presented earlier in this chapter.

For each indicator in the checklists, the user (e.g., program, supervisor, practitioner) is asked to indicate whether (Yes/No) the practices used are present or absent. Space is provided for noting examples of practices that can be examined not only in terms of presence or absence but also consistency or inconsistency with the practice standards. The checklists also include a section for the program or practitioners to develop a plan for making desired improvements in their practices. The checklists can be used for a number of different purposes. First, they can help a program plan for and implement the key characteristics of evidence-based teaming practices in early childhood intervention. Second, team leadership and supervisors can use the checklists as observational tools for determining the extent to which the program implements a PSP approach to teaming. They can be used to provide feedback and guidance about which practices are consistent or inconsistent with the practice indicators and what the team members can do to improve their practices. The team leadership and/or supervisor can use the Program Planning section with the team to develop strategies for changing practices to better mirror the practice indicators. Third, a practitioner can use the checklists to conduct a self-assessment to examine their use of PSP teaming practices. A self-assessment could be accomplished by the practitioner reflecting on their practices as a team member and determining whether the practices are consistent or inconsistent with each practice indicator. The Program Planning section can be used to develop plans for changing practices and identifying the supports needed to make practices consistent with the indicators. Fourth, the checklists can be used for program evaluation purposes by monitoring consistency in the use of the practices and improvements over time.

CONCLUSION

This chapter described the research supporting the implementation of a PSP approach to teaming. The research falls into three areas: 1) a defined team, 2) a PSP as the team liaison to the family, and 3) team support for the PSP. We used this research to further delineate specific characteristics and implementation conditions required for effectively using this teaming approach. Due to

Checklists for Implementing a Primary Service Provider Approach to Teaming

Team or practitioner's name: _____   Date: _____

Checklist Descriptions

These checklists include practice indicators of the key characteristics of a primary service provider approach to teaming in early childhood intervention. A **primary service provider** approach to teaming is using a multidisciplinary team in which one member is selected as the primary service provider, receives coaching from other team members, and uses coaching with parents and other primary care providers to support and strengthen parenting competence and confidence in promoting child learning and development and obtaining desired supports and resources.

The four checklists describe different areas of primary service provider teaming practices: 1) preparing for a team-based approach, 2) using a primary service provider, 3) coordinating joint visits, and 4) conducting team meetings. Each section contains indicators of a specific area of a primary service provider approach to teaming practices. For each indicator, determine whether the program is adhering to the aspect of the practice described. Space is also available for notes or examples of adherence.

Use of the Checklists

The four checklists include 30 indicators that are the foundation for implementing a primary service provider approach to teaming. The checklists can be used for a number of different purposes.

- They can be used to help a program learn and master the key characteristics of evidence-based teaming practices in early childhood intervention.

- Team leadership and supervisors can use the checklists as observational tools for determining the extent to which the program implements a primary service provider approach to teaming. They can be used to provide feedback and guidance about which practices are consistent or inconsistent with the practice indicators and what the team members can do to improve their practices. The team leadership and/or supervisor can use the Program Planning section with the team to develop plans for changing practices to better mirror the practice indicators.

- A practitioner can use the checklists to conduct a self-assessment to examine his or her use of a primary service provider approach to teaming practices. A self-assessment could be accomplished by the practitioner reflecting on his or her practices as a team member and determining whether the practices are consistent or inconsistent with each practice indicator.

- The Program Planning section can be used to develop plans for changing practices and identifying the supports needed to make practices consistent with the practice indicators. They can be used for program evaluation purposes by monitoring consistency in the use of the practices and improvements over time.

(continued)

Figure 2.1. Checklists for implementing a primary service provider approach to teaming. (From The Family, Infant and Preschool Program [FIPP] Center for the Advanced Study of Excellence [CASE], part of the J. Iverson Riddle Developmental Center [JIRDC] in Morganton, NC; reprinted by permission. Copyright © 2013 Family, Infant and Preschool Program.)

Figure 2.1.   *(continued)*

Team or practitioner's name: _____   Date: _____

	Are practices characterized by the following?	Yes	No	Examples/notes
Preparing for a team-based approach	Program leadership determines the number and specific location of families served by the local program.	Y	N	
	Program leadership determines the fewest number of teams necessary to cover the program area based on the premise that a team of four full-time practitioners can serve approximately 100–125 families when drive time does not exceed 30–45 minutes for a one-way trip.	Y	N	
	Program leadership identifies the geographic area that each team will cover based on family distribution within a given catchment area, geographic region (e.g., county), zip code, portion of a school district, and so forth.	Y	N	
	Program leadership ensures that each team minimally consists of an early childhood educator and/or early childhood special educator, occupational therapist, physical therapist, and speech-language pathologist.	Y	N	
	Program leadership ensures that the role of service coordination is fulfilled either by one of the disciplines previously listed (i.e., blended model) or by an individual solely responsible for service coordination (i.e., dedicated model).	Y	N	
	Custodial family members are always members of their child's team.	Y	N	
	Program leadership assigns available practitioners to teams beginning with those who are employed or contracted with the program for the greatest amount of time.	Y	N	
	Teams have an identified team leader.	Y	N	
	Program leadership assigns each new referral to the team responsible for the geographic area in which the child resides.	Y	N	

	Are practices characterized by the following?	Yes	No	Examples/notes
Using a primary service provider	All therapists and educators on the team are available to serve as a primary service provider.	Y	N	
	One team member is selected to serve as the primary service provider to the family and other care providers.	Y	N	
	The primary service provider is selected based on four factors: 1) parent/family, 2) child, 3) environmental, 4) practitioner.	Y	N	
	The primary service provider assigned to a family uses a coaching interaction style to build the capacity of the parents and other care providers to support child learning as well as to identify and obtain needed resources and supports.	Y	N	
	The primary service provider receives coaching support from other team members through ongoing formal (planned) and informal interactions.	Y	N	
	The primary service provider for a family changes as infrequently as possible (i.e., rarely changes).	Y	N	

(continued)

Team or practitioner's name: _____   Date: _____

	Are practices characterized by the following?	Yes	No	Examples/notes
Coordinating joint visits	Team members support the primary service provider through joint visits.	Y	N	
	The primary service provider and other team members conduct joint visits at the same place and time.	Y	N	
	The primary service provider along with the parents and/or other care providers predetermine questions, expected outcomes, and specific actions to be taken during the joint visit.	Y	N	
	The primary service provider and other team members define their roles for the joint visit based on questions, expected outcomes, and specific actions to be taken as related to the priorities of the primary service provider and parent.	Y	N	
	The primary service provider debriefs the joint visit with the parents and/or other care providers to evaluate the usefulness of the joint visit and determine next steps.	Y	N	
	The primary service provider and other team members debrief the joint visit to evaluate the usefulness of the joint visit and determine next steps.	Y	N	

	Are practices characterized by the following?	Yes	No	Examples/notes
Conducting team meetings	The team leader ensures that the purpose of the team meeting is to share information among team members as families move through the early intervention process and for primary service providers to receive coaching from their team members.	Y	N	
	All team members attend the weekly team meeting.	Y	N	
	All team members are present for the entire team meeting.	Y	N	
	The primary service provider informs the parents of the dates and times of team meetings when their name is on the agenda and invites them to attend if they desire.	Y	N	
	The primary service provider invites the parents to send questions or updates to the team meetings via the primary service provider and ensures timely feedback.	Y	N	
	The team leader ensures that the team meeting is led by a competent and consistent facilitator. The team meeting facilitator may or may not be someone other than the formal team leader.	Y	N	
	The team meeting facilitator develops a meeting agenda with time limits that have been prepublished.	Y	N	
	The team has clearly defined roles of the facilitator and other meeting participants.	Y	N	
	Program leadership compensates team members for team meeting time.	Y	N	

(continued)

Figure 2.1. *(continued)*

Team or practitioner's name: _____ Date: _____

Program Planning

Prepare a plan for making changes and/or ensuring sustainability based on analysis of the primary service provider approach to teaming practice indicators. Describe the specific action steps that will be taken and identify the particular experiences and opportunities that will be used to make the needed programmatic changes.

Preparing for a team-based approach	**Needed change**
	Action steps (i.e., what will be done; by when):

Using a primary service provider	**Needed change**
	Action steps (i.e., what will be done; by when):

Coordinating joint visits	**Needed change**
	Action steps (i.e., what will be done; by when):

Conducting team meetings	**Needed change**
	Action steps (i.e., what will be done; by when):

the complexity, confusion, and controversy often related to using PSP teaming practices, claims of using this approach must be further explored to ensure that the evidence-based characteristics and implementation conditions are actually present. Defining the characteristics and providing the implementation conditions based on available research provides accountability and ensures systematic operationalization of the practices. The operational definition provided in this chapter can serve as a foundation for further research of the benefits and outcomes when this teaming approach is implemented.

Although the research contained in this chapter establishes a strong base of support, additional research is needed. More specifically, further comparison of child and family outcomes of teams using a PSP approach with other common models of team interaction would be helpful. Further study would also yield beneficial information regarding team caseload size, effective use of distance technology, frequency of team meetings, minimum and maximum number of members necessary for effective teaming and supports to families, level of program leadership support required, effective technical assistance to support implementation and fidelity, and fiscal implications for state and local programs.

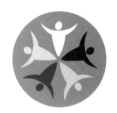

A Pilot Study of the Use of Geographically Based Early Intervention Teams Using a Primary Service Provider Approach to Teaming

The purpose of this study was to collect pilot data on the effectiveness of using a primary service provider (PSP) approach to teaming. More specifically, the study was designed to examine whether children with disabilities served by a geographically based early intervention team using a PSP, coaching interaction style, and strategies to promote parent-mediated child learning 1) met individualized family service plan (IFSP) outcomes more rapidly, 2) achieved higher ratings on developmental evaluation, and 3) received services at an overall lower cost than those provided to children with disabilities in other service delivery models.

METHODS

Two geographically based early intervention teams were formed in a suburban/rural district as part of a Part C statewide program that agreed to participate in the study. The early intervention coordinator in the district identified practitioners and service coordinators willing to participate in the study as well as form two geographically based teams that used a PSP approach to teaming, a coaching interaction style with families and colleagues, and natural learning environment practices. The two teams consisted of an early childhood special educator, an occupational therapist (OT), a physical therapist (PT), a speech-language pathologist (SLP), and a service coordinator. One nutritionist was shared by both teams. All newly referred children to the designated catchment areas served by the two early intervention teams were invited to participate in the study as members of the experimental group. If the children were determined to be eligible for Part C and the family was willing to participate in the study, then the children were included. Twenty-five children were enrolled in the study. The following criteria were established to identify matches (i.e., control group) for the 25 children in the experimental group: 1) child age at entry into the study, 2) child diagnosis, 3) length of time served by the program, 4) simultaneous participation in the program, and 5) family socioeconomic status. Matches were identified for 20 of the 25 children in the experimental group. The five children without matches were excluded from the study.

PARTICIPANTS

Participants were divided into experimental and control groups. Children in each group were matched pairs based on demographic information and length of enrollment in the program.

Children's Experimental and Control Groups

Fifteen of the 20 identified pairs of children were matched by gender. Children in both groups had diagnoses that included developmental delay, seizure disorder, cerebral palsy, Down syndrome, visual impairment, severe disabilities, and autism/pervasive developmental disorder (PDD). Nineteen of the 20 pairs were matched exactly by diagnosis. In one pair, a child with PDD was matched with a child with autism. The mean chronological age of the children upon entry into the study was 12.35 months ($SD = 9.70$) for the experimental group and 12.85 ($SD = 9.01$) months for the control group. Upon exit, the mean chronological age of the experimental group was 19.95 months (SD = 8.41) and the control group was 21.84 months (SD = 8.19). The differences between the matched ages at the first and second evaluations were not significant $t(19)$ = –0.499, p = .623 and second evaluation $t(18)$ = –1.315, p = .205. Fifteen of the 20 pairs were matched by socioeconomic status.

Practitioners' Control Group

Limited data were available on the practitioners in the control group due to the retrospective nature of this study. The state early intervention system participating in this study used a brokered-type system, whereby service coordinators procured services for children matched to child impairments identified during the evaluation process. For example, a child demonstrating delays in the areas of communication and motor may have an OT, PT, and SLP assigned for ongoing services on the IFSP. Individual practitioners in the control group decided the frequency and intensity of service provision with little to no interaction between service providers assigned to a particular child and family. The study placed no parameters on the type, amount, or manner in which the services were provided, and no team meetings occurred among practitioners in the control group. The control group consisted of practitioners representing disciplines identified on the IFSP, including six early childhood special educators, eight OTs, 11 PTs, and nine SLPs. Four of the 34 practitioners were male and 30 were female. The number of children served by practitioners in the control group was as follows: one practitioner served three children; nine practitioners served two children each; and 24 practitioners served only one child each.

Practitioners' Experimental Group

Data were collected on nine practitioners in the experimental group, which included two early childhood special educators, one nutritionist, two OTs, two PTs, and two SLPs. See Table 2A.1 for specific information about the practitioners and Table 2A.2 for caseload information.

The practitioners in the experimental group participated as two teams in a 2 1/2 day workshop focused on implementing evidence-based practices with a 9-month follow-up component. The practices taught and used by the teams consisted of 1) focusing on promoting child participation within everyday activities as the intervention, 2) using coaching as the interaction style with parents, and 3) using a PSP approach for teaming. No restrictions were set regarding the amount of service provided to each child. Required team meeting time was one meeting per week with no limitation placed on the amount of team meeting time. The follow-up support included monthly conference calls with the authors for coaching and discussing questions regarding implementing the evidence-based practice model, reviewing coaching logs written and submitted by team members, reviewing other documentation, and scheduling a 1-day on-site follow-up visit to discuss implementation issues and use of the practices.

Practitioner Fidelity

Data were collected to ensure that practitioners in the experimental group were adhering to the practices as delineated during the training institute. The practitioners in the experimental group

Table 2A.1. Characteristics of practitioners in the experimental group

	Minimum	Maximum	Mean	Standard deviation
Years of experience in major area of study	8	20	14.50	4.751
Total number of years working in the program	1	10	4.92	3.012
Practitioner age at time of survey	30	54	41.25	7.226

Table 2A.2. Practitioner caseload in the experimental group

Practitioner	Gender	Discipline	Number of children
1	F	Nutrition	1
2	F	Occupational therapy	1
3	F	Early childhood special education	1
4	F	Speech-language pathology	2
5	F	Physical therapy	5
6	F	Occupational therapy	4
7	F	Physical therapy	3
8	F	Speech-language pathology	2
9	F	Early childhood special education	1

were asked to maintain coaching logs written after each visit to document coaching and natural learning environment practices. The coaching log serves as a recollection or transcript of the conversation with notation of the actions that occurred. The transcript that was written on the log included any questions asked by the practitioner, responses of the parent, information shared by the practitioner, description of modeling by the practitioner, actions taken by the parent, and feedback provided by the practitioner. Space was provided for coding the presence of the characteristics of coaching (joint planning, observation, action, reflection, and feedback); types of reflective questions asked by the practitioner (awareness, analysis, alternatives, or action); and the types of feedback provided to the parent by the practitioner (affirmative, informative, directive, or evaluative). Space was also provided for the practitioner to reflect on their practices to self-assess how closely the practices matched coaching and natural learning environment practices.

The practitioners were required to attend team meetings, document the team meeting discussions, and identify the amount of time spent at each teaming meeting supporting individual families in order to document the adherence to a PSP approach to teaming. Data were also collected on the total number and length of each visit and number of joint visits.

Data were collected on control group practitioners by using billing documents provided by the program. These data captured the number, length, and costs of visits. Control group practitioners were not members of teams, did not participate in joint visits, and engaged in business-as-usual practices with no control measures or restrictions placed on their practices.

Child Developmental Outcomes

Due to the initiation and conclusion dates of the study, data were collected over a range of 6–46 weeks for individual children with a mean of 20.8 weeks. The data collected for both groups included all developmental testing and an IFSP written and implemented over the course of the project period. Developmental scores were charted for each child across five domains of development (i.e., adaptive, motor, cognitive, communication, personal-social) for all available testing during the data collection period. Mean age-equivalent scores were then computed using all domain areas. The scores used were those closest to the entry and exit of the data collection period. Furthermore, the researchers obtained data regarding who completed the initial and follow-up evaluation and was involved in ongoing service delivery for each child.

Service Costs

The billed units for all services on each child's IFSP were collected and reviewed. Data collection for the experimental group also included team meeting minutes, team meeting time for each team member, and documenting joint visits between team members.

Individualized Family Service Plan Outcomes

IFSP documents were reviewed to determine the number of outcomes that were met, not met, or ongoing. A child's IFSP is subject to review when a goal on the IFSP is met, a team member requests a review, or minimally at 6-month intervals as mandated by federal law. The difference between the expected number of IFSP reviews (minimal number as determined by federal regulations) and the actual number of IFSP reviews held due to IFSP outcome achievement was determined for each child in the study.

DATA ANALYSIS AND RESULTS

The data analyzed included practitioner fidelity, service cost, individualized family service plan outcomes, and child development outcomes.

Practitioner Fidelity Data

The coaching logs were used to document coaching and natural learning environment practices and were coded by the researchers using the Coaching Log Coding Tool. The purpose of writing and coding was to document the extent to which practitioners were interacting with parents using coaching and natural learning environment practices to build the parents' capacity to promote their children's growth and development.

The Coaching Log Coding Tool is a 17-item instrument that measured the extent to which the content of each interaction with the parents reflected natural learning environment practices, and the process of the interaction demonstrated the presence of the five characteristics of coaching: 1) joint planning, 2) observation, 3) action and practice, 4) reflection, and 5) feedback. The Coaching Log Coding Tool was used in this study as a process and outcome measure to examine practitioner adherence to and use of coaching and natural learning environment practices. Items related to natural learning environments practices examined five dimensions: 1) child learning, 2) parenting support, 3) community resources, 4) family-centered practices, and 5) child and parent outcomes. These dimensions are based on an integrated framework for providing early childhood intervention and parent support (Dunst, 2004). Items that measured coaching practices included indicators related to the characteristics of coaching practices as identified in research on the effectiveness of coaching to promote behavior change (Bowman & McCormick, 2000; Bruce & Ross, 2008; Homa et al., 2008; Kurtts & Levin, 2000; Peterson et al., 2007; Tschantz & Vail, 2000). Each indicator in both measures within the Coaching Log Coding Tool was rated using a Likert-type scale ranging from 1, indicating *not at all consistent* with the practices, to 5, indicating *completely consistent*. A rating of 0 was used if the content was not discussed or the coder was unable to determine whether the content was discussed. The indicators were selected by a group of five experts in the use of coaching and natural learning environment practices. Measurement of interrater reliability among the researchers and one independent reviewer on the coding tool yielded a Cronbach's alpha of .853 and was significant at the .05 level.

The adherence to natural learning environment practices was analyzed for the nine practitioners in the experimental group. During the data collection period (the first 6 months the practitioners used the new practices), one practitioner was rated as 4 (*mostly consistent*), five practitioners were rated as 3 (*somewhat consistent*), and three practitioners were rated as 2 (*mostly not consistent*).

Coaching practice adherence was also analyzed for the nine practitioners in the experimental group. Results indicated that one practitioner was rated as 5 (*completely consistent*), two practitioners were rated as 4 (*mostly consistent*), five practitioners were rated as 3 (*somewhat consistent*), and one practitioner was rated as 2 (*mostly not consistent*).

Adherence to a PSP approach to teaming was analyzed for both teams in the experimental group across all nine practitioners. Analysis of the IFSP for each child in the experimental group revealed selection of a PSP with joint visits provided by other team members. No children were being seen by multiple providers on different days at different times. The number of joint visits that occurred during the data collection period varied by child based on length of time the child had been enrolled in the program and the additional need for support identified by the PSP. Joint visits across both teams accounted for 11% of the total number of visits. The PSPs remained constant for 17 of the 20 children during the data collection period. The rationale for changing the PSP for one child was documented as a personality conflict between the PSP and parent. The PSP changed for the two other children because a team member returned from maternity leave. Results indicated that both teams met weekly during each week of the data collection period. All practitioners attended every team meeting during that time period, with the exception of one practitioner missing one meeting.

Service Cost Data

The total number of actual hours of service received by each child across all disciplines, including team meeting time for the experimental group, was calculated by analyzing and triangulating billing documents submitted to the early intervention program, coaching logs, and team meeting minutes. The service data compare the means of 13 variables between the experimental and control groups (see Table 2A.3). These variables measure the number of hours that a type of practitioner (e.g., SLP, OT, PT, early childhood special educator, nutritionist) spent with a given child. Because the children in the experimental group were served by teams, the number of hours of service provided can be measured as the service hours excluding team meeting time or the number of hours including team meeting time. Comparing these means yields Cohen's *d* statistic and an associated magnitude of effect (Rosenthal, 1994). Measurable differences were identified between the experimental and control groups for the amount of service provided even when teaming time was added. Only small effect sizes were noted within speech-language pathology and ECSE between the control and experimental groups, which could be due to a lack of availability and/or low utilization of these disciplines for children in the control group. The treatment effect on the number of hours of nutritional services that were provided was not calculated because these services were not made available to any child in the control group. The box plots in Figure 2A.1 illustrate the

Table 2A.3. Descriptive statistics of service hours per child by group

	Experimental mean	Control mean	Experimental standard deviation	Control standard deviation	Cohen's *d*	Magnitude
Total number of service hours (all disciplines) including team meeting time	18.24	21.80	7.71	15.03	−0.30	Small
Total number of service hours (all disciplines) excluding team meeting time	11.21	21.80	4.54	15.03	−0.95	Large
Total number of physical therapy service hours including team meeting time	5.87	9.01	5.58	10.10	−0.38	Small
Total number of physical therapy service hours excluding team meeting time	4.35	9.01	5.45	10.10	−0.57	Medium
Total number of occupational therapy service hours including team meeting time	4.17	7.80	4.77	11.11	−0.42	Small
Total number of occupational therapy service hours excluding team meeting time	2.65	7.80	4.41	11.11	−0.61	Medium
Total number of speech-language pathology service hours including team meeting time	3.92	2.84	3.87	4.66	0.25	Small
Total number of speech-language pathology service hours excluding team meeting time	2.40	2.84	3.74	4.66	−0.10	Small
Total number of early childhood special education service hours including team meeting time	2.48	2.15	3.70	4.90	0.08	Small
Total number of early childhood special education service hours excluding team meeting time	1.02	2.15	3.62	4.90	−0.26	Small
Total number of nutrition service hours including team meeting time	1.79	0.00	2.43	0.00	NA	NA
Total number of nutrition service hours excluding team meeting time	0.80	0.00	2.41	0.00	NA	NA

Key: NA, not applicable.

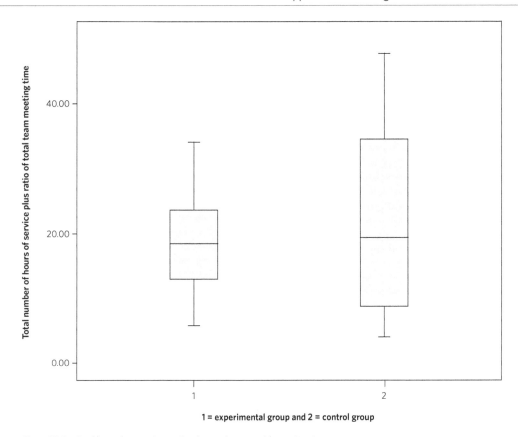

1 = experimental group and 2 = control group

Figure 2A.1. Total hours for experimental and control groups with teaming time.

distribution of total hours for both the control and experimental groups (including teaming time for the experimental group).

The mean number of total service hours with teaming time was lower for the experimental group than the control group. This (paired) difference is not significant at a .05 significance level, $t(19) = -1.27$, $p = .219$. The box plots demonstrate the extent to which the variability of the number of hours was lessened for the experimental group. The mean number of total service hours without teaming time is lower for the experimental group than the control group. This (paired) difference is significant at a 0.05 significance level, $t(19) = -3.57$, $p = .002$ (Figure 2A.2). Here the difference in variability between the groups is even more pronounced.

Individualized Family Service Plan Outcome Data

In all cases, the differences in the expected and actual number of IFSP reviews were positive, indicating that the federal IFSP review requirements were met for all children in the study. Table 2A.4 contains the percentage of children who had 0, 1, or 2 IFSP reviews *in excess* of the expected number. These data indicate a significant difference between groups for more IFSP reviews than is mandated by federal regulations, x^2 (2, $N = 40$) = 11.613, $p = .003$.

Child Developmental Outcome Data

Considerable care was taken to match the children on a variety of criteria. Table 2A.5 demonstrates the extent to which the matched children's developmental data were similar. The average developmental age calculated from the five separate developmental domains—adaptive development,

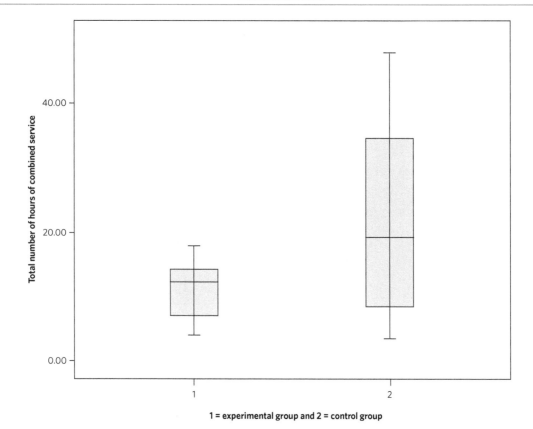

1 = experimental group and 2 = control group

Figure 2A.2.   Total hours for experimental and control groups without teaming time.

cognitive development, communication, motor development, and personal-social development—is presented in the table and also used as the unit of analysis. The mean overall proportional change index (PCI) values were compared for the treatment and control groups using a PCI formula recommended by Wolery (1983). The overall PCI was calculated for each child using the following formula.

$$\text{Subject overall PCI} = \frac{(DA_{\text{Exit}} - DA_{\text{Entry}}) / (CA_{\text{Exit}} - CA_{\text{Entry}})}{DA_{\text{Entry}} / CA_{\text{Entry}}}$$

Whereas *CA* is the subject's chronological age, *DA* is the subject's mean developmental age across the five domains.

Overall, both groups made developmental progress beyond that accounted for by maturation; however, no differences were found between groups. Caution should be exercised when interpreting these indices as they are based on the assumption that children develop at a steady rate in the

Table 2A.4.   Difference between expected and observed individualized family service plan reviews by group

	Zero more than expected	One more than expected	Two more than expected
Experimental	55%, *n* = 11	35%, *n* = 7	10%, *n* = 2
Control	100%, *n* = 20	0%, *n* = 0	0%, *n* = 0

Table 2A.5. Child developmental outcome data

	Experimental mean	Control mean	Experimental standard deviation	Control standard deviation	Cohen's d	Magnitude
Developmental age at entry	7.31	7.26	6.95	6.29	0.01	Small
Developmental age at exit	13.47	14.87	8.72	8.78	−0.16	Small
Overall proportional change index	1.49	1.59	1.67	1.32	−0.07	Small

absence of intervention (Lee & Kahn, 2000). This assumption has not been empirically justified and has been shown to be inappropriate for children with severe disabilities.

Further analysis was completed to examine the possibility of practitioner bias related to child developmental data. Practitioners in the control and experimental groups involved in ongoing service delivery were often responsible for evaluating developmental progress. At least one evaluator was present at both the initial and follow-up evaluation events (i.e., evaluator match) for 13 of the 20 children in the experimental group and 14 of the 20 children in the control group. In order to address the concern that an evaluator present on both occasions would bias the scores, an univariate ANOVA procedure was performed on the log-transformed PCI scores to determine if a group by evaluator match interaction occurred. Of the 40 participating children, two children in each group did not have scores recorded and one child in each group had a score of 0, which is undefined when transformed. The group by evaluator match interaction was not significant, $F(1,28) = 0.912$, $p = .348$. Similarly, at least one practitioner was involved in the follow-up evaluation (i.e., practitioner match) for 11 of the 20 children in the experimental group and 17 of the 20 children in the control group. The group by practitioner match interaction was not significant, $F(1,28) = 0.766$, $p = .389$. Although these results provide some evidence that the PCI scores were not influenced by the relationship the evaluators had to the children being evaluated, true interactions may be undetected due to the low power of the test resulting from small sample sizes.

DISCUSSION

The study findings confirmed and expanded current knowledge of a PSP approach to teaming. The findings were organized based on practitioner fidelity, service cost, IFSP outcomes, and child development outcomes.

Practitioner Fidelity Data

The analyses of the coaching logs and team meeting documents revealed that natural learning environment practices were more difficult for practitioners to master than coaching and PSP teaming practices. Six of the nine practitioners in the experimental group achieved a rating of 3 or above (*somewhat consistent* or *mostly consistent*) on the Coaching Log Coding Tool for the natural learning environment practices within the first 6 months following the initial training. Eight of the nine practitioners achieved a rating of 3 or higher (*somewhat consistent, mostly consistent,* or *completely consistent*) for adherence to coaching practices during the same time period. Both experimental group teams (i.e., all nine practitioners) demonstrated completely consistent adherence to PSP teaming practices during the 6 month data collection period. Although a higher rating of fidelity would be preferred with all nine practitioners achieving a rating of 5 (*completely consistent*) in natural learning environment practices, coaching practices, and PSP teaming practices, the data revealed progress toward adherence for each practitioner. The coaching logs showed that each practitioner made an effort to implement the practices and provided documentation of their practices with families to achieve the intended outcomes. The outcomes are notable considering that the experimental group practitioners were learning new practices and could be exhibiting their worst performance during data collection for adherence.

Service Cost Data

The service cost data in this pilot study were analyzed considering total service hours with and without teaming time for those children in the experimental group. This dual calculation illustrated the number of service hours for the children in the experimental group was less than the children in the control group, both with and without teaming time added. Children in the control group did not have teams. Thus, no teaming time was accrued by the practitioners supporting the children in the control group. Teaming is a required characteristic when using a PSP. Even though teaming time adds to the total number of service hours, the total number of service hours for the experimental group was less than the control group. Teaming time can be a specified and limited amount of time each week for every practitioner on the team.

Teaming time is currently not a billable service for third party reimbursement. The responsibility for payment for teaming time rests with the early intervention program as a required component for efficient and effective service delivery. No child in the experimental group received the maximum allowable billable units; yet, they made progress at least equal to the progress made by the children in the control group. The team process used in the experimental group provided an internal check and balance system for determining the level of service delivery for each child. No individual provider could decide in isolation the amount of intervention needed for a particular child.

The children in the experimental group had access to a team that included an early childhood special educator, nutritionist, OT, PT, service coordinator(s), and SLP. No children in the control group had access to a nutritionist. Team members in the experimental group used joint visits whenever necessary, thereby providing the family and child access to providers from multiple disciplines. Fewer service hours were needed for the children in the experimental group, even with the use of joint visits. Most third party payers do not reimburse for two practitioners providing services to a child/family at the same date and time. For this pilot study, the data demonstrate that payment of practitioners for joint visits costs less than the control group in which multiple practitioners see the same children on different days and times. Even though most third party payers deny payment for joint visits, the cost savings from not having multiple practitioners seeing children on different days and times could be used by programs and states to cover the costs of the joint visits.

The data illustrate implications for early intervention administrators in costs related to the number of contracts/people to manage and subsequent budgeting, billing, training, and monitoring requirements. Administrators using a PSP approach to teaming either hire or contract with the minimum number of practitioners necessary to support children and families in the designated catchment area. This teaming model not only decreases the number of people to manage, but it also provides for reduction in the magnitude of training and monitoring duties. For example, nine practitioners across two teams supported 20 children in the experimental group compared with 34 practitioners supporting 20 children in the control group. It is critically important to note that the 20 children in the experimental group represent only approximately 20% of a full caseload for a team. These numbers were low due to data collection procedures required for the study. Practitioners in the control group determined their own caseload based on the number of hours they were willing to contract with the program. Using a PSP approach can allow program administrators more predictability in budgeting as the variability of the services is decreased compared with a model without teams.

Individualized Family Service Plan Outcome Data

A difference was present between the groups regarding achievement of IFSP outcomes and reviews. The children in the experimental group achieved IFSP outcomes in a shorter period of time, which resulted in more frequent IFSP reviews than required by federal regulations and received by the children in the control group.

Child Developmental Outcome Data

The child developmental outcome data from this study are representative of how well the experimental and control groups were matched to limit variability. Both groups made developmental progress beyond that accounted for by maturation; however, no differences were found in the amount of developmental progress between groups. As expected, the amount of developmental progress is indicative of the short time period of data collection and is also minimized because means were obtained for groups that contained children with mild disabilities who reached chronological age level at exit as well as children with severe disabilities who actually showed regression in developmental scores. Both groups making progress with no differences is, in fact, a substantive issue because services for the experimental group in this pilot study 1) cost less, 2) required fewer resources, and 3) yielded IFSP outcome achievement in a shorter period of time.

LIMITATIONS AND DELIMITATIONS OF THE STUDY

Although this pilot study provides useful, comparative data on two different approaches of service delivery in early intervention, several limitations of the study exist. The small sample size is the first limitation of the study. The sample size of 20 pairs ($n = 40$) was limited by the logistics of the study. As the authors were implementing a matched pairs study and accepting all interested new referrals into the study, exact matches relevant to age, diagnosis, and enrollment in the program were limiting factors. The short period of data collection due to obtaining pairs enrolled in the early intervention program within 6 months of one another to ensure the most consistency as possible was also a limitation of the study. If the data collection period was longer, then the possibility of obtaining group differences might have been heightened.

A strength of this study was that the sample contained a group of children with diagnoses that were representative of natural proportions of the types and levels of disabilities seen within a typical early intervention program. The variety and level of disability was actualized as a limitation, however, in terms of looking at differences in child developmental outcomes between groups. A larger sample would have provided the opportunity to group children by type and level of disability, enabling us to identify child developmental outcome differences between groups. For example, one would anticipate that a child with a severe type of cerebral palsy would not make discernible progress over time, especially a short period of time, but a child with a developmental delay or language delay would most likely show developmental progress. The developmental gains of individual children are diluted by those individual children with more severe disabilities when means are obtained across the large group. The fact that no significant differences were noted between groups regarding child developmental outcomes in this study is indeed a credible finding.

Additional limitations of the study are that demographic information of practitioners in the control group or detailed descriptions of interventions they implemented for children were not available for analysis. Documentation for billing purposes was available, but it was not detailed enough to analyze types of interventions and practices used to implement the IFSP.

Finally, the learning curve of the practitioners involved in this study is another limitation. All practitioners in the experimental group were actively engaged in learning new practices and skills because data collection began immediately following the training. Although experimental group practitioners demonstrated adherence to the PSP approach to teaming practices and showed progress related to adherence to coaching and natural learning environment practices, outcomes could be different with stronger fidelity data across practitioners.

Strengths of this study include the robust matching of child pairs between the control and experimental groups, yielding an increased generalizability of data. Threats to the validity of the study were minimized because factors such as age, severity and type of disability, and socioeconomic status were controlled. The availability of detailed, comprehensive documentation practitioners' activities in the experimental group is another strength of the study. The practitioners in the experimental group provided team meeting documentation at the child level by time, content, and outcomes of discussions that occurred during each team meeting. Attendance of each practitioner at team meetings was also recorded to factor into the time contribution and overall cost of the team meetings. Practitioners in the experimental group also recorded the number and length of each visit, all joint visits, and adherence to natural learning environment practices, coaching practices, and a PSP approach to teaming. We received billing records, which provided the amount of time spent by control group practitioners for assessment of their direct service hours, strengthening the analyses of service costs.

RECOMMENDATIONS FOR FUTURE STUDIES

A larger sample size and extended data collection period would enable detection of differences between groups of children by type of developmental disability. Future study should include collecting baseline data for practitioners in the experimental group to allow time for developing competence in implementing new practices and documenting and analyzing control group practitioner demographics and the practices they implemented. Obtaining video samples from home visits and team meetings from both groups would also strengthen the study. Future study should include parental measures regarding capacity to support child growth and developing and examining the use of alternative payment strategies for team meeting time (e.g., payment of stipends by the program to the practitioners, assigned cost for teaming time by child). Including these strategies as a component of data analysis would allow more precise cost comparisons with programs not using a PSP approach.

STUDY CONCLUSION

The service delivery data indicate that the children in the experimental group received fewer service hours, including team meeting time, than the control group, which had no team meeting time. IFSP outcomes were met more often by children in the experimental group. No differences were noted between the groups for child developmental outcome data. Early intervention services and supports provided by the program using the PSP approach were less expensive than those services provided using a multidisciplinary approach. Practitioners in the experimental group not only met all federal requirements for Part C, but also exceeded time frames for reviewing IFSP documents. Finally, fewer practitioners were involved in the lives of families, resulting in less disruption to family life. This pilot study of using geographically based early intervention teams using a PSP demonstrates promising data regarding efficient use of resources for early intervention programs.

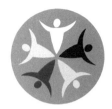

A Pilot Study of the Characteristics of Effective Team Meetings When Using a Primary Service Provider Approach to Teaming

Although Part C clearly indicates that a team of professionals from multiple disciplines should be used for purposes of evaluation, assessment, and intervention for infants and toddlers with disabilities and their families, the field of early intervention lacks research and guidance on how to conduct effective team meetings. This study was intended to identify strategies and supports for effective meetings for teams using a primary service provider (PSP) approach to teaming in an attempt to fill the gap between current research and practice.

More specifically, we conducted this study to identify the characteristics of meetings to address three basic research questions:

1. Is the current team meeting structure providing the supports needed by team members?

2. What are the characteristics of an effective team meeting when using a PSP approach to teaming?

3. Would specific guidelines for presenting information and providing coaching in the team meeting be seen as useful to meeting participants?

PARTICIPANTS

The participants for this study consisted of a convenience sample of 25 practitioners in an early childhood intervention program in a southeastern state in the United States. All participants were females. The participants included two occupational therapists (OTs), six teachers licensed in birth to kindergarten education, one psychologist, eight Early Head Start home visitors, two speech-language pathologists (SLPs), three physical therapists (PTs), and three nurses. The team members attended a scheduled weekly meeting for 1 hour. The program used a PSP approach to teaming; therefore, the primary purpose of the team meeting was to provide opportunities for individuals serving as PSPs to receive support related to their work with individual families as well as provide support to other team members based on their experiences and area of expertise. Team members also used the meeting for quarterly updates on families, which consisted of a brief overview of the current plan for supporting the family, status of the plan, and next steps. In addition, participants announced new children and families recently assigned to PSPs along with the reason for the referral, transitions of families to other programs, and closures (e.g., graduation, disenrollment).

DATA COLLECTION PROCEDURES

Data were collected prior to and following the intervention by observation, survey, and individual interviews. The observation data were collected for 4 weeks prior to the intervention and 6 weeks postintervention. Observational data were collected and coded by the second author and an independent observer. The authors developed the coding system, practiced coding with an independent observer prior to initiating the study, and came to consensus on the ratings as part of the independent observer's training. They continued to use consensus rating through the preintervention stage. Observers coded the type of staffing (e.g., primary coaching opportunity, quarterly update, transition, closure, welcome to the program), the order in which other team members responded to the team member presenting, and the type of response (e.g., advice, information, reflective question, confirmation of an action plan). All observations were made and coded by both observers during the team meeting.

The authors and a research associate generated survey and interview questions for team members using existing literature on effective teaming characteristics (Bell, 2007; Daniels, 1993; Doyle & Straus, 1993; Holpp, 1999; Kayser, 2011; Larsson, 2000; Pell, 1999; Weaver & Farrell, 1997). This process resulted in 21 survey questions that asked individuals about the ideal frequency, timing, organization and membership size for the meeting, level of co-worker expertise, and individual preferences for participating in teamwork. Open-ended questions were used to seek more detailed information from participants, such as determining whether participants had a shared understanding of the purpose of the meeting, deciding the role of the facilitator in the meeting, and exploring factors within the meeting that might support or detract from individual participation.

The research associate scheduled interviews with PSP meeting participants after they signed informed consents to participate in the study. All initial interviews occurred within 2 weeks of signed consent, and second interviews occurred within 2 weeks of the end of the 6-week intervention period. One interviewer conducted all interviews in one of two offices where participants could be assured their responses were confidential. Participants completed a 21-question survey with a 5-point Likert-type scale ranging from 1 (*not at all true*) to 5 (*extremely true*). Immediately after participants completed the survey, the interviewer asked if they wanted to elaborate on any responses. The interviewer then asked 12 standardized open-ended questions. The interviewer recorded answers and probed with both preset and interviewer-identified follow-up questions to obtain elaboration when answers were nonspecific or limited in scope.

All PSP meeting participants agreed to complete the survey and participate in the interview, resulting in 14 initial interviews. Supervisors were excluded from interviews because they were not the recipients of support in the team meeting, but rather only participated to provide support. Four participants from the meeting whose jobs did not involve regular home visiting were dismissed from the meetings as part of the study. These four participants were not included in the final interview process, resulting in 10 interviews at the end of the intervention period.

INTERVENTION

The intervention focused on the characteristics of the team meeting because the program was already implementing a PSP approach to teaming. The intervention phase of this study was developed based on the results of the team member surveys and interviews in conjunction with the available literature on effective meetings. The intervention included three components: logistics, facilitation, and participant interaction style.

Logistics

The meeting was extended from 60 minutes to 90 minutes and moved from 4:00 p.m. to 10:30 a.m. on Fridays. The new meeting time was determined by providing the individuals who attended the team meeting with the parameters for decision making (i.e., the meeting must occur weekly, all necessary team members must be available to attend in person, day/time should coordinate with other meetings that team members need to attend) and then allowing them to come to consensus on the day/time without supervisory or administrative staff present. Meeting agendas were pre-published (Daniels, 1993) and posted to a location on the program's intranet in order for individual meeting participants to post agenda items prior to the meeting. Therefore, the meeting facilitator could assign times to each item on the agenda when preparing for the meeting (Holpp, 1999; Kayser, 2011; Pell, 1999). Two items included on the team meeting agenda prior to the intervention (transitions and closures) were moved to optional discussion items at the discretion of the person who added the item to the agenda and if time permitted. Written instructions were also provided for how and when to post items to the electronic version of the agenda. Furthermore, meeting participants were assigned seats in order to assist all participants with immediately determining what human resources (people and disciplines) were available when the meeting started.

Facilitation

Although the team participating in this study had an individual responsible for facilitating the meeting prior to initiation of the study and during the data collection period prior to the intervention phase, the role of facilitator was assumed by the second author during the intervention phase. The second author has 18 years of experience in small-group facilitation in a variety of contexts, including team meetings, strategic planning meetings, task group meetings, and regular meetings. He had been mentored by one of the coauthors of the book *The Complete Guide to Facilitation: Enabling Groups to Succeed* (Justice & Jamieson, 1998). Written guidelines for the role of the facilitator were also developed using literature-based recommendations (Doyle & Straus, 1993; Holpp, 1999; Kayser, 2011; Weaver & Farrell, 1997). The facilitator was responsible for assigning times to each agenda item and ensuring that meeting participants remained within the designated time (Holpp, 1999; Kayser, 2011; Pell, 1999). A volunteer who would be interested in being mentored by the second author to become the team's permanent facilitator was sought from among team meeting participants during the intervention phase of the study. One individual volunteered and was selected to serve as the permanent meeting facilitator. She had been with the program for 3 years.

Participant Interaction Style

The interaction style of participants was modified by implementing written guidelines to prepare participants (Holpp, 1999; Weaver & Farrell, 1997) to present information in the PSP team meeting as well as guidelines for providing coaching to other team members during the PSP team meeting. The meeting facilitator was responsible for ensuring that all participants adhered to the written guidelines. Only staff members who provide direct support to children and families enrolled in the early intervention component of the program and their supervisors were invited to attend as regular meeting participants (Bell, 2004; Daniels, 1993; Doyle & Straus, 1993; Kayser, 2011; Larsson, 2000; Pell, 1999). Care was also taken to ensure that the meeting participants represented all necessary disciplines (e.g., early childhood education, early childhood special education [ECSE], nursing, occupational therapy, physical therapy, speech-language pathology). Other individuals were invited as needed for specific situations based on their knowledge and expertise.

DATA ANALYSIS AND RESULTS

Results were based on the analysis of data collected from direct observations during team meetings and interviews with participants.

Findings From Observations

Prior to the intervention, 23 staff members attended the team meeting, with 17 members (74%) actually participating on a regular basis. Participation as part of the observation of team member behavior was defined as asking a question or sharing information with the person requesting a primary coaching opportunity or presenting a quarterly update. Following the intervention, 16 staff members (94%) attended the team meeting on a regular basis, with all members regularly participating (see Figure 2B.1).

Of those team members participating, the mean number of talking turns per person was 4.7 before the intervention and 6.4 after the intervention. A *talking turn* is defined as the number of times during a meeting in which a team member asked a question or shared information. The mean number of talking turns per person prior to the intervention ranged from 0 to 36 per meeting. The mean number of talking turns after the intervention ranged from 0.33 to 17.5 talking turns per

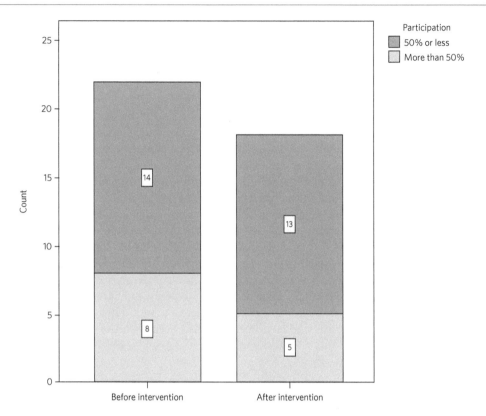

Figure 2B.1. Counts of meeting attendees who participated in more than 50% of the meetings attended.

person per meeting. Three individuals were identified as "high talkers" during the preintervention phase. The high talkers averaged 12.7, 15.7, and 36 talking turns per meeting. The next closest mean number of talking turns per meeting was 5, which were attributed to the person acting as the meeting facilitator. The highest talker was a regular team member, whereas the next two highest talkers were supervisors. Postintervention, four individuals were identified as high talkers, with mean number of talking turns per meeting of 14.5, 14.6, 15.2, and 17.5. Consistent with the preintervention data, two of the highest talkers were supervisors. The other two high talkers were different regular team members than those during the preintervention phase. The individual who was the highest talker during the preintervention phase did not attend the team meeting during the intervention phase.

Team member participation in the discussion was coded as either advice giving, information sharing, asking an open-ended question, asking a closed-ended question, or making a statement to a person in the team meeting other than the person who was seeking a primary coaching opportunity or sharing a quarterly update, transition, closure, or welcome to the program. Otherwise, all comments and questions coded were directed to the presenter. Advice giving was coded if the team member told the person what they should do in the given situation prior to anyone asking the person a reflective question or the person sharing what they had previously done, what worked/did not work, and/or what ideas they had regarding the issue or question being raised. Advice giving involves the team member who is responding to the presenter making an assumption about what they believe should be done without first allowing the presenter an opportunity to reflect on their actions or how to close the gap between the current state and desired future state. Information sharing was coded if the input was provided after at least one reflective question had been asked by team members. An open-ended question was coded by the observer if the question was phrased

Table 2B.1. Type of team member question or comment

	Advice giving	Confirm plan	Give information	Open-ended question	Closed-ended question	Statement to other team member	Process question or statement	Total
Preintervention count	3	6	156	67	30	36	0	298
Percentage of use preintervention	1.0%	2.0%	52.3%	22.5%	10.1%	12.1%	.0%	100.0%
Postintervention count	2	18	214	148	10	94	8	494
Percentage of use	.4%	3.6%	43.3%	30.0%	2.0%	19.0%	1.6%	100.0%
Postintervention p value associated with difference in proportions		.1947	.0136	.0219	P<.0001	.0105		

in such a way as to yield any response other than "yes" or "no," whereas a closed-ended question was coded only when a yes/no question was asked. Meeting participants used a mean number of 74 comments or questions per week prior to the intervention. Participants used 81 comments or questions per week after the intervention phase. A comparison by type of comment or question before and after the intervention is included in Table 2B.1.

The team meeting prior to the intervention was scheduled for 60 minutes from 4:00 p.m. to 5:00 p.m. The mean length of the actual team meetings before the intervention was 45 minutes due to earlier meetings running into the team meeting time, waiting for late arriving team members, and side conversations delaying the start of the meeting. The time of the meeting was changed to 10:30 a.m., and the length of the meeting was extended to 90 minutes based on feedback from meeting participants. The mean length of meetings after the intervention was 61 minutes.

The amount of time for each staffing opportunity was also coded by the observers. The mean length of time for each primary coaching opportunity prior to the intervention was 12 minutes. The mean length of time for primary coaching opportunities after the intervention was 25 minutes. The mean length of time for each quarterly update prior to the intervention was 3 minutes, and after the intervention it increased to 8 minutes. Discussion of transitions prior to the intervention averaged 2 minutes each and closures averaged 1 minute. Team members were given the option of sharing transitions and closures as part of the intervention. No transitions were shared during the meeting following the intervention. Closures following the intervention averaged 1 minute. Sharing of basic information about families newly referred to the program (i.e., Welcome to the Program presentations) averaged 1 minute prior to the intervention and 2 minutes after.

Findings From Initial Interviews

Fourteen team members participated in the initial interview. The authors and research associate read and coded interviews for content separately and then met to reach consensus about coding and create themes. The majority of participants shared a similar understanding of the purpose of the meeting—to share information, knowledge, resources, and strategies and receive support from fellow team members. Themes for other comments fell into four categories: content details found valuable or not valuable to include in the meeting, organizational requests to make the meeting more effective, time of meeting difficulties, and interaction styles that team members found either helpful or not helpful to accomplish the purpose of the meeting.

Content details included discussion about keeping or removing agenda items such as required reporting of families leaving the program, making the transition to other programs, or introducing other team members to families entering the program. An example of content details from participant 1 was, "Take out pieces (remove agenda time spent on) transitions, closings, and welcomes." The two predominant themes in the category of content details were 1) to discontinue or revise how components, including discussion of transitions, closures, and families entering the program, were discussed and 2) to keep and allow more time for urgent agenda items.

Organizational requests included discussing methods to standardize the process that would assist individual participants to prepare for and stay focused on the content during the meeting. An example of an organizational request from participant 16 was, "The meeting would be more effective for me if the way in which staffing is brought up (could be) more systematic." Themes in this category included sign up for staffing in advance, allow more time for the meeting, participants should come prepared, a need to keep people on track, a need for guidelines to be more systematic in presenting time-sensitive family or staff needs, and supervisors should attend.

Time of the meeting came up in most interviews. The PSP team meeting occurred at 4:00 p.m. on Fridays before the intervention was implemented. An example comment about time from participant 14 was, "A different time might help us be more attentive." Scheduling the meeting at a different time of day was the theme that predominated this category.

Interaction styles included discussion from participants about the kinds of conversations that occurred during the meeting that participants found unhelpful. Participant 8 said, "Sometimes we give too much advice, (and) sometimes we are put on the spot and that's not helpful for getting support." Themes from the interaction styles category included feeling judged or interrogated, advice giving/coaxing, talking too much, and receiving too many questions with not enough information sharing. One question on the Likert-type scale survey asked participants whether they felt too many people attended the meeting. The average for this question was 1.8 before the intervention, with 1 labeled *not at all true* and 2 labeled *a little true*. The intervention did include reducing the number of staff who attended the meeting for other reasons, and the average was 1.3 ($p = .08$) when participants were asked the same question at the end of the intervention. When asked during the open-ended questions if they would like to expand on their answers to any of the survey questions, many participants commented that they liked having supervisory staff in attendance. Reasons for this were varied. Participant 1 stated, "I think supervisory staff give us expertise we don't otherwise (have access to)." Others wanted supervisors present to know what challenges staff experienced, which was expressed by participant 24: "Supervisory staff are helpful so (they can) know what's going on, what we are doing, what challenges we face." When talking about including supervisors, some (e.g., participant 10, participant 7) stated they felt it worked because "they are respectful and helpful," and others (e.g., participant 17) expressed that supervisors "would benefit from attending to learn how to better support staff," including how to coach staff more effectively.

The interviewer also asked whether interviewees found the team meeting to be engaging. The answers were split, with seven individuals saying it was not engaging in its current format, six saying it was engaging, and one person refraining from giving an answer.

Finally, one open-ended question asked team members why and how often they chose to get help directly from peers rather than bring a question to the team meeting. All team members used the technique of getting support from peer colleagues, ranging in frequency from every day to once every other week. Reasons for going directly to one person included getting to talk longer about the issue, getting immediate feedback or support in the case of a stressful situation, getting answers related to a specific content area, and refining a skill already discussed in the large-group setting. Newer team members reported using individual support more often to get assistance in using the conceptual framework for providing supports they were learning to implement. Some people stated they felt more comfortable talking one to one about concerns because they felt it was less stressful to go to a person identified as comfortable to talk with about issues they felt they should already know about or that they could not get off their minds.

Findings From Final Interviews

After all participants completed surveys and interviews, the survey responses from a Likert-type scale were entered into Excel and evaluated for significant change. Participants rated five questions *significantly improved* as a result of the intervention, reporting increased satisfaction with organization of the meeting to cover everything on the agenda and with the facilitation of the meeting. The average rating for the question "staffing meets my needs" also improved significantly, from *somewhat true* (2.79) to *very true* (3.9) on a scale from *not at all true* to *extremely true* (1–5).

Following the same procedure as the initial interviews, the authors and research associate read and coded final interviews for content separately and then met to reach consensus about coding and to create themes. Participants' understanding of the purpose of the meeting did not change, but new themes emerged. Themes for comments in these interviews fit into three categories— improved organization, greater sense of control, and improved process of facilitation.

Improved Organization

The final interviews included comments about the effectiveness of interventions that addressed content and organizational concerns. The majority of participants found that a written agenda posted ahead of time and written guidelines for preparing content and the coaching process was helpful. Some participants found having a smaller meeting was helpful. Participants reported the new requirement to be prepared affected participation, helping their participation when they were prepared and deterring participation when they were not.

Greater Sense of Control

Many participants expressed a greater sense of personal control. Some expressed they felt more comfortable asking questions and sharing because clear guidelines were established for how questions were to be presented in the meeting. Others expressed feeling control through the flexibility in the level of detail individuals shared in order to get their questions answered. Participant 10 stated, "I know what I am supposed to share, and if other people start asking other questions, I can choose not to answer."

Improved Process of Facilitation

The majority of participants found the new guidelines for facilitation kept the meeting on track. Participants indicated the guidelines assisted the team member bringing a question and the rest of the team members in offering information and support in a measured manner, rather than the questioner getting bombarded with questions or receiving too much information at once. Participant 17 said the defined role of the facilitator assisted the meeting by "keeping conversations efficient." Participant 8 stated that it was helpful "to ensure the person getting help has a plan (to implement with a family)."

All team members continued to seek assistance directly from others after the intervention period, with almost all reporting they used this method of assistance more than once each week. No team members reported feeling uncomfortable taking questions to the PSP team meeting after the intervention, but rather reported they used peers if they desired immediate information, needed support, felt it was a less intense issue, or felt the question was very topic specific. Participant 6 used peers when she felt questions were "not important enough for the team meeting," and Participant 17 used that technique because she did not have to plan as much.

DISCUSSION

The first research question for this study was whether the existing team meeting structure provided the supports needed by team members. The first step to answer this question was to assess perceptions of the purpose of the meeting via the surveys, initial interviews, and follow-up interviews. Results indicated that participants' perceptions were consistent with one another as well as program management. The purpose of the meeting is to provide and receive support related to working with families and gaining access to needed resources to ensure families are receiving comprehensive care. Many participants indicated during the preintervention interviews that they did not get their needs met during the meeting; therefore, the intended purpose of the meeting was not fully realized. Several members told the interviewer they did not feel like the group had enough time to pose issues and questions they would like to have discussed. The follow-up interviews after the intervention phase of the study revealed that meeting participants' needs were being addressed and they were satisfied with the new organization of the meeting and facilitation.

Individuals participating in the team meeting prior to the intervention indicated that the right number of people attended; therefore, they did not believe this contributed to not having their needs met during the team meeting. As part of the intervention, only individuals whose primary role within the organization was direct support of families through regular home-based or community-based visits continued to attend the team meeting on a regular basis. As a result, the number of people attending the meeting was reduced from 23 to 17. The exception to this ground rule was the continued participation of supervisors (four people). Although somewhat of a surprise to the authors, team members indicated in the interviews that they wanted supervisors to attend team meetings to provide needed information and observe team member participation. The intervention allowed for any team member not identified as having to attend the team meeting on a regular basis to attend the meeting on the request of any regular meeting attendee or if the nonregular team member needed input of the regular meeting attendees. The follow-up interviews indicated that the new number of individuals attending the team meeting was the right number, provided for full participation by all team members, and enabled team members to have their needs met. All of the team members participated following the intervention as opposed to only 74% of meeting attendees prior to the intervention. This could be attributed to having the right people and right number of people regularly participating in the team meeting as similarly found in the teaming literature (Bell, 2004; Daniels, 1993; Kayser, 2011; Larsson, 2000; Pell, 1999).

Interviewees indicated that the 60-minute length of the meeting prior to intervention was inadequate and did not allow them to feel as if they could fully participate and receive the supports needed. In actuality, the meetings were only lasting 45 minutes by the time participants arrived and the meeting was called to order. The meeting length was scheduled for 90 minutes as part of the intervention; however, the mean length of the meeting during the intervention phase was 61 minutes, which resulted in a net gain of 16 minutes. The mean length of time for primary coaching opportunities increased by 13 minutes (52%), and the mean amount of time for quarterly updates increased by 5 minutes (62.5%) as a result of this modest increase in the amount of meeting time. The amount of time saved by making presentation of closures optional does not account for the increased time available to spend on primary coaching opportunities and quarterly updates. The increased amount of time available for primary coaching opportunities and quarterly updates may be attributed to more efficient facilitation of the meetings with written guidelines, prepublishing the agenda, and written guidelines for how to share information in the team meeting and how to provide support to the presenting team member by using a coaching interaction style.

The number of individuals determined to be high talkers during the team meeting increased from three to four individuals, although no high talkers following the intervention reached the previously high number of talking turns during the preintervention phase. The two supervisors who were identified as high talkers before the intervention continued to be high talkers after the intervention, even though their mean number of talking turns compared with talking turns of other participants was discussed with them. Other meeting participants, however, did not indicate during the interviews that the number of talking turns by the supervisors was excessive, nor did it inhibit or limit their ability to participate in the meeting.

The mean number of comments by meeting participants increased by seven comments from the preintervention to the postintervention phase. The amount of advice giving was less than expected during the preintervention phase (1% of all comments) and decreased only slightly (0.04%). Somewhat surprisingly, the amount of information sharing decreased from 53% of comments to 47% following intervention. This could be attributed to the team members' prior experience with using coaching practices and trying to promote the other person's reflection rather than immediately telling the other person what to do. Open-ended questions, which are more appropriate than closed-ended questions when using a coaching interaction style, increased from 23% to 31%, whereas closed-ended questions decreased from 10% to 2% following intervention. This could be attributed to the written guidelines for coaching one another during the team meeting as well as intervention of the facilitator. Statements directed to team meeting participants other than the person who was presenting a question or issue as a primary coaching opportunity or a quarterly update increased from 13% of comments in the preintervention phase to 20% of comments following the intervention. This could be attributed to the facilitator's lack of enforcement of the team meeting guideline related to directing information and questions to the person presenting rather than other team members, members clarifying the teaming process, or members obtaining support from supervisors during the meeting.

The second research question was related to identifying the characteristics of a team meeting when using a PSP approach to teaming. Based on the results of the interviews and observational data, three characteristics were identified that led to increased meeting effectiveness: 1) using a meeting facilitator, 2) clearly defining roles of the facilitator and other meeting participants, and 3) adopting a prepublished agenda. Participants indicated during the follow-up interviews that having a facilitator with a clearly defined role helped to ensure the meeting ran smoothly and everyone's needs were met, which is consistent with the literature on effective team meetings (Doyle & Straus, 1993; Holpp, 1999; Kayser, 2011; Weaver & Farrell, 1997). Participants reported that having the prepublished agenda (Daniels, 1993) caused them to be better prepared for the meeting. Lack of preparation of some team members was expressed as an issue during the initial interviews.

The third research question was whether specific guidelines for presenting information and providing coaching in team meetings would be seen as useful by meeting participants. The publication of guidelines (Holpp, 1999) for meeting participants was requested during the initial interviews in combination with an effective meeting facilitator. Results of the follow-up interviews with meeting participants indicated that the meeting guidelines provided a greater sense of meeting participants' sense of control over the meeting. Participants reported that they knew what their roles were during the meeting and how they were to interact and support one another. They found that they could help monitor one another's behavior to ensure that the meeting guidelines were followed. This finding is consistent with Bell (2004) and others (Borrill et al., 2001; DeDrue & West, 2001; Erez et al., 2002) as related to the need for effective teams to have at least some degree of self-management. The participants also found the facilitator helpful in keeping people on track and helping the person speaking with formulating a question they want the team's help in answering.

LIMITATIONS OF THE STUDY

This study had several limitations that should be considered when generalizing the results to other teams. First, the study used a convenience sample from the program in which the authors are affiliated. Second, all of the participants had been working on the same team and participated in team meetings for a minimum of 1 year. Third, only one team was included in the study, rather than multiple teams from other similar organizations.

RECOMMENDATIONS FOR FUTURE STUDIES

The authors have a number of recommendations for researchers interested in duplicating or expanding on the present study. More data is needed across programs and teams in order to make broader generalizations of the data. Future study participants should have varying levels of experience with teaming and participating in team meetings. Follow-up observations and interviews at least 3 months after the intervention phase of the study would provide evidence of the extent to which the team meeting participants have become acculturated to the interventions. The team meetings should be videotaped for coding or minimally for cross-checking the coding that occurred during the actual team meeting in order to ensure greater accuracy of the observational coding.

STUDY CONCLUSION

Using a meeting facilitator, clearly defining roles of the facilitator and other meeting participants, and adopting a prepublished agenda led meeting participants to report that the team meeting better met their needs and accomplished the purpose to provide and receive support related to working with families and gaining access to needed resources to ensure families are receiving comprehensive care. The team participating in this study met weekly and adhered to the characteristics of the PSP approach to teaming, including using an identified team of individuals from multiple disciplines with one team member serving as PSP to the care provider(s) and allowing the PSP to receive coaching from other team members through ongoing planned and spontaneous interactions.

Checklists for Implementing a Primary Service Provider Approach to Teaming

Team or practitioner's name: _____   Date: _____

Checklist Descriptions

These checklists include practice indicators of the key characteristics of a primary service provider approach to teaming in early childhood intervention. A **primary service provider** approach to teaming is using a multidisciplinary team in which one member is selected as the primary service provider, receives coaching from other team members, and uses coaching with parents and other primary care providers to support and strengthen parenting competence and confidence in promoting child learning and development and obtaining desired supports and resources.

The four checklists describe different areas of primary service provider teaming practices: 1) preparing for a team-based approach, 2) using a primary service provider, 3) coordinating joint visits, and 4) conducting team meetings. Each section contains indicators of a specific area of a primary service provider approach to teaming practices. For each indicator, determine whether the program is adhering to the aspect of the practice described. Space is also available for notes or examples of adherence.

Use of the Checklists

The four checklists include 30 indicators that are the foundation for implementing a primary service provider approach to teaming. The checklists can be used for a number of different purposes.

- They can be used to help a program learn and master the key characteristics of evidence-based teaming practices in early childhood intervention.

- Team leadership and supervisors can use the checklists as observational tools for determining the extent to which the program implements a primary service provider approach to teaming. They can be used to provide feedback and guidance about which practices are consistent or inconsistent with the practice indicators and what the team members can do to improve their practices. The team leadership and/or supervisor can use the Program Planning section with the team to develop plans for changing practices to better mirror the practice indicators.

- A practitioner can use the checklists to conduct a self-assessment to examine his or her use of a primary service provider approach to teaming practices. A self-assessment could be accomplished by the practitioner reflecting on his or her practices as a team member and determining whether the practices are consistent or inconsistent with each practice indicator.

- The Program Planning section can be used to develop plans for changing practices and identifying the supports needed to make practices consistent with the practice indicators. They can be used for program evaluation purposes by monitoring consistency in the use of the practices and improvements over time.

(continued)

Team or practitioner's name: _____ Date: _____

	Are practices characterized by the following?	Yes	No	Examples/notes
Preparing for a team-based approach	Program leadership determines the number and specific location of families served by the local program.	Y	N	
	Program leadership determines the fewest number of teams necessary to cover the program area based on the premise that a team of four full-time practitioners can serve approximately 100–125 families when drive time does not exceed 30–45 minutes for a one-way trip.	Y	N	
	Program leadership identifies the geographic area that each team will cover based on family distribution within a given catchment area, geographic region (e.g., county), zip code, portion of a school district, and so forth.	Y	N	
	Program leadership ensures that each team minimally consists of an early childhood educator and/or early childhood special educator, occupational therapist, physical therapist, and speech-language pathologist.	Y	N	
	Program leadership ensures that the role of service coordination is fulfilled either by one of the disciplines previously listed (i.e., blended model) or by an individual solely responsible for service coordination (i.e., dedicated model).	Y	N	
	Custodial family members are always members of their child's team.	Y	N	
	Program leadership assigns available practitioners to teams beginning with those who are employed or contracted with the program for the greatest amount of time.	Y	N	
	Teams have an identified team leader.	Y	N	
	Program leadership assigns each new referral to the team responsible for the geographic area in which the child resides.	Y	N	

	Are practices characterized by the following?	Yes	No	Examples/notes
Using a primary service provider	All therapists and educators on the team are available to serve as a primary service provider.	Y	N	
	One team member is selected to serve as the primary service provider to the family and other care providers.	Y	N	
	The primary service provider is selected based on four factors: 1) parent/family, 2) child, 3) environmental, 4) practitioner.	Y	N	
	The primary service provider assigned to a family uses a coaching interaction style to build the capacity of the parents and other care providers to support child learning as well as to identify and obtain needed resources and supports.	Y	N	
	The primary service provider receives coaching support from other team members through ongoing formal (planned) and informal interactions.	Y	N	
	The primary service provider for a family changes as infrequently as possible (i.e., rarely changes).	Y	N	

(continued)

Team or practitioner's name: _____ Date: _____

	Are practices characterized by the following?	Yes	No	Examples/notes
Coordinating joint visits	Team members support the primary service provider through joint visits.	Y	N	
	The primary service provider and other team members conduct joint visits at the same place and time.	Y	N	
	The primary service provider along with the parents and/or other care providers predetermine questions, expected outcomes, and specific actions to be taken during the joint visit.	Y	N	
	The primary service provider and other team members define their roles for the joint visit based on questions, expected outcomes, and specific actions to be taken as related to the priorities of the primary service provider and parent.	Y	N	
	The primary service provider debriefs the joint visit with the parents and/or other care providers to evaluate the usefulness of the joint visit and determine next steps.	Y	N	
	The primary service provider and other team members debrief the joint visit to evaluate the usefulness of the joint visit and determine next steps.	Y	N	

	Are practices characterized by the following?	Yes	No	Examples/notes
Conducting team meetings	The team leader ensures that the purpose of the team meeting is to share information among team members as families move through the early intervention process and for primary service providers to receive coaching from their team members.	Y	N	
	All team members attend the weekly team meeting.	Y	N	
	All team members are present for the entire team meeting.	Y	N	
	The primary service provider informs the parents of the dates and times of team meetings when their name is on the agenda and invites them to attend if they desire.	Y	N	
	The primary service provider invites the parents to send questions or updates to the team meetings via the primary service provider and ensures timely feedback.	Y	N	
	The team leader ensures that the team meeting is led by a competent and consistent facilitator. The team meeting facilitator may or may not be someone other than the formal team leader.	Y	N	
	The team meeting facilitator develops a meeting agenda with time limits that have been prepublished.	Y	N	
	The team has clearly defined roles of the facilitator and other meeting participants.	Y	N	
	Program leadership compensates team members for team meeting time.	Y	N	*(continued)*

Team or practitioner's name: _____ Date: _____

Program Planning

Prepare a plan for making changes and/or ensuring sustainability based on analysis of the primary service provider approach to teaming practice indicators. Describe the specific action steps that will be taken and identify the particular experiences and opportunities that will be used to make the needed programmatic changes.

Preparing for a team-based approach	**Needed change**
	Action steps (i.e., what will be done; by when):

Using a primary service provider	**Needed change**
	Action steps (i.e., what will be done; by when):

Coordinating joint visits	**Needed change**
	Action steps (i.e., what will be done; by when):

Conducting team meetings	**Needed change**
	Action steps (i.e., what will be done; by when):

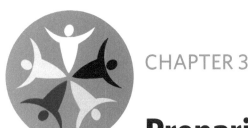

CHAPTER 3

Preparing for a Team-Based Approach

A state's, agency's, or program's decision to use a PSP teaming approach requires thoughtful consideration. The motivating reason for programs to move to this approach should be based on the *Mission and Key Principles for Providing Services in Natural Environments* (Workgroup on Principles and Practices in Natural Environments, 2007b), the DEC Recommended Practices in Early Intervention/Early Childhood Special Education (2014), as well as the evidence and supporting documentation provided in Chapter 2. That is, considering the purpose of early intervention and the intended roles of family and service providers and the use of geographically based teams made up of individuals from multiple disciplines, with one member serving as the key liaison working most closely with the family, is the most effective teaming strategy to meet the needs of children and families in early intervention. Other reasons programs choose to use a primary provider often involve perceived reduction in the costs of services and/or lack of or limited availability of personnel in specific disciplines (e.g., occupational therapy, physical therapy, speech-language pathology). These motivating factors are misleading because costs may be reduced depending on the existing program model and resources (see Chapter 2). Service delivery costs may be reduced for programs that have providers who currently maximize allowable billable services for all children enrolled in the program. The service delivery costs could increase for those programs that provide limited services to most enrolled children, especially with the added costs of team meeting time and joint visiting. If programs choose to use a primary provider because they lack availability of needed disciplines, then they often perceive that all children can be served by a developmental specialist or educator with therapists available to consult, provide instruction to the primary provider, and develop home programs for families to implement. This is inconsistent with the characteristics and implementation conditions of an evidence-based PSP approach to teaming and does not address the availability issue of needed disciplines.

FACTORS TO CONSIDER

Several factors exist when deciding to use a PSP approach to teaming. This teaming approach requires establishing a logistical and fiscal infrastructure to support the implementation, which includes establishing a team of the necessary members and operationalizing a process for teaming; leadership, staff development, and ongoing support for implementing new practices; and procedures to incorporate the use of team meetings.

 Remember

Following are the best reasons programs choose a primary service provider (PSP) approach to teaming.

- *Mission and Key Principles for Providing Early Intervention in Natural Environments*

- DEC Recommended Practices in Early Intervention/Early Childhood Special Education

- Research evidence to support the effectiveness of using a PSP

Identification and Availability of Resources

Program administrators need to consider the available resources and the time required of team members to participate in team meetings, joint visits, and staff development when identifying resources to support a geographically based team. This teaming approach is effective when team members are employees and/or contractors. If team members are salaried staff, then payment is not an issue; however, if team members are contract providers, then their contracts will most likely need to be reconfigured to include these activities. If specific disciplines are currently unavailable or give a limited amount of time to the team, then the program will need to consider providing additional incentives for existing contractors and/or recruiting new team members in order to obtain the needed amount of time from all disciplines to serve as a primary provider and support the team.

Consider the following scenario in which Kim, a district early intervention coordinator (EIC), needs more contract time from an OT on one of the area's geographically based teams. The numbers for the area indicate a minimum need of a half-time OT (20 hours), but Kim has only been able to recruit Sandy, an OT who is able to give 4 hours each week to the team. The purpose of this conversation is for the EIC to articulate the program's need for increasing the amount of OT support available, explain the constraints on the team given the current time the OT has available, and explore with her the possibility of increasing available time on the team.

> **Kim:**   Sandy, thank you for making some time to talk with me this morning.
>
> **Sandy:**   No problem, Kim. I appreciate you rearranging your schedule for my availability.
>
> **Kim:**   As you know Sandy, your availability is actually the topic of this meeting. You've made it pretty clear in our past conversations that all you have time for in your schedule is 1 half-day each week for early intervention. Does that continue to be the case?
>
> **Sandy:**   Yes. I wish I did have more time. Because I knew we were going to talk about this, I tried to see if I could rearrange my days and add a few more hours.
>
> **Kim:**   I appreciate that. As you know, we currently hold our team meetings on Tuesday afternoons because that is the only day you are available. The team meetings are always an hour long, and sometimes we need even longer. So, that leaves just a few hours for you to do joint visits with other team members and see the few families for whom you serve as PSP.
>
> **Sandy:**   You're right. I always feel rushed and agree that more time is needed.
>
> **Kim:**   I'm really interested in contracting with an OT for at least 20 hours each week, and you currently are available for 4 hours. I agree with you. Our current situation is not meeting the needs of the other team members or children enrolled in our program. I'm not only concerned about the lack of time you have for us in terms of the quantity of the hours, but also the limitation on the day and time of the week—Tuesday afternoons. It really limits your flexibility. How is it working with the FAB scheduling concept we discussed a few months ago—the idea of being flexible and activity based and using bursts of support for scheduling visits with children and families? (See Chapter 5 for more information on FAB scheduling.)
>
> **Sandy:**   Well, I'm just really not able to use the FAB scheduling approach. I basically have about 2 hours left each week following our team meeting when I include the drive time. I can only do joint visits during that time, and I can only schedule to see the families I serve as PSP during those late Tuesday afternoon activity settings. I know that it isn't ideal, but I really do squeeze a lot into those few hours.
>
> **Kim:**   I understand your situation. How do you think your scheduling approach matches with the practices we are now implementing in our program?

Sandy: Well, I know it doesn't match, but I've scheduled this way a long time. I think I can make it work.

Kim: How do you think your inability to use a more flexible approach to scheduling affects your other team members?

Sandy: Well, I know it is difficult to fit in the joint visits we need to do.

Kim: Yes, we all talk about that openly during team meeting. It does inhibit our ability to fully implement the PSP approach to teaming. What effect does it have on your implementation of natural learning environment practices?

Sandy: What do you mean?

Kim: What I need you to know is that the FAB scheduling approach is not only essential for our team to be implementing, but it also ensures that we are using natural learning environment practices. I am going to need to focus on recruiting an OT who can give us more time across a variety of days and time slots each week.

Sandy: Are you unhappy with my contributions to the program?

Kim: No, on the contrary. I'm very pleased with all other aspects that you bring to our team. The only problem is your limited availability.

Sandy: What about another part-time OT? That would help, wouldn't it? I might be able to talk to an OT I know at the hospital.

Kim: I appreciate you thinking of other options. I just have to think about the duplication for the program regarding managing the contracts as well as the ongoing training and technical assistance needs. To be quite frank, if I contracted with another part-time OT, then they would have to work on Tuesday afternoons to accommodate your schedule and attend team meetings. Then I have an additional tight schedule with another team member. I really feel like it is more constraining to the rest of the team and program than it is helpful.

Sandy: I really haven't thought about it that way. I do hear what you're saying. Maybe I could have a discussion with our department head at the hospital to see if I could work longer days there.

Kim: How much more time do you think that might free up for early intervention?

Sandy: Four hours at the most. I was thinking about all day on Tuesdays.

Kim: I appreciate you thinking this way, but that's just not going to be enough time. Expanding to a full day on Tuesdays adds the complicating factor of those times during the day that aren't very popular with most families for home visits, such as 8:00 a.m. If you were able to increase your time, then I would need it to be more flexible so that you could use FAB scheduling.

Sandy: I see your point. It sounds like I'm losing my contract.

Kim: Sandy, we do enjoy having you on the team, but the amount of time you have available doesn't meet our needs. I will be actively recruiting for another OT who does have the time to contract for what we need. Is there anything that I can do to entice you to change your mind?

Sandy: Well, I have worked really hard on learning these new practices, and I do enjoy working on this team. If I could make up the difference in my contract for the hours I would lose at the hospital, then I could consider decreasing my hours there.

Kim:	So, increasing your contract hourly rate? Is that what you're asking?
Sandy:	Is that possible?
Kim:	I don't have much room in our contract budget, but it would be worth it to me to take a look at the budget considering our investment in you and how well you work with the team. I could go over those numbers and give you a call this evening. How would that work with your schedule?
Sandy:	I appreciate you considering my request.
Kim:	I'm glad we were able to talk about this openly. If this does work out, how many additional hours are you thinking would be feasible?
Sandy:	Well, I've heard you say you need 20 hours each week and that I need to be available different days and times of the week. I need to talk with my supervisor and look at my schedule. I'm not sure that I can jump to 20 hours right away, but I could possibly increase my availability over the next few months. Would that be an option?
Kim:	Give me an example of what you're thinking.
Sandy:	Well, if I could contract for the morning time 1 day a week right away, such as 9:00 a.m. to 1:00 p.m., then I could work on expanding other late afternoon and evening options. That's just off the top of my head, what do you think?
Kim:	I like the sound of that. Those early evening options would probably work well with a lot of families. Okay, I appreciate your flexibility. I need to take a look at our budget. Do you have any questions for me?
Sandy:	No, I don't think so. I'll be expecting your call this evening. If the contract adjustment is not a possibility, then would you let me know before you start heavily recruiting for another OT? I'd like to talk about this with my husband to see if we have any other options.
Kim:	Definitely. Once I look at the budget and we talk, we can plan our next steps. How does that sound?

Kim and Sandy then arranged the time for their telephone call later that day. Kim was able to review their budget and talk with the fiscal manager. They agreed that they could offer a $5.00 per hour increase and decided to go with a weekly range in the contract agreement of 16–24 hours per week. Sandy accepted the contract offer and was able to shift her schedule over the next 12 weeks to regularly be available 18–20 hours each week. This scenario provides an example of a program administrator being upfront with contractors regarding the amount of time needed to efficiently and effectively participate on a team using a PSP approach. Although this is not an easy conversation, these open, honest discussions are essential to ensure that the needs of children, families, other team members, and the program are met.

Program leadership will need to develop a plan for redistributing personnel resources over time for programs with higher numbers of a particular discipline than will be needed on a geographically based team or team members that serve in more of an assistant-type role. For example, if a program currently has four full-time developmental specialists, one full-time SLP, and one half-time OT, then the program would need to recruit a PT, either increase the amount of time provided by the current OT or recruit another half-time OT, or recruit an OT that could work full time in order to establish a core team. The situation with the developmental specialists would need to be reconsidered as there are more developmental specialists than needed. One possibility would be that the developmental specialists receive training and fill the role of service coordinator. The team needs the fewest number of people (employees or contractors) who will give the most amount of time to support children and families in order for this teaming approach to be most effective. If the numbers of children enrolled in the program increase and additional team members are needed, then another SLP is typically the preferred option due to the high number of referrals received by most programs based on language or communication needs. If the team's caseload continues to expand, then additional team members are added to maintain a balanced complement of disciplines and prepare for the possibility of dividing the existing team into two smaller teams serving designated sections of the current geographic area.

Buy-In of Program Leadership

Supporting implementation of new practices not only requires the attention of program leadership during initial phases, but it also ensures ongoing fidelity over time. Teaming in this manner requires a strong leader not only for logistical management but also to promote the use of the practices and facilitate team members' ability to effectively work with one another. Leadership at all levels must be committed to using the practices and the significant role of the team in the program's organizational structure.

How to Structure the Start-Up

Deciding how to structure the start-up is key for all program leadership when considering this teaming approach. Two factors to consider are how to 1) transition currently enrolled children into this teaming approach and 2) approach programwide implementation. The expectation when teams initially implement a primary provider approach to teaming is that all newly referred children will be assigned a team and a primary provider. This team will be responsible for supporting the children and families from the point of initial referral to transition. The responsibilities within this team include initial contact (intake), evaluation, assessment, IFSP development, intervention, and transition. Individuals who only perform one function (e.g., intake service coordinators or evaluation) are now integrated into the team and serve multiple functions along with other team members to maximize the team's efficiency and resources. For example, service coordinators perform intake and ongoing functions, which eliminates a change in service coordinators for newly enrolling families. Many programs, especially those that receive a high number of referrals on a regular basis, establish separate evaluation teams in an attempt to meet the Part C, 45-day time line requirement from referral to IFSP implementation. Typically, the evaluation team determines eligibility and provides recommendations for services to be included on the IFSP. The core team members are able to meet the time lines when children are assigned to geographically based teams because scheduling and communication are supported through regular team meetings. This also enables teams to meet the Part C stipulation that a member of the evaluation team and team member involved in ongoing service delivery participate in the IFSP meeting.

Programs often have questions related to children and families currently enrolled in the program, especially those receiving services from multiple providers. If the child is within 6 months or less of transition from Part C early intervention, then the team most likely will maintain the current service delivery approach to support the child through this process. For those children who are not approaching transition, the next scheduled IFSP is a logical opportunity for the service coordinator to discuss the PSP teaming approach with the family and strategies for identifying the PSP. The IFSP review should include reexamining the outcome statements to assess the extent to which they are functional, participation based, and include a meaningful context that has been prioritized by the family (see Chapter 4 for more information on writing functional, participation-based IFSP outcome statements). The team should also consider those children who currently have only one provider. Revisiting the IFSP earlier than the next scheduled review may be an option as the transition to the new teaming approach will not substantially alter the child's existing plan of service delivery. The team should also discuss the children who currently have multiple providers and consider the components of role expectation, role gap, role overlap, and role assistance in order to support the parents in identifying the best possible PSP and which of the current practitioners are needed to serve as SSPs.

Start-up questions also arise regarding whether to begin implementation with just one team serving a defined catchment area or fully use the teaming approach programwide (full or partial implementation). The answer to this question is based on a program's (local/state) resources and ability to provide the necessary initial and ongoing training and support as teams make the transition to and use this approach. We recommend that statewide programs identify pilot sites that are geographically diverse (i.e., urban, suburban, rural, remote) to initially implement the PSP teaming approach in order to identify systemic issues, which may include but are not limited to state policies and procedures, fiscal challenges, and/or availability of resources. In contrast, we recommend programwide implementation at start-up for individual programs and agencies to ensure that all families served are treated equitably, maximize program resources, and minimize the stress on individual practitioners when required to operate in different teaming configurations.

Implementation of Team Meetings

Team meetings within this practice approach are new and different for most programs. Because all team members must participate in every meeting from beginning to end, a new culture around the importance of the meeting must often be established by program leadership. Depending on the size of the catchment area and location of team members, leaders have to consider creative mechanisms for linking team members. In addition to face-to-face meetings, participation using technology such as conference calls and web-based meetings in real time may be viable options. See Chapter 7 for more detailed information about team meetings.

 Remember

Following are the factors to consider when making the decision to use a primary service provider approach to teaming.

*   Logistical and fiscal infrastructure
*   Identification and availability of resources
*   Buy-in of program leadership
*   How to structure the start-up
*   Implementation of team meetings

ESTABLISHING GEOGRAPHICALLY BASED TEAMS

Establishing geographically based teams to support families and their children is the first step in moving to a PSP approach to teaming. Teams are not child specific in this approach, but they consist of representatives from a variety of disciplines that are assigned to provide supports within a given catchment area. A *catchment area* is defined as a geographic region (e.g., town, county, multiple counties), zip code, portion of a school district, or health district.

A core team can serve approximately 100–125 families when drive time does not exceed 30–45 minutes for a one-way trip to visit a child in their home or community setting. A core team using a dedicated service coordination model must minimally include one full-time equivalent of an early childhood educator or early childhood special educator, OT, PT, SLP, and approximately three (full-time equivalent) service coordinators. Team members representing these disciplines are considered core because they are the most commonly available, frequently referred for, associated with parent priorities, or required by Part C. The team must include a service coordinator who may be a dedicated service coordinator or another discipline that also provides service coordination (blended role), depending on the state's or program's guidelines. Service coordinators do not function as PSPs in a dedicated service coordination model. They may serve as both service coordinator and PSPs in a blended model in which practitioners are also responsible for service coordination. If practitioners are also responsible for the role of service coordination or situations that require extensive travel times, then the number of families supported by the core team will be less than that of a team using a dedicated service coordination model.

Custodial family members (including foster parents) are always members of the child's team, as well as any other people the family would like to include. In situations in which the child has a noncustodial parent(s), the noncustodial parent(s) could be a member of the team. If the child is spending time with custodial and noncustodial parents, then the same PSP should support all parents involved with the child across the child's natural environments.

Other core team members might also include audiologists, nurses, dieticians, psychologists, social workers, teachers of children with vision or hearing impairments, mobility specialists, physicians, assistive technology specialists, and so forth. Circumstances specific to a particular child may require additional team members such as Early Head Start teachers, Parents as Teachers home visitors, child care providers, and any other individuals parents deem important in the child's life.

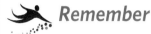

Remember

A core team serving 100–125 families using a dedicated service coordination model must minimally include

- One early childhood educator/special educator

- One occupational therapist

- One physical therapist

- One speech-language pathologist

- Three service coordinators

Individuals serving in a support role, such as aides, assistants, and paraprofessionals, are not members of the core team. Based on a scarcity model of practitioner availability, assistants sometimes work under the direction of one of the aforementioned disciplines for the sole purpose of providing a specific traditional therapy regime to the child (e.g., a PT assistant goes to the child's home to practice walking with a walker). A PSP approach to teaming uses natural learning environment practices to promote parent competence and confidence in using everyday activities as opportunities for child learning. This approach requires the expertise of and accessibility to the supervising therapist or educator to maximize just-in-time learning opportunities and continue the ongoing conversation to support the parent or other care providers rather than using an assistant to implement an approved exercise program or standard set of activities. A limited number of state licensure laws allow autonomous practice of therapy assistants. Assistants could be considered as members of a core team in these circumstances, but the assistant should never be substituted for a licensed therapist.

If a team is responsible for serving less than 100–125 families, then the amount of time needed from each of the required core team members may be less than full time. All team members, however, must be available to serve as a PSP, participate in joint visits, and attend team meetings. The number of teams needed by a program may vary depending on the size of the catchment area and location of the families and other team members. For example, a program in a catchment area that serves 100–125 families but has geographic barriers (e.g., mountains, large bodies of water) and/or families who are widely dispersed across a rural or remote region may be better served by more than one team supporting fewer families.

The team must have a designated leader who is minimally responsible for facilitating the team meetings and whose role is also to prepare the team meeting agenda, guide the discussion during the team meeting, and prepare the team minutes. Other responsibilities of the team leader might include coordinating referrals, assigning evaluators, reviewing documentation, supervising, and so forth. The team leader might be a program administrator, service coordinator, or other team member, depending on the assigned duties. For consistency, the team leader role should be filled by the same person and not rotated among team members (Borrill et al., 2001; Erez et al., 2002). Appointing a team leader based on title alone (e.g., program manager) should be avoided, if possible, and maximizing participative decision making for all team members will result in better performance (Bell, 2007). The team leader, whether appointed or allowed to emerge over time must, however, have skills in group facilitation and demonstrate organizational skills and the ability to manage the regularly scheduled team meetings required by this approach. See Chapter 7 for more information about the role of facilitating team meetings. The team leader is responsible for guiding the team, whereas each PSP is responsible for supporting individual families.

PREPARATION CHALLENGES AND SOLUTIONS

Many challenges exist for a program that is considering using a PSP teaming approach. This section describes the most commonly identified challenges and misperceptions that can contribute to a programs' or individual team members' lack of success with implementation. Each identified challenge includes solutions that have been effectively implemented by teams across the country as well as internationally.

Support of Program Leadership

Support of program leadership at all levels within the organization is one of the most important considerations when using a PSP approach. Agreement is important among leaders and managers across agencies in systems using a service coordination model in which the service coordinators are employees or contractors of an agency separate from the organization responsible for providing intervention services. Lack of support or ambivalence at any level can interfere with the process of moving from conversation and discussion to planning and implementation. Using a PSP approach to teaming can be perceived as a controversial move by all that are affected by the change (e.g., families, practitioners, referral sources, funders, other community partners).

A program leader must possess a detailed understanding of the practices and clearly articulate the vision and competently address any and all questions and concerns. A visionary leader expects resistance when changes are implemented and assists other members of the management team to join the vision. For example, consider a highly respected, large urban program in which the executive director decided that the program would move to using a PSP approach to teaming. The program participated in planning, training, and ongoing support to implement the approach in spite of objections from the existing team members and cautiously optimistic support from the team supervisors. The concerns and objections from practitioners (within and outside of the team) began to surface and erode the confidence of the team supervisors once implementation was in process. As a result, the practices were not being implemented with fidelity, leading to further questions about the teaming approach. The executive director observed the unrest and soon realized that the team supervisors were either not in support of the new approach or lacked the skills to appropriately manage the transition. She met with team supervisors to share her observations in order to ensure implementation. One of the supervisors expressed lack of support for the approach and resigned her position. The other team supervisor expressed an inability to respond to questions and concerns as well as frustration with her own lack of competence with the practices. She did, however, express belief in the approach and a desire to continue to learn and support the team, but she needed intensive support. The executive director refocused her energies on the management team and assumed the vacant team supervisory role until a new supervisor could be appointed for one team and the existing supervisor prepared to lead the other. She attended every team meeting and confidently and competently answered questions and addressed concerns as they surfaced and assisted team members in maintaining fidelity to the practices. She also met regularly with the leadership team to ensure they had the necessary skills to support the teams. In retrospect, the executive director could have initially focused more time and energy on the team supervisors to ensure that they were ready to meet the challenge of implementing a PSP teaming approach.

Conversely, in another program, the team supervisor was the impetus for moving to a PSP approach to teaming and had initial approval from the program director. The team participated in

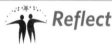
Reflect

- If you are an administrator of a program considering using a primary service provider (PSP) approach to teaming, what are some examples of how you can demonstrate support for your team(s)?

- If you are an administrator of a program currently using a PSP approach to teaming, what are some examples of how you demonstrate support for your team(s)?

- If you are a team leader, what do you do daily to demonstrate support of your team's use of a PSP approach to teaming?

- If you are a team member, what support do you need from your team leader and/or program administrator to implement a PSP approach to teaming?

training and ongoing support to implement the approach and was making positive strides toward full implementation in their district. The parent of a child currently enrolled in the program expressed concern to the program director about having a primary provider instead of the three providers she was accustomed to working with her child and preferred bringing her child into the center for therapy rather than having the primary provider come to her home to support her and her child. The program director agreed with the parent on the grounds of parent choice and individualized services. The team supervisor in this scenario had gained approval of the program director, but not her full understanding of the approach and practices. In retrospect, the team supervisor could have spent time with the program director to prepare her for possible questions and concerns and enhance her ability to support the team in implementing the new approach.

Brokered System Approach

Using a brokered system model to identify service providers to implement the IFSP is another challenge when preparing for a team-based approach. Typically, state programs using brokered systems fall into two categories: 1) the service coordinator serves as the broker and is responsible for assembling evaluators, IFSP development, and identifying ongoing service providers from among a list of approved agencies and/or individual providers; and 2) the program completes the evaluation and IFSP and the service coordinator identifies possible disciplines (e.g., ECSE, OT, PT, SLP) that the family selects from a list of approved providers. A team is nonexistent in both situations because providers work independently with the child and family. It is possible to implement a PSP teaming approach for states or programs that primarily use contracted personnel. Preparing for the approach involves distributing the contract providers among the identified geographically based teams (the fewest number of providers who give the most time). Because these contract providers most likely do not work in an office together, the program may need to plan ahead and provide the infrastructure necessary for teaming to occur (e.g., meeting space, conference call technology) and support the team by providing or identifying a team leader. See Chapter 6 for more specific information about covering the costs of joint visits, and see Chapter 7 for more information about team meeting logistics, including fiscal support of team members' time to meet.

Lack of Providers

The lack of providers to serve on the team is one of the most commonly verbalized challenges when considering the move to a primary provider teaming approach. A specific discipline is either completely unavailable or inadequate numbers exist to meet the needs of enrolled children and families. Limited availability or shortages of a particular discipline in these circumstances are most likely a challenge regardless of the teaming approach being implemented. Unfortunately, some areas have chronic shortages of particular disciplines due to the location, level of compensation, and hiring or contracting issues of the program. In these situations, targeted recruitment, competitive compensation packages, and serving as a fieldwork site for university internships and practicum experiences for all disciplines may increase the availability of needed practitioners. The shortage for programs using a multidisciplinary or interdisciplinary model of team interaction may be due to multiple providers serving the same child on a regular basis. Resources are maximized and supported through team meetings and joint visits when programs implement a PSP approach.

Referring Outside of the Early Intervention Program

Programs often inadvertently sustain practitioner shortages within their own program by referring to a hospital or private clinic for a specific type of therapy that is believed to be unavailable through the early intervention program. This thereby sustains the practitioner in the other program who most likely is interested in working with infants and toddlers rather than providing impetus for the practitioner to work directly for early intervention via a staff or contract position. If the practitioner in the hospital or private clinic setting is willing to serve children and families in their natural environments, then they would probably be agreeable to attending team meetings and participating in joint visits as stipulated in the contract with adequate compensation. If individuals or programs refuse to provide supports and services within natural environments and participate in team meetings, then this is not early intervention under Part C, based on federal regulations, and a referral to practitioners in these settings for early intervention services would be inconsistent with evidence-based practices in early intervention. When possible, the team should examine what is needed and how that area of expertise can be obtained through the team or another resource.

Listen in on a team meeting in which a new geographically based team using a PSP approach is challenged by the competing, multiple needs of a child and family enrolled in the early intervention program. Ed, an early childhood special educator and PSP, is presenting a quarterly update and has concerns about the team's ability to meet the child's needs. Pay particular attention to the way in which the EIC explores with the team the reason for the need to refer to services outside of the early intervention program and the role assistance needed from other team members to support the PSP.

Carolee (EIC):	Let's start out reviewing where we are with this family. We've been supporting them about 8 months, correct?
Allen (service coordinator):	Yes, Carolee. The child, LaRoy, is 18 months old. They moved here from out of state and contacted us right away. At the time LaRoy enrolled, he did not have a diagnosis, but all involved knew that he had a lot of needs. We all thought Ed would be the best PSP because of his experience working with children with intense challenges.
Carolee:	So Ed, share with us the support you've been providing.
Ed (early childhood special educator):	Well, we're pretty sure LaRoy has a significant visual impairment and some hearing loss, but we still don't have a definite diagnosis. He's not made any real progress with his motor skills because of the issue of his uncontrolled seizures. I really think he needs more of a medical model type of support.
Carolee:	Ed, I'm going to interrupt. How does the information you're presenting match with how we present our quarterly updates?
Sharon (SLP):	Here, let me try. Ed, what are the activity settings you've been using as the focus of your support?
Ed:	Thanks, you're right. I was focused on LaRoy's problems or impairments. I'm just really worried about him.
Carolee:	We understand, Ed. We're going to address your concerns. I promise.
Ed:	Well, we've really been focused on mealtimes. LaRoy has a tough time eating and keeping down food. Allen, Sharon, and Tracy have all given LaRoy's mother and me lots of support related to eating. Caley also helped out with some positioning ideas. We've also tried some new things at bath time. We need to spend more time on that, but his recurring hospitalizations due to seizures have really been an issue. We also need to address his car seat, and we've made some nice progress with bedtime routines. He is now sleeping in his own bed. We're using one of those reflux wedges and it seems to be helping.
Carolee:	So, mealtimes, bath time, car rides, and bedtime. You've described progress with bedtime, but still have challenges in the other activity settings. Is that accurate?
Ed:	Yes.

Carolee:	Okay. You've also described some support you've received from other team members. So let's focus on what assistance you need from us now. You mentioned that you feel LaRoy needs more of a medical model type of support. Explain to us what you mean by that statement.
Ed:	I've been talking to the other team members and I'm pretty convinced that we need to refer LaRoy to the feeding clinic at Children's Hospital. He just needs some intense medically focused therapy. Mrs. Moore spoke to the SLP at the clinic during LaRoy's last hospitalization and the SLP indicated that he would be a good candidate for their feeding clinic.
Caley (PT):	Ed, what does the feeding clinic offer that we can't provide? I'm not sure I understand what you mean when you say medically focused therapy.
Ed:	I just feel that LaRoy needs a lot more support than I can provide.
Caley:	Why?
Ed:	Well, it's both about time and expertise. I really feel like LaRoy needs more intensive support around his ability to manage foods.
Sharon:	How can I help? Feeding really is my area of expertise.
Ed:	I know we shouldn't change the PSP, but I feel like I need a lot of help. I just thought that the feeding clinic made more sense.
Carolee:	This question is for all of you. What would the ideal support for LaRoy and his mom look like? Let's not limit ourselves to the notion of medical versus educational. What would the best support possible look like considering what we know about evidence-based practices?
Tracy (OT):	That's a good question, Carolee. I'm not sure we're all on the same page. This discussion should help with that. I'll start. I feel like this is a situation in which we typically would have provided service from all team members on a regular basis. I know, though, that we would have had a lot of cancellations due to LaRoy's health issues.
Caley:	I don't disagree, Tracy, but we have all seen LaRoy and his family and provided support. Isn't this one of those situations in which all of us going to the home separately would have just added to the confusion?
Tracy:	You're probably right. Sharon, what do you think?
Sharon:	I'm worried that I haven't been available enough for you, Ed. Is that how you feel?
Ed:	No. I know I can ask for your help. I guess I'm just feeling overwhelmed. When Mrs. Moore mentioned the feeding clinic, well, it just seemed like a good solution.
Carolee:	What are some of the pros and cons of the feeding clinic?
Ed:	Well, one of the pros is that we could just transfer our problems with feeding to the therapist at the hospital.
Sharon:	How would that work? I think we would still be responsible for supporting mealtimes being successful. Wouldn't we, Carolee?
Caley:	I'll jump in. Yes, we would. The feeding clinic won't be contextualized with what happens at home. Plus, how in the world would LaRoy's mom be able to get him to the clinic? We have the problems with the car seat and his overall health. I just can't imagine how that would be helpful.

Ed:	Actually, Mrs. Moore was already asking herself those same questions. She wanted to know what I thought. It sounds like the positive benefit was more for me than LaRoy and Mrs. Moore.
Allen:	Ed, that takes a lot to admit. I appreciate your honesty. How often have you been seeing LaRoy?
Ed:	Well, that's probably a big part of my problem. We've been focused on lunchtime because it's convenient for both of us. I've probably averaged weekly visits. I need to go more often, don't I? Don't answer. I know I do. I just find it difficult to flex my schedule.
Sharon:	Ed, what would help?
Carolee:	Good question, Sharon. How can we help?
Ed:	It sounds like we agree that the feeding clinic is out and that I need to increase the frequency of my visits.
Carolee:	What about the time of day of your visits. How will that change?
Ed:	I think I need to talk with Mrs. Moore about really buckling down and tackling mealtime. I'm going to take a hard look at my schedule and think about this very seriously. I probably need to review my scheduling with all families. Sharon, would you be available for some high-intensity joint visiting soon with LaRoy?
Sharon:	Sure. I can't go until the end of next week, but by then I can rearrange some visits and we can go a few days in a row if needed.
Ed:	Let's plan on that, but I'll need to call Mrs. Moore first.
Caley:	Ed, I also feel like you've been waiting on some of the other support you might need around car rides and bath time. What can we do to help with that?
Ed:	You're right about that. You know what, I think we should call Mrs. Moore right now and see if she could talk with us. I'll call her first and then we can put her on speakerphone if she has time and is okay with that. What do you think?
Carolee:	Great idea, Ed. First, how can we put to rest this issue of medical versus educational supports? I want to ensure that we're all confident that our team can meet the needs of all of the children and families we serve. If not, I want to identify those areas of role gap so I can support you in obtaining the information that you need.
Tracy:	To me, this conversation demonstrates that our teaming is working. I think we are going to have doubts along the way, but we'll be fine as long as we can talk openly about our questions and concerns.
Caley:	I agree. I just don't want anyone worrying unnecessarily. Ed, why didn't you bring up your concerns sooner?
Ed:	I've been thinking about that. I don't really know the answer as to why, but now I am going to be more aware and sensitive to this feeling I had and bring it up right away.
Carolee:	Excellent. I think that Ed has just shared some information for all of us to consider.

Ed telephoned Mrs. Moore, who was available and eager to talk with the team. They put a plan in place to address all of the activity settings over the next few weeks with intensive support from Sharon and Caley via joint visits with Ed.

The PSP in this scenario was feeling pressure in terms of availability and expertise to support a child and family with high needs. The EIC demonstrated leadership in assuring the PSP that the team was available to support him and used coaching to support all team members to develop a plan. The team recognized that Ed's artificially invoked dichotomy of medical versus educational therapy was not really the issue, but rather an underlying need for more intensive support from Ed to the family and the team to Ed. The other team members used coaching to support one another and explore the options available to them to ensure a cohesive plan to support the child and family.

Lack of Specific Expertise

A core team may occasionally lack a specific area of expertise. For example, a team may lack a member with in-depth experience and expertise with assistive technology, feeding, or working with children with visual or hearing impairments. Teams in these circumstances can gain access to resources external to the team and/or develop their own skills over time through ongoing training and technical assistance. If teams gain access to resources external to the team, then the expert should be considered an ad hoc member of the team and provide evidence-based early intervention services. For example, referring a child for therapy at the feeding clinic of a regional medical center does not meet the natural environment provisions of Part C. If, however, the feeding specialist would be willing to meet with the team or support the child, family,

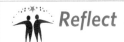

Reflect

How does your team gain access to needed areas of expertise to support the children and families served by your team?

and PSP during a joint visit, then this would be considered an appropriate early intervention service. Many states have regional consultants who are available to early intervention programs to serve in this capacity with expertise including, but not limited to, the areas of assistive technology, autism, positive behavior supports, vision, and hearing.

Acceptance of a Primary Service Provider Approach to Teaming

Getting team members, families, referral sources, and other community agencies to accept a PSP approach to teaming is another common challenge faced by programs. A general lack of understanding of the teaming approach is one of the most common challenges. Practitioners express concerns regarding licensure, liability, and practice act violations due to misperceptions about using a PSP. The practitioner feels that will be asked to take on or give away skills typically associated with a particular discipline. For example, a PT may claim liability issues if she believes that she must teach a development specialist to make a seat insert for a child's highchair or learn how to teach a child speech sound placement for correct articulation. Yet, when using a PSP approach to teaming, the PT would most likely be considered the expert on the team for making seat inserts; therefore, she would either be the PSP for the child or would accompany the PSP on joint visits to fabricate the seat insert. Similarly, the SLP is the team's expert on articulation and would either serve as the PSP or as a secondary provider to support the parents' and child's ability to learn correct placement for speech sound production.

All team members are responsible for having the knowledge necessary to support families in the areas of child development across all domains, parenting, and resource identification, acquisition, and evaluation (i.e., role expectation). Therapists and educators are also responsible for understanding and sharing information about basic child development and answering parenting questions. More specifically, teachers working in early intervention should know how to help a child with cerebral palsy grasp a spoon, SLPs must know how to position a child correctly in a stroller or highchair, PTs need to be able to support parents and other care providers in promoting parent–child communication within the context of everyday activities, and OTs should know answers to common questions parents ask about child growth and nutrition. These are a few examples of knowledge and expertise required of therapists and teachers working in early intervention that may extend beyond traditional discipline expectations. Yet, they would not be considered out of the scope of practice of an individual on an early intervention team using a PSP approach and are necessary to help parents and care providers of young children.

A PT expresses her concerns about using a PSP approach to teaming to her EIC in the following conversation. Specifically, she feels that she should serve as the PSP for all children with torticollis (a contracture of the neck muscles present at birth) as she believes her PT licensure law and code of ethics is violated if she teaches the ECSE stretching exercises for the child. Notice how the EIC delves more deeply into the PT's concerns related to building the capacity of her teammates while also maintaining her professional identity.

John (EIC):	Sophia, thank you for agreeing to meet to talk with me about your comments during team meeting this afternoon.
Sophia (PT):	Sure. I know that you disagree with me about my stance on kids with torticollis.
John:	This really isn't about whether we agree, but how your comments match with the characteristics of the practices we are now implementing in our organization.
Sophia:	What do you mean? I just don't believe in one-size-fits-all approaches. There are exceptions to every rule.
John:	Talk to me about your thoughts of how our practices are one size fits all.
Sophia:	Well, how you think that this teaming approach will work for all children. That is one size fits all.
John:	What is your understanding of the characteristics of the PSP teaming approach?
Sophia:	Well, we have to choose only one person to work directly with the child and the rest of us have to consult. I know that children with torticollis need direct PT services.
John:	What are the other characteristics of the approach?
Sophia:	Team meeting . . . and well, I don't recall the exact wording.
John:	Okay, let me clarify. This teaming approach is not about only one person serving the family, but identifying a team liaison that works with the child and family on a regular basis. This person is selected from a defined team, and the primary provider receives ongoing support from the other team members as needed. How does this help?
Sophia:	I understand that it isn't only one person. I misspoke. I just feel like there are certain children that need direct physical therapy.
John:	I agree. Of course some children need a PT to serve as the primary service provider, and we can do that. What are you thinking of when you say that children need direct physical therapy?
Sophia:	Well, I just can't be teaching everyone stretching exercises—the other team members—it's just not safe.
John:	What does the research tell us? Let's just focus on children with torticollis.
Sophia:	Stretching is an evidence-based strategy that is effective for children with torticollis but not for children whose muscles have spasticity. They need longer, more sustained stretching such as braces or night splinting.
John:	Okay, how do we consider that information in light of the *Mission and Key Principles for Providing Services in Natural Environments*?
Sophia:	Using context and helping families, but stretching works.

John: Right. We've established that stretching can be effective in this situation. What other strategies are helpful in this type of circumstance?

Sophia: Well, my approach has to be individualized, but generally it is really important to take a look at the child's day and routines as well as what is motivating to the child—what he or she is interested in. After you know that, then you help the care providers understand how to support the child in actively strengthening and stretching the child's neck throughout the day.

John: Would you mind giving me an example?

Sophia: Say the child has an older sibling that he really likes to watch and be with. I can show the parents how to hold the child and encourage him to watch and look at the older sibling in ways that work against the tightness in his neck. We can also switch sides for nursing or bottle feeding, we can change the position of the child in his crib, and we can move the car seat so the child looks out the window away from the tightness. There are lots of things we can do that really work.

John: So, in the specific situation earlier today in team meeting, how is what you are describing different than what Teri would do as the early childhood special educator on our team in her role as the PSP?

Sophia: No. I know she knows all of these things. It's the stretching exercises that I'm worried about.

John: Okay, that is helpful to understand. What would the stretching exercises look like?

Sophia: The exercises should be part of the family's routine, such as when they hold the infant or after the infant's bath. The stretches are very gentle and require the adult to place their hands in a specific position in order to increase the child's range of motion. It's not cranking on the child's neck by any means, but we need to be cautious because the head and neck area is delicate.

John: Is the PT the only person who can do this? I guess what I mean is, do you feel you need to be the one performing the stretches every time the stretches are needed?

Sophia: No, of course not. I would teach the parents how to do the stretches.

John: That makes sense for when you are the PSP. How will that look when you are not?

Sophia: I would need to make sure that the rest of the team knows how to support the parents in doing the stretches.

John: What would help you be more comfortable in supporting others around the specific strategy of stretching?

Sophia: Well, I know for sure I wouldn't be comfortable teaching them without seeing the child.

John: That makes sense. How would you increase your comfort level?

Sophia: I feel like I'm going to need to do joint visits, and probably not just one or two.

John: Okay, so serving as the SSP during a joint visit is an evidence-based strategy. I agree. How will you know when the coachee or PSP is competent in supporting the family to implement the strategy?

Sophia: I think it will be different for all of the team members. Won't it make sense for me to be the primary in some situations?

John:	Yes. I'm sure it will. Let's review why Teri was identified as the best and most likely primary provider for this particular child and family.
Sophia:	This child has global delays, but the parents are really young, and we all agree that working with parents who are teenagers is one of Teri's strengths.
John:	I also recall that you felt that this child's torticollis was short term, positional, and not related to other issues. Is that correct?
Sophia:	Yes. So the long-term view, right?
John:	Right. That's what I was thinking, too. Sophia, how were you imagining your support of Teri to look?
Sophia:	I actually wasn't thinking about that. I was thinking that this is a child I would typically see. I'm worried that I won't get to use my expertise. I guess I'm having doubts about my continued role.
John:	Can you be more specific?
Sophia:	I really like being a PT. Does that sound silly? I just don't want to lose my skill base.
John:	I'm hearing you say that you're concerned about your specific role as a PT on our team. Is there anything else?
Sophia:	I am a bit worried about some of the other team members' abilities when it comes to this type of thing.
John:	You mean the stretching?
Sophia:	Yes, I do.
John:	Again, how can you increase your comfort level with this aspect of your role assistance for your team members?
Sophia:	Is it okay for me to do a lot of joint visits?
John:	I am very willing to support joint visits for any and all team members. I just need to know that we have a plan for how you are going to build their capacity and your sense of confidence in their abilities.
Sophia:	That's a good point. I know that it just can't be about me. I think I'd like to start with one situation at a time. I'll go talk with Teri right away. I probably need to apologize to her about my reaction earlier today.
John:	Well, that's up to you, but I do want to know how you can use your coaching skills to develop a plan with Teri.
Sophia:	Right, it can't be my plan. I think I need to ask her the same questions you asked me about comfort level and confidence. This has been really helpful. It was also somewhat cathartic to talk about all of the strategies that I typically use that aren't just focused on stretching and are about participation in daily activities. I have a lot of confidence in my team members around those strategies. They've taught me a lot about how to promote participation.
John:	I'm glad you feel that way. I've enjoyed observing the sharing of information between team members during the team meetings.
Sophia:	So, I'm going to start out with having a coaching conversation with Teri about our plan with the child we discussed earlier today. I'm also going to apologize and make

sure that I didn't hurt her feelings. Is it okay if I start out with an explanation of where I was coming from at the next team meeting? I guess I'm asking for some time in the team meeting to do some planning.

John: I can absolutely support that plan. Also, if I hear signs of drifting from the plan in future team meetings, would you be comfortable with me bringing it up in the context of the team meeting?

Sophia: Yes. I am. I've got to be willing to share my feelings in a way that helps us move forward. I need to get better at that.

John: I really appreciate your openness and your commitment to the team. Would you like to plan a time outside of team meeting to talk about this again?

Sophia: How about we touch base on this topic when we meet next month to go over documentation?

John: That sounds like a great plan. Thanks again.

The EIC noted behavior in the team meeting that did not match the characteristics of the practices being implemented by the team. He requested a conversation with the PT who was having difficulty with the concept of PSP for certain children and families. John used a coaching conversation to approach the issue and develop a plan for getting and staying on track with evidence-based practices. He assisted the PT in exploring her concerns related to supporting other team members around the issue of torticollis. As she reflected, the PT realized that supporting other team members was very similar to her approach for assisting parents and other caregivers, was well within her scope of practice as a PT, and does not violate her licensure law or code of ethics.

Misperception of Limiting Services

The notion of limiting services is another common misperception about a PSP approach to teaming. Individuals believe that less service is being offered and/or access to needed services is being withheld because a PSP is identified and is the only practitioner who sees the child and family. This is not true. In fact, a core team is required for every child and family when using a PSP approach to teaming. More than one discipline participates in the evaluation, assessment, and development of the IFSP. All disciplines are present at every team meeting and participate in service delivery decisions and ongoing intervention through joint visits whenever needed by the PSP and family. Frequency and intensity of visits is not dictated based on the use of the primary provider, but it is determined on an individual family basis. Going from four different disciplines on a regular basis to a PSP does not necessarily reduce the amount of service delivered by the primary provider. In contrast, gatekeeping of services occurs in a multidisciplinary or interdisciplinary model of team interaction, which limits the types of disciplines involved based on the child's identified impairments or areas of need. For example, if a child presents initially with only motor delays, then an educator would most likely not be involved. Similarly, if a child's area of delay is only related to communication, then speech services would most likely be the only service identified on the IFSP. When working with infants and toddlers, dividing the child's needs into discrete areas is virtually impossible because of the overlap of one developmental area with another. In early intervention, if a child meets the state's eligibility criteria, then that child qualifies for any services identified by the IFSP team needed to meet the child's outcomes. The child is not merely eligible for services in the identified areas of delay. The PSP is selected by the entire team as the best long-term match to support the family in achieving the IFSP outcomes and promoting timely access to other team members as and how they are needed (see Chapter 5 for more details on how the PSP is identified).

Misperception of Early Intervention Practitioners Serving as Generalists

The view of all early intervention team members as generalists demonstrates a lack of understanding for the PSP approach to teaming. A team of individuals representing multiple disciplines and areas of expertise ensures that children and families have access to the specialized knowledge and skills necessary to meet IFSP outcomes. An everyone is a generalist approach implies a watered-down version of service delivery in which all team members have similar knowledge, skills, and method of intervention and the specialized training of therapists and educators is not used or needed. In a PSP approach to teaming, careful consideration of the best team member for each individual child and family is emphasized during every step of the IFSP process. Specialized knowledge and expertise needed to support achievement of the IFSP outcomes is one of the primary considerations for selecting the primary provider. The need for joint visits from secondary providers is also based on specialized knowledge and skills needed by the PSP and family.

Misperception That Primary Service Provider Approach to Teaming Is Indirect Treatment

Another misunderstanding is that using a PSP results in an indirect treatment or service delivery model because a single provider could or should not implement all of the needed direct interventions for a particular child and family. Using a PSP approach to teaming is not an issue of direct or indirect intervention, but how a team organizes resources to efficiently and effectively support individual children and families. The primary provider works closely with parents and other care providers to mediate their ability to support the child's learning and development. The primary provider will use natural learning environments as the context for intervention and coaching as the interaction style with parents and care providers. Interaction may include hands-on assessment, modeling, direct teaching, and sharing information within their scope of practice. If, and when, direct contact by a team member (not the primary provider) is needed by the PSP, child, and/or family, then this contact is encouraged and happens through a joint visit with the PSP.

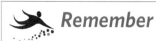 **Remember**

Using a primary service provider approach to teaming is not an issue of direct or indirect intervention, but how a team organizes resources to efficiently and effectively support individual children and families.

Misperception That More Direct Service Is Better

More therapy and services is a commonly held belief for serving children with disabilities; therefore, direct practitioner–child therapy from providers of multiple disciplines is often viewed as higher quality services that result in accomplishing IFSP outcomes faster. Increasing the child's participation in everyday activity settings and routines provides more opportunity for learning and development to occur. The role of the PSP is to focus on the naturally occurring learning opportunities to maximize child participation. Visits occur within the context of real-life activities, which naturally crosses developmental domains, and parents and other care providers are supported by their PSP to become confident and competent in promoting child learning within and across these activities even when the primary provider is not present. Having more team members directly involved tends to result in therapist–child interventions that are decontextualized. Multiple practitioners may lead to interventions and ideas that conflict with one another, homework for the care providers, potential duplication of efforts, and loss of valuable time that the child could be spending participating in real-life activities that occur frequently and naturally and have development-enhancing qualities.

Misinterpretation of Family Choice

Another misunderstanding about the PSP approach is that families' choices are restricted when they are assigned a designated team instead of selecting from a matrix or list. Actually, having parents choose their providers from a matrix tends to restrict the family to the limited disciplines identified as needed based on child impairments rather than providing them with immediate and ongoing access to a team of individuals from multiple disciplines, thus coordinated and comprehensive. Families are actively involved in deciding who the PSP is going to be and why, thereby making an informed decision about their child's and family's services and supports. Parents may request a change of PSP any time they feel unhappy with their choice.

Team Culture

Developing a team culture is another challenge programs face when implementing a PSP approach to teaming. For many programs, practitioners enter early intervention after working in a different setting, such as private practices, therapy clinics, hospitals, and rehabilitation centers. Practitioners can work somewhat independently in these settings and rely solely on their professional training and preferred practice patterns to develop and implement treatment plans. In Part C, however, practitioners are guided by federal law and regulations as well as recommended practices and current research related to early childhood intervention. The federal regulations require using a team consisting of multiple disciplines and all intervention be based on current research to achieve the intended outcomes for young children and their families (IDEA 2004). Working on a team requires individuals who are agreeable, conscientious, intelligent, competent in their area of expertise, high in openness to experience, mentally stable, like teamwork, and have been with the organization long enough to be socialized (Bell, 2007). Teams need ground rules that outline how team members will work together and participate during team meetings. A team's ground rules should promote open and honest communication, trust, respect (for all team members, including families who may not always be physically present), and inquiry. A few examples of team ground rules include

- Arrive at team meetings and joint visits on time

- Avoid using a cell phone during team meetings

- Be open to the perspectives of other team members

- Share the air time during team meetings

- Be prepared to give and receive support during team meetings

- Use the Worksheet for Selecting the Most Likely Primary Service Provider (Appendix 5E)

- Use the Joint Visit Planning Tool (Appendix 6A)

- Share individual family information when families are not present in the same manner as if the family was sitting at the team table

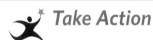

Take Action

Work with your team members to establish ground rules for how you will work together and participate during team meetings. Have each team member sign a copy of the ground rules and post them during team meetings. Revisit the ground rules when a team member leaves or joins the team.

Programs that contract with service providers must be aware that these individuals are acculturated to the setting in which they spend or devote the greatest amount of their time. Early intervention team leaders and program managers must expect to spend time acculturating new staff and contracted service providers to early intervention in terms of federal and state regulations, evidence-based practices, and working with other team members to most effectively support infants and toddlers with disabilities and their family members and care providers. Certain cultural aspects from settings other than early intervention are threats to the fidelity of practices within a team-based environment, including professional autonomy, billing requirements, productivity levels, physician prescriptions, and perceived professional hierarchies. Practitioners in many environments are completely autonomous. They have no supervision, make independent decisions (e.g., the need for a particular service, frequency, intensity, type of intervention used, discharge criteria), and can have little to no access or use of individuals from other disciplines, resulting in limited experience and a narrow view of teaming. Many of these practitioners are accustomed to a strict fee-for-service billing structure in which the number of visits is determined by third party payers or the consumers' ability to pay for the out-of-pocket expense for the service. In addition, many environments require a minimum productivity level for each practitioner in order to maximize efficiency and are driven by the prescriptions received from physicians. Most of the environments outside of early intervention that employ therapists are medical in nature, with the exception of public schools. A hierarchy often exists within the medical community in which physicians are the gatekeepers for services. Educators and service coordinators are typically not a part of these environments and therefore are not recognized as medically necessary service providers. In these instances, new team members from the medical community may need additional orientation about the important role that educators and service coordinators fulfill on the team.

The cultural influences of outside settings combined with limited experience in early intervention under Part C can initially affect the team culture. Practitioners are interdependent in a PSP approach to teaming. Team members rely on one another for information, coaching, and expertise in order to ensure that services are comprehensive, coordinated, and effective. No one team member dictates the frequency, intensity, and services for a particular child or family. Parents can choose to participate in early intervention or decline services, but the services identified on the IFSP are based on the entire team's input. Similarly, prescriptions from physicians are required to bill for services but do not delineate the type, frequency, and intensity of services a child and family receive. The input from the physician is included as part of the team decision-making process. Frequency and intensity of the identified service cannot be based on what and how much is billable, but instead it must be based on what the team decides is most appropriate to meet the IFSP outcomes. As opposed to some settings, early intervention law and family-centered practice place the burden of inconvenience on the program and practitioners instead of the family and other care providers. For example, all meetings must be held at a time and location convenient for the family, and services are provided in natural environments, including child care and other community-based settings. Therefore, program managers and team leaders must be diligent to ensure that all team members receive an in-depth orientation and necessary ongoing support to establish the foundation for effective teaming and developing the early intervention team culture.

The role of the service coordinator is also related to team culture, especially in systems in which the service coordinator must assemble child-specific teams from lists of available practitioners. Service coordinators in these systems have been responsible for making many independent decisions. Service coordinators are equal team members in a PSP approach to teaming and share decision-making responsibilities. The ongoing collaboration required between the service coordinator and the PSP is another complication for teams that use a dedicated service coordination model. Although the PSP may be the team member with the most direct interaction with the family, the service coordinator continues to have important responsibilities related to family support, IFSP time lines, transition, and access to necessary informal and formal resources. Service coordinators who are knowledgeable and effective serve as a resource to other team members, just as a therapist or educator would function on a team. Service coordinators who have a limited view of their role as completing and managing the necessary paperwork and meeting time lines may risk being marginalized by other team members.

Billing for Services

Funding is a major challenge, regardless of the teaming approach used by an early intervention program. Most programs are required to use multiple funding streams, with early intervention funds as the payment of last resort. All early intervention programs in an economy with level or decreased funding are challenged to maximize and effectively use available resources. The cost of a PSP approach to teaming has yet to be empirically determined largely due to the existing variations in teaming across programs, lack of implementation fidelity, and other confounding variables. For example, a program identifying experimental and control groups would simultaneously conduct two different service delivery models. A study of two different programs would introduce differences such as practitioner experience, leadership support, third party reimbursement, team culture, and so forth. Several early studies, however, indicated that choosing a PSP as the liaison to support children and their families may indeed be more cost effective (see Chapter 2; Barnett & Escobar, 1990; Barnett et al., 1988; Borrill et al., 2001; Eiserman et al., 1990; Tarr & Barnett, 2001; Warfield, 1995). Program administrators preparing to use a team-based approach must consider mechanisms to ensure payment for services, team meetings, joint visits (more than one practitioner) with the child and family, and colleague-to-colleague coaching conversations when the family and child are not present.

Payment for Services

Regardless of the teaming approach being used, administrators of programs required to gain access to third party payments for early intervention services must be aware of the specific requirements of Medicaid and other private insurers. All programs must have a mechanism in place for paying providers of services that are deemed necessary by the IFSP team but are not allowable costs by public and private insurers. For example, educational services are not a billable service in some states. Educators in these situations, however, serve as PSPs and are paid using early intervention funds (salary or contract).

Successfully billing a third party payer for the services provided by the individual practitioners on the team is one of the factors used for considering the most likely PSP (see Chapter 5 for more information about how to select the most likely PSP). Any primary provider may find themself in a situation in which a particular visit in part or whole may not be billable to a third party payer. For example, when the PT as PSP assists a parent in exploring resources for child care, this portion of the visit would most likely not be billed as a physical therapy service. Program administrators need to budget accordingly for these situations. If the program in the previous example uses a blended service coordination model, then, in many cases, the portion of the visit spent discussing child care resources would have been billable under case management.

In all circumstances, individual practitioners billing third party payers are responsible for determining the amount of time during each visit that is billable based on their discipline, licensure requirements, and third party payer allowable costs. For some services (e.g., speech-language pathology services in some states), the event is billable in its entirety compared with being billed in units of time. In these circumstances, the SLP must determine if the visit required the discipline-specific expertise and knowledge to bill for the services provided on that date.

Payment for Team Meetings

Identifying a mechanism to pay for team meeting time is something administrators need to consider when preparing to use a PSP approach to teaming. Granted, this is potentially the most expensive aspect of using this teaming approach because this is an added cost, as most programs do not require practitioners to meet together beyond the IFSP meeting. Team meetings, however, are a required implementation condition for this approach, and administrators must identify a funding stream (see Chapter 7 for more information about team meetings). As previously stated, programs using geographically based teams identify the fewest number of team members needed to serve the children and families in a particular catchment area. Only these team members attend team meetings, as opposed to having every practitioner on a program's provider or vendor list participate. For example, the program in the study described in the Chapter 2 appendices reduced the number of providers serving children and families in a designated geographic area from 45 to 9, which saved substantial funds and time regarding contract management, provider training, and cost for attendance at team meetings. Administrators using contract providers should consider requiring team meeting attendance as part of written contracts. Team meeting time will not be an added expense for those programs using salaried employees, but, in most circumstances, the time required to meet will be nonbillable.

Payment for Joint Visits

Joint visits are also a required implementation condition when using a PSP approach to teaming. In most states, two practitioners cannot bill for a service provided on the same date at the same time. Joint visits, however, need to occur on the same date at the same time (see Chapter 6). Practitioners participating in joint visits should determine which person will bill the third party payer and who will bill the early intervention program. Administrators must identify a mechanism for paying contracted team members to conduct joint visits because salaried employees' time will already be covered.

Payment for Colleague-to-Colleague Coaching
Support When Children and Families Are Not Present

Identifying funds to support colleague-to-colleague interactions outside of team meetings and joint visits is another consideration for program administrators contemplating using a PSP approach to teaming. As noted in the team meeting study in Chapter 2, team members frequently gain access to one another for colleague-to-colleague support, which is described as effective, efficient, and necessary by team members and should be encouraged by team leadership. In fact, colleague-to-colleague conversations may decrease the need and costs for joint visits. These interactions are most often brief, targeted, and are conducted face to face, by telephone, and via e-mail. Administrators should consider multiple strategies for tracking these activities and develop fiscal policies to delineate fair and equitable reimbursement for team member time. As with team meeting time, if team members are salaried employees, then colleague-to-colleague interactions are absorbed as a component of daily activities.

 Take Action

Work together as program leadership and team members to identify possible funding mechanisms to support team meetings, joint visits, and colleague-to-colleague coaching opportunities.

Professional Development

The need for initial and ongoing training and support is another challenge when considering implementing a PSP teaming approach. Research indicates that therapists and educators use the practices with which they are most comfortable, not necessarily current practices that are supported by evidence in early childhood intervention. In fact, many practitioners will defend the use of their expert opinion and experience rather than empirical data and dispute existing evidence in order to support their strongly held beliefs (Bruder, 2010; Campbell & Halbert, 2002; Dunst, 2009; Malone & Gallagher, 2010). Teaming approaches are either not a part of preservice training or the inclusion of the content is highly variable from program to program. If teaming content is included, then students receive didactic information but do not routinely have opportunities to develop skills for collaborating with other disciplines with whom they will be required to work closely in a PSP teaming approach (Bruder, 2010; Bruder & Dunst, 2005). Program administrators will need to provide basic level training, skill-building opportunities, and follow-up support for practitioners who lack preparation for working on a team, experience with teaming, belief in a PSP approach, and understanding of the characteristics and implementation conditions. These types of training and follow-up support activities may occur through team meetings, joint visits with more experienced team members, new team member orientation, colleague-to-colleague

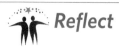 **Reflect**

How do you ensure the use of evidence-based practices by all team members?

coaching, and other just-in-time learning opportunities that occur as part of program implementation.

CONCLUSION

The thoughtful consideration required by program leadership to move to a PSP approach to teaming involves identifying new resources, using available resources, achieving buy-in of all program leadership, structuring the start-up process, establishing geographically based teams, and implementing team meetings. This chapter provided a road map for developing the infrastructure necessary to successfully plan this transition. The process for preparing to use a team-based approach is typically not without its share of challenges. This chapter included possible solutions to some of the common misperceptions and barriers to implementation. The next step for many programs as they prepare to move forward with implementing a PSP approach requires a critical examination of the current process for developing IFSPs, including using participation-based outcome statements as well as service delivery statements that support the use of a PSP.

 Take Action

Develop a team training and support plan to address role assistance needs for all team members related to using evidence-based practices, parent and parenting support, and adult interaction/adult learning. Be sure to address role gap of individual team members as well as the team as whole.

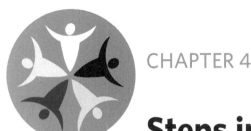

CHAPTER 4

Steps in Early Intervention

Gathering Information, Evaluation, Assessment, and Individualized Family Service Plan Development

An entire chapter on the early intervention process in a book on teaming may seem curious to some. Understanding the process for gathering information, conducting evaluation and assessment, and writing functional, participation-based outcomes is critical for implementing a PSP teaming approach. Individual practitioners have traditionally been responsible for conducting separate evaluations and then developing and implementing discipline-specific IFSP outcomes based on the child's impairments in developmental skills. For example, if a child had a delay in communication skills, then the SLP would do an evaluation, identify specific child impairments, and write outcomes to remediate the current impairment or promote achievement of the next developmental milestone. A sample outcome written in this manner might be that "Mike will use two-word utterances 90% of the time." In contrast, Mike's parents share that mealtimes are also very challenging because they do not know what Mike wants to eat and he often becomes very upset. In this situation, a functional outcome such as, "Mike will choose what he wants to eat and drink for mealtimes and snacks using his words," will not only address the concerns about his delays in language, but also enable his family to enjoy a mealtime together without tantrums, as well as promote Mike's development across multiple domains including motor, cognitive, social-emotional, and adaptive. The functional outcome related to mealtime provides the opportunity for other team members to be involved compared with the deficit-based outcome that most likely limits the options to the SLP. This chapter is designed to provide a simple framework for a program using a PSP approach to teaming to initiate the early intervention process from referral to development of the IFSP in an effective, efficient, and timely manner. Once the outcomes are written (usually three or four at the most), the IFSP team members decide what supports are necessary to accomplish the outcomes in a way that maximizes the care providers' confidence and competence. Selecting the primary provider and writing service delivery statements are discussed in detail in Chapter 5.

A TEAMING FRAMEWORK FOR THE INITIAL STEPS IN THE EARLY INTERVENTION PROCESS

An early intervention program should follow three basic steps prior to implementing a PSP approach to teaming: 1) gather information by identifying family and care provider priorities as they relate to child participation (i.e., learning) in everyday activity settings and/or parent/family support; this is followed by an evaluation to determine eligibility unless the child has a condition

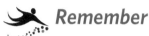

Remember

The three steps to developing participation-based individualized family service plan outcome statements are

1. Gather information

2. Observe

3. Document the outcome statements

that automatically qualifies for Part C of IDEA services; 2) observe families and their children engaged in real-life, everyday activities across settings and with important people in their lives; and 3) document participation-based outcome statements on the IFSP. All three steps occur in conjunction with the team meeting process and as a part of the initial visit, evaluation, assessment, and IFSP meeting, which occur in the child's and family's natural environment (see Appendix 4A for a detailed description of the process).

The Checklists for Developing Participation-Based IFSP Outcome Statements (see Appendix 4B) include practice indicators of the key characteristics for writing participation-based IFSP outcomes in early childhood intervention. Each individual checklist contains indicators for the three steps: gathering information, observing families and children in context, and documenting participation-based IFSP outcomes. The checklists may be used by administrators, individual practitioners, service coordinators, or teams to assess adherence to writing quality outcomes.

Gather Information

Initial conversations with family members and other care providers are critical. The service coordinator involves the parents in a conversation about family, community, and early childhood program activity settings; child interests; and resources needed by the family. Activity settings and interests are the foundation on which the early intervention team and family promote the child's participation. Child participation in meaningful activities provides opportunities for the child to practice existing skills and learn new abilities (Dunst et al., 2006). Those practitioners who have no knowledge of the activities important to the family and the child tend to focus on skills to be taught, strategies to use to teach those skills, and activities in which the strategies can be embedded. Practitioners and parents who use this type of traditional approach target the desired skills and strategies rather than support the child's participation in the activity. Instead, the focus should remain on the child's participation in the activity, which provides increased opportunities for skill development and practice.

The process for gathering information begins with identifying child and family activity settings, routines, interests, current participation, and desired participation or possibilities for successful child involvement in real-life situations and settings as well as needed parent supports. Once the family indicates an interest in moving forward with the IFSP process, the service coordinator begins to identify family and care provider priorities by using strategies and tools that incorporate interview, discussion, and observation of these priorities as they are reflected across everyday activities with important people in the life of the child and family.

The service coordinator gathers information and listens for possible IFSP outcome statements during conversations with family members and care providers as they share their priorities, questions, challenges, and ideas. When discussions revolve around daily life, parents and care providers are able to share insightful information about the child's current abilities and participation in everyday activity settings. Parents and care providers often state desired outcomes as they describe their interactions, observations, and questions. If a child spends time in a child care setting or substantial time with an extended family member or friend, then these care providers should be included in the process as soon as possible, with the parent's permission. Great potential exists for IFSP outcome statements to be different based on the environment and the people involved.

When parents and other care providers make statements related to delayed skills, practitioners should be ready to probe further into how the delay influences child participation in existing or desired activity settings or routines. Family members may contact an early intervention program because their child has not yet achieved a specific developmental milestone or because their child has recently received a diagnosis of a condition or disability that causes delayed skill development. These types of priorities often lead to a focus on skill development, yielding IFSP outcome statements that are skill based (e.g., I want my child to talk; Parents want Kendall to stop biting). For example, if a parent states that their priority is for the child to be able to walk, then early interventionists should be prepared to discuss the implications of not walking on everyday activities. Asking the family to imagine a specific activity setting (e.g., playing in the backyard with the puppy) in which the child who cannot walk would look or change if the child could indeed walk on their own can be an effective strategy. A parent might say, "Instead of carrying him down the steps off the porch, he could walk down on his own, and I could carry out the toys we would play with," "I'd like him to be able to explore some on his own instead of me always deciding where we go and what we do," or "He could go after the puppy when she wanders off, instead of screaming and crying." Each of these parent statements could be written as an IFSP outcome statement. In addition to walking, each of these outcome statements involve elements of play, communication, social interaction, cognition, and motor development that could be expressed and enhanced during the activity setting of playing in the backyard with the puppy.

Observe Families and Children

Evaluation and assessment are opportunities to observe the child and family functioning within an environment in which they are comfortable (e.g., family's home, other familiar setting). Evaluation is used to determine eligibility and is conducted by members of the core team rather than a separate evaluation team with members who never serve as a PSP. Results of the evaluation should be provided to the family during this visit, unless extenuating circumstances exist. Assessment is differentiated from evaluation and ideally is conducted at a separate visit by the most likely PSP and other team members, if necessary, and within the context of everyday activities to assist in developing participation-based IFSP outcomes. Assessment and development of the IFSP are conducted during the same visit. Assessment is used to analyze the child's current level of participation within identified activity settings and the existing degree of parent or care provider responsiveness to the child. Practitioners plan with parents and caregivers when, where, and how observations of children, family members, and other care providers engaged in real-life activities and situations can happen in a timely manner. Based on the information gathered about family and care provider priorities,

 Take Action

The following tools are particularly effective in gathering information about family and care provider priorities related to child participation in everyday activity settings and needed or desired resources and supports. Choose at least one of the tools to capture information about child and family activity settings and interests with the next new family you support.

- The *Interest-Based Everyday Activity Checklists* (Swanson et al., 2006) consist of three different checklists—one for children birth to 15 months of age, one for children 15–36 months of age, and one for children 36–60 months of age. These assessment/intervention tools are designed as checklists, which are used to identify interest-based child learning opportunities occurring as part of everyday family and community life and increase child participation in the activities. It is available at https://fipp.ncdhhs.gov/wp-content/uploads/casetools_vol2_no5.pdf

- *The Roadmap for Assessing Meaningful Participation (RAMP)* (Rush et al., 2020) is a process for helping early intervention team members gather information about child interests and everyday activity settings; conducting a participation-based assessment within the context of a real-life activity; and developing participation-based IFSP outcomes and strategies to support the child's involvement within and across everyday activities.

- The *Routines-Based Interview (RBI)* (McWilliam & Stevenson, 2019) is a conversational process that replaces a discussion of passes and failures on test protocols for deciding intervention priorities to instead devise a plan to help parents and care providers focus on their priorities for their children. The interview process involves six steps that begin with talking about the day-to-day life of the child and family. By talking about everyday situations, the family members and care providers are asked to choose the things that are most meaningful to them. It is available at http://eieio.ua.edu/uploads/1/1/0/1/110192129/rbi_checklist_with_ecomap_with_edits_12.23.19.pdf everyday activity settings, child interests, current participation, and desired participation, early intervention practitioners thoughtfully plan for these observations to happen prior to the IFSP meeting. The practitioner(s) conducting the assessment observes the child across different settings, people, and times of day, which yield information inherently important when developing participation-based IFSP outcome statements. Observing during activity settings in which the child is successful, as well as when the child is challenged, provides information directly applicable to writing quality IFSP outcome statements.

Involving parents and other care providers in the observations with the child is critical for obtaining authentic information. Observation in real-life activity settings more often involves the early interventionists stepping back and allowing family members and other care providers to demonstrate how things currently happen, what they usually do, and what they have already tried in similar situations. The practitioner and parent may try a variety of strategies to assist the child to participate in activities that they want and need to do more fully. For example, if the child needs to get in and out of the bathtub, then the practitioner and parent may try a number of different ways of assisting the child to discover the most viable option. In contrast, evaluation determines a child's initial and ongoing eligibility, whereas assessment is an ongoing process that is difficult to differentiate from intervention when done well. Assessment in natural settings requires the following: 1) a comfort level with watching others as they go about what they would typically be doing if the practitioner was not present, 2) knowledge of typical child development, 3) knowledge of responsive parenting and teaching, 4) ability to perform task analysis and think on one's feet while observing others, and 5) a willingness to be open to the possibilities of how families and care providers go through their everyday lives.

Document Quality Individualized Family Service Plan Outcome Statements

The IFSP outcome statements should be based on identified priorities of the family and other care providers, according to Part C. The outcomes reflect statements of what the family would like to occur and identify the expected result (Dunst & Deal, 1994). IFSP outcomes are family-worded, positive statements that are action oriented and indicate changes the family wants to see, rather than a description of a need (Cripe et al., 1997; Rosin et al., 1996). Outcome statements can be categorized into two broad categories—family focused and child focused. A particular priority may be better represented by one category versus the other; however, in most instances, a specific priority can be stated as family focused or child focused depending on the family's preferences or desired focus. Table 4.1 provides examples of family priorities that can be stated as family- or child-focused outcomes. Writing these types of outcome statements is further explained in the following sections.

Table 4.1.   Examples of family- and child-focused individualized family service plan (IFSP) outcome statements

Child-focused IFSP outcomes	Family-focused IFSP outcomes
Jimmy will have fun playing with his toys and his brother while positioned comfortably throughout the day.	Dana and Barbara will learn a variety of new strategies, including positioning, that they can use to make Jimmy's play time more enjoyable.
Mark will gain weight so that he will be consistently healthy.	Dorothy and Roger will ensure that Mark has daily access to the nutritional and medical resources he needs in his home and community so that he will be consistently healthy.
Sally will feed herself using her fingers and a spoon during mealtime and snack time daily.	Miss Fern (at child care) will feel comfortable letting Sally learn how to feed herself.
LaKeisha will put on her own shirt and pull up her pants by her third birthday.	LaKeisha's grandma will know strategies for helping LaKeisha dress herself without a fuss.
Robbie will enjoy his favorite activities of book reading and having snacks while riding in the grocery cart during shopping trips with his father.	Robert Sr. and Robbie will complete their grocery shopping trips within 30 minutes, with Robbie being content and remaining in the grocery cart.

Family-Focused Outcome Statements

The child's parent or caregiver is identified as the actor or learner when writing family-focused outcomes, and the statements can cover three content areas: 1) parent/family support (e.g., identifying and obtaining family supports and resources), 2) child learning (e.g., promoting the child's participation within family life related to child learning); and 3) parenting (e.g., toileting, bedtime routines, nutrition). Parent/family support outcome statements represent areas of interest or need identified by family members to promote the stability and/or growth of the family in ways that directly or indirectly meet the needs of the eligible child. The focus of child learning or parenting outcomes centers on the parents' or care providers' ability to promote the child's participation in activity settings (e.g., Mike and Pat will learn new ways of helping Joey join the family for meals at the dinner table) or targets learning regarding specified parenting topics (e.g., Mike and Pat will both be comfortable putting Joey to bed for naps and at bedtime).

 Remember

The following are characteristics of family-focused, participation-based individualized family service plan outcome statements.

- Family member or care provider is the actor or learner
- Based on family priority
- Based on desired resource
- Based on support related to child learning and/or parenting

Child-Focused Outcome Statements

Child-focused, participation-based outcomes are written with the child as the actor or learner and address family and care provider priorities related to enhancing a child's participation within an existing or desired activity setting or routine to promote learning, growth, and development. Outcome statements that are child focused and participation based can target interest-based activity settings (e.g., Joey will help his parents water the garden and houseplants) or focus on new activity settings and situations that the parents and care providers are interested in the child experiencing (e.g., Joey will join the family for meals at the dinner table on Friday and Saturday nights).

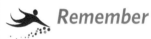 **Remember**

The following are characteristics of child-focused, participation-based individualized family service plan outcome statements.

- Child is the actor or learner
- Based on family priority
- Based on child participation in everyday activity settings
- Based on child interests

Capturing Family Priorities as Outcome Statements

Early interventionists should know the answers to questions such as, "What are your concerns?" "Where would you like us to focus?" and "What are your goals?" by the time the IFSP meeting takes place. No need exists to restate these questions just because they appear on most IFSP documents. Best practice at the IFSP meeting is to summarize the information gathered and double check with families to make sure no priorities are going unaddressed. Parents and other care providers know what they would like to see when they are engaged in a conversation about everyday activities and ideas about how the child's participation might prove to be more successful or helpful to the family members.

IFSP outcomes naturally flow from conversations with parents and other care providers when team members obtain information about child participation in current and desired activity settings as the sources of children's learning opportunities or needed parent supports. Because the conversation is contextualized around 1) child participation in current and desired activities rather than limited to identifying impairments and parental concerns or 2) resources needed by the parent related to the child's growth and development, parents know what they want the child's participation and family life to look like within and across those activities, which become

Remember

Context is the benchmark for how the child's participation will be enhanced and/or developed within and across activity settings.

potential outcomes on the IFSP. For example, if the mother must carry the child around the home with her or lay him down in order to do her household chores, but she has expressed a desire to have him play with his toys to entertain himself while she does her chores, then this could be the outcome. In contrast, because the child is unable to sit independently, a more traditional skill-based outcome would be for the child to sit independently for at least 5 minutes.

Context is the benchmark for how the child's participation will be enhanced and/or developed within and across activity settings. The outcome statements of targeted activity settings serve as the measuring stick or snapshot of success. Rather than focusing on only the activity setting delineated in the outcome statement, the practitioners concentrate on the breadth and depth of the supports assisting the family members and care providers to encourage and challenge the child's participation, growth, and development within and across activity settings. Some examples of the content of family-focused, parent/family support outcome statements include, but are not limited to, employment, education, housing, insurance, medical care, transportation, utilities, food, clothing, child care, counseling, and crisis intervention. Outcome statements for some of these examples might include, "Mr. Reynolds will find child care for his daughter Maria before Christmas"; "John and Darla will find an affordable apartment of their own by Margaret's second birthday"; and "Lorrie will choose a new doctor who accepts Medicaid for Isaac before his next immunizations are due."

Guidelines for Writing Participation-based IFSP Outcome Statements

The following guidelines or guardrails are helpful when documenting participation-based IFSP outcome statements, which are discipline free. For example, an IFSP document should not contain separate occupational therapy goals, physical therapy goals, speech-language therapy goals, or education-based goals. The outcome statements are identified by family priority and based on child participation in current or desired activity settings or a needed family resource or support. IFSP outcome statements are jargon free and should be written in words that all team members can understand and as close to how the parent or care provider actually stated the outcome. All team members can then engage in further conversation in order to share a common understanding of what progress toward the outcome would look like. This exchange of information is the insurance for a shared understanding of the "How will we know when we get there?" measurement that many states have adopted on their IFSP documents. The family measures progress on the IFSP outcome statements. Practitioners often express a concern regarding measurability of participation-based outcomes. Many practitioners have had prior experience with writing individualized education program (IEP) outcomes that have historically required specific measurability criteria (e.g., 3 of 5 times for 5 consecutive days; 100% of the time; within 6 months; every time she wears her coat to school). When writing quality IFSP outcome statements, the parents determine whether the IFSP outcome has been achieved. When developing the outcome statement, it is important to discuss the outcome so that everyone involved feels comfortable with how progress will be measured. A special occasion or life event can serve as the time line on an IFSP outcome statement, including a birthday or culturally relevant holiday or a real-

Remember

Words that describe action, engagement, enjoyment, and involvement are required for quality, child-focused individualized family service plan outcomes to reflect enhanced participation.

life point in time such as when grandma visits this summer or by the time school starts this fall (for the siblings). This strategy can assist parents and other care providers to think in real time about the possibility of achieving outcomes within the context of the big picture of their family life. The time period of 6 months is meaningful to most early interventionists because it is the maximum time period allowed between reviews of IFSP documents. This 6-month time period can be ambiguous for most family members and care providers, however.

The "third word rule" is an additional concept to consider when writing child-focused, participation-based outcome statements. This concept only applies to child-focused outcome statements and sometimes is a phrase, rather than just a single word, but the notion is that the third word (or phrase summarizing the concept) is a function rather than a specific skill. The application of the third word rule can often serve as a litmus test regarding the focus of the outcome statement. For example, consider a situation in which a particular family shared with the early intervention team that their daughter, Vianne, does not like taking a bath. They further describe bath time as a really rough time for the entire family. The family feels that Vianne's inability to sit makes her uncomfortable and frightened so that she cannot enjoy her bath. A possible outcome statement for Vianne could be, "Vianne will sit in the bathtub during her bath." The third word is *sit* in this IFSP outcome statement. Sitting is a skill that Vianne does not currently possess. Sitting is certainly an important skill, but the focus could be placed on the act or skill of sitting instead of Vianne's enjoyment of bath time. In contrast, "Vianne will play with her toys and be happy during bath time while sitting up in the tub" has *play* as the third word, which is a contextualized activity that requires a variety of different skills. When the third word is a skill (e.g., sit, walk, say, use, reach, behave), practitioners may have a tendency to decontextualize the intervention by working directly on the skill listed in the outcome statement. The third word rule does not hold true 100% of the time, but it is an effective filter to use when developing IFSP outcome statements. Examples of third words that meet this standard include, but are not limited to, *play, go, help, be, do, join, enjoy, tell, get*, and *move*. Words that describe action, engagement, enjoyment, and involvement are required for quality, child-focused IFSP outcomes to reflect enhanced participation.

The following words should be avoided when writing child-focused, participation-based IFSP outcome statements: *tolerate, receive, increase or decrease, improve*, and *maintain*. These words are not congruent with functional, meaningful outcome statements. These words are generally descriptors of passive types of activities (e.g., tolerate a certain position, tolerate something being done, receive a specific service or treatment, maintain range of motion, maintain eye contact) or are reflective of some type of skill enhancement or physical trait (e.g., increase range of motion, decrease spasticity, improve behavior, increase attention span, decrease tantrums, increase oral-motor control).

Practitioners responsible for obtaining reimbursement from third party payers may be concerned about writing IFSP outcomes in the manner described in this chapter. The concern stems from the third party payers' focus on the child's skill-based impairments and the required justification for a specific type of therapy to be provided to remediate the identified delay as part of a plan of care. Remediation of the child's skill-based impairments occurs

 Reflect

Review the following child-focused, participation-based outcome statements and compare with outcomes for the children you currently serve.

- Jack will take at least one, 1-hour nap each day while placed in his crib.

- Taylor will help feed the horses by holding the feed bucket.

- Julie will go fishing with her family and hold the fishing pole by spring break.

- René will eat her meals with the rest of the family while sitting in her highchair.

- Myka will play with the puppy by throwing the ball while being held by Dad.

- Joel will go visit grandma and ride in his car seat all the way home by Thanksgiving day.

- Sondra will play with her toys so grandma can cook breakfast and get the older kids off to school.

- Bonita will go to the park with Aunt Judy and will hold her hand and stay close by her when she visits this summer.

- J.D. will play together with his brother and express himself without hitting.

- Cara will sleep through the night by her birthday.

- Matt will help with cleanup after dinner by bringing dirty dishes to the sink.

- Marcus will play in the backyard, getting around on his own using his walker.

- Cami will be line leader at school.

- Greg will go to the library with Auntie Nell and pick out books to read.

- Vyonda will make some friends at storytime at the library.

- José will eat enough food to gain weight and not have to have surgery.

(continued)

Reflect (continued)

- Timika will go on vacation with her family to the beach.

- Charley will be happy and relaxed when his mom leaves him at child care.

- Ahmet will get to eat what he wants during mealtimes by pointing or looking at the choices his parents provide.

- Sana will play happily with her sisters while Mrs. Y cooks dinner before the new baby is born.

- Rose will join the family on short hikes at Upper Creek Falls while riding comfortably in her infant carrier.

- Sam will go boat riding with his family at the lake while wearing his life vest.

by implementing interventions that focus on child participation as delineated in the IFSP. IFSP outcomes were never intended to serve as the therapy goals on a plan of care, but rather guide an individual practitioner in designing a plan of care to meet the requirements of the third party payer. For the previous example, "Vianne will play with her toys and be happy during bath time while sitting up in the tub," the team determined that the OT would serve as the primary provider. The child's delays in sitting, reaching, and being bathed by her parents were described on the plan of care with specific OT goals for sitting with support, reaching for a toy, and tolerating a 10-minute bath. Justifying the need for the occupational therapy service was also described with recurrent descriptions of progress related to the three goals on the OT's plan of care. Intervention to support Vianne's IFSP outcome would focus on her parents feeling comfortable and having success assisting Vianne in playing with her toys in the tub while sitting comfortably and enjoying bath time. The role of the OT would be to identify strategies that Vianne's parents have already tried, brainstorm new ideas, model, teach implementation of the ideas, and support the parents in successfully using the ideas during the bath time routine. Vianne's participation in a more enjoyable bath time will accomplish both the IFSP outcomes and the OT's goals on the plan of care for the third party payer.

Monty Finch-Sawyer

This case study provides information gathered from the family by the early intervention team to develop IFSP outcome statements that are based on family priorities and are functional and participation based. In addition to background information about the family, the case study also includes excerpts from the child's IFSP (see Figure 4.1). A completed copy of the Checklists for Developing Participation-Based IFSP Outcome Statements is provided to assess the extent to which the team developed outcomes that are consistent with the practice indicators for writing effective IFSP outcome statements (see Figure 4.2).

Marcus and Lian have one child, Monty, who is 20 months old. They live in a suburban neighborhood and both work full time. Monty attends child care 30–40 hours per week at the local YMCA. Monty enjoys playing with trains and has a train table in his room. He spends up to 20 minutes at a time pushing the trains, pulling up and down stop signs on the tracks, and loading and unloading things in the train cars. His parents say he jabbers in what appears to be sentences, but they rarely understand any words. He plays with his trains typically before leaving for child care and most evenings before bed. He enjoys looking at books and hearing stories. He can sit for a very short time while looking at books and, if sitting, prefers to be on his parents' laps and turn pages while they read together. He will also listen to stories while playing with trains or moving around the room. When they ask, Monty will point at or get the book he wants to read and bring it to his parents.

Typical evenings include coming home for dinner, bath, play time, and then going to bed. They occasionally go out to eat before coming home, but Marcus describes this as a difficult activity, so they rarely do it. If they go out to eat, then they will play in the play area at the fast-food restaurant where they are or at a park on the way there or the way home. Monty enjoys running and climbing at the park or indoor play area. He will sit in a swing by himself and loves to be pushed fast and high. He also enjoys sitting on his father's lap on a swing. He can climb the stairs of the full-size slide and enjoys sliding fast as well.

Monty sits in a booster seat at the table at home. He uses a spoon some but spills frequently and prefers to feed himself with his fingers. He is described by his parents as a picky eater, preferring pizza, cheese cubes, dry cereal, crackers, and chicken nuggets or chicken fingers. His parents place other foods on his plate at all meals, but only rarely will he take a bite of anything else. He does not name or point at the foods he wants, but his mother says she can read his nonverbal cues to understand his food preferences. After meals, Marcus plays with Monty in his room until time for bath and bed. Monty can remove all his clothes himself except his shoes. He lifts his arms for his parents to put on a shirt and lifts his leg while a parent holds him up and puts on his pants. He is not yet putting on any clothes himself. His parents also say they have a hard time brushing his teeth. He falls asleep easily when he gets into bed.

His parents express concern about Monty becoming upset on the weekend whenever they leave the house. He enjoys going to the park and on picnics when there are few people around and seems to like adults, but they becomes upset easily when there are a lot of adults or children around. This is worse when they try to take him shopping, out to eat, or anywhere else in the community on weekends. When he is upset he wants to be held, he will not walk on his own, he cries, he rocks, and sometimes repeatedly hits his head with his hand.

Monty tends to play alone at child care. Monty's idea of playing with other kids is taking their toys. His parents say his teacher is concerned that he hits other children and other children in his class avoid being near him. Monty tends to stay very close to his teacher during his time at child care, sometimes holding on to her leg and walking around with her rather than playing with toys. His teacher notes that this tends to happen when the classroom is busy or there are loud noises either from outside the classroom or when more than one child is being loud in the classroom. She also notices that Monty wants to be held much more than other children his age. She is concerned about his language, difficulty soothing himself, and difficulty interacting with other children.

CONCLUSION

Families identify outcome statements that are visions of what they would like to see for themselves or their child in order to participate in real-life activity settings or events within existing or desired environments, as well as obtain necessary family resources and parent supports. This chapter provided a simple framework for writing functional, participation-based outcome statements that are family focused and child focused. Early in the IFSP process, a team member listens to families and other care providers discuss everyday successes and challenges as well as

 Reflect

Review the following family-focused, participation-based outcome statements and compare with outcomes for the children you currently serve.

- Will's parents will feel comfortable holding and playing with him.

- Donnie's parents will give him a bath and know that he enjoys bath time.

- Rhoda's parents will learn what makes her smile.

- Chad's mom will recognize new ways to include him in home-school activities.

- Mrs. Stillwater will go grocery shopping while Arlie rides contentedly in the shopping cart.

- Norman's mom will keep the house clean and safe so he can stay with her for a 30-minute visit.

- Denny's sister will feel comfortable helping her get ready for bed each night.

- Grandpa Bill will understand what Madelyn says so he can take care of her while Tiffany goes out on a date.

- Mr. Brainard will get his GED so he can apply for a job at the distribution center.

- Danny and Alice will be able to answer questions about Teri's diagnosis of Down syndrome.

- Uncle Larry and Cori will eat a meal at the drive-in restaurant at least once a week.

- Mr. Tanaka will feel comfortable changing Hiroshi's diapers.

- Bill and Reba will know that Sharon's development is on track.

Take Action

Use the Checklists for Developing Participation-Based Individualized Family Service Plan (IFSP) Outcome Statements (see Appendix 4B) with the next child and family assigned to your team or program to check your adherence to the three-step process.

observes them and the children in their care during real-life activities. The child and family IFSP outcome statements are written to include the family's real-life contexts and serve as the focal point for intervention and the benchmarks for measuring progress.

Individualized Family Service Plan (IFSP)

Child/Family Routines and Activities

Where does your child spend the day? Who is involved? How would you describe your child's relationship(s) with you and the people he or she spends the most time with in different settings?

Monty wakes up happy and babbles to let his parents know when he is awake. When Lian is in town, she feeds him soon after he gets up. Monty sits at the table in a booster seat. He will not tolerate being strapped in and likes to get down and back up several times during most meals. He prefers toast and cheese cubes or dry cereal and sits in a booster seat. When his dad is home alone, Marcus dresses him before breakfast so he can get Monty to the car as soon as Marcus is ready to go. They make Monty's lunch most days as he is a very picky eater and will not eat most lunch foods at child care. Lunches are mostly finger foods—cheese cubes, crackers, cut apples or grapes, and raw cut vegetables.

Monty spends weekdays at the YMCA child care near the family home. He mainly spends time with the teachers, and he seems very comfortable with them. He hugs them and seeks them out for comfort. Marcus picks Monty up from school every day, and Monty usually runs to and hugs him when he comes into the room.

Marcus often cares for Monty by himself weekday evenings because Lian travels out of town for work 3–5 days each week. Monty is always excited to see his Mom when she gets home from a trip, and she spends all her time with him when she is home. Monty cuddles with his parents and child care teacher, but tends to avoid strangers, especially men. He warms up to women quickly and smiles at women who say hello or wave to him when they are out in the community.

What are the things your child enjoys most (including toys, people, places, activities)?

Monty loves playing with trains. He has Thomas and many of the other trains in the Thomas the Train books. He has a train table in his room and can spend as much as a half hour at a time playing at the train table. He pushes cars and likes putting together and taking apart tracks. Monty also likes sitting on and pushing riding toys.

Monty enjoys storytime at child care and at church and reading books with Mom and Dad, but he doesn't sit for more than 2 minutes in most situations. If the teacher at the YMCA holds him and asks him to turn every page, then he can sometimes sit through an entire story. His nursery caregiver, Rose, notes he loves to play with the train in the nursery and with the plastic animals.

What does your family enjoy doing together and why? Who is involved? When does this occur?

Marcus, Lian, and Monty enjoy going to the park together, playing at home outside in the backyard, and playing with trains in Monty's playroom weekday evenings and on the weekends. They also enjoy going on family picnics most weekends, either alone as a family or with friends from church who have two girls that are older than Monty. Lian and Monty go to church on Sundays and Monty goes to child care at church.

What activities and relationships are going well?

Monty likes to see and play with his grandparents, although he doesn't see them often. He also enjoys going to church. Lian explains Monty really likes the playtime there, especially the trains. He gets along with adults well in these places, although he doesn't listen as well if there are a lot of noises or other children present. He does best if the teacher is right next to him all or most all of the time when he is away from his parents.

What, if any, routines and activities do you find to be difficult or frustrating for you or your child?

Going out to restaurants or shopping at stores with loud music, loud noises, flashing lights, or large crowds is very difficult. Monty cries, screams, takes his parents by the hand and tries to pull them away, and hides under the table at restaurants.

Visiting close friends and his grandparents is hard because they have larger dogs or cats and Monty cries, climbs on his parents, and tries to leave if he sees or hears them.

Monty seems to avoid other children. Marcus is concerned that even when Monty is really having fun, such as playing with trains at church or attending a recent swimming class at the YMCA, he moves himself physically away from other kids his age. He will sometimes play near them but not with them.

What are the activities and routines your family currently does not do because of your child's needs, but is interested in doing now or in the near future?

The family doesn't eat out much because Monty can't sit still, tries to run away, and hides under the table. They would like to eat out as they did before Monty began acting this way, which was two to three times each week. The family would also like to take Monty to Disneyland, but currently feel this is impossible. They would love to take Monty to amusement parks or places that have rides because they think he would like the rides, but they are worried about how he will handle the crowds and noise.

(continued)

Figure 4.1.   Monty Finch-Sawyer's individualized family service plan (IFSP).

Family Concerns, Resources, and Priorities

Summary of family concerns (based on challenges in everyday routines and activities):

Generally, Monty's parents worry about the way he gets upset when there are more than three or four people near him and how he gets upset around noises, music, and flashing lights. He has a hard time feeling or touching things gently; he plays hard when he does touch other kids and that often upsets the other children. Monty gets in trouble at child care for hitting other children, but Monty's parents don't think he hits on purpose. He gets frustrated quickly and kicks, hits, screams, and cries when adults can't guess what he wants. Monty's parents are very concerned about his language skills and their ability to understand what he says. They feel that his lack of ability to talk and use words contributes to the challenges he has playing and interacting with other children.

Priorities of the family (based on concerns previously identified):

- Would like Monty to be able to go out to eat, to a store, or to some place he'd enjoy, such as an amusement park, without getting upset when there are other people, noises, or lights

- Would like for him to have friends and play with other children

- Would like for him to be able to talk clearly enough so that other people can understand him and he can tell us what he wants without crying, screaming, rocking, kicking, and throwing things

Strengths and resources that the family has to meet their child's needs (include family, friends, community groups, and financial supports that are helpful to you):

- Monty's child care teacher is very willing to do anything she can to help him. Marcus and Lian both work full time, and Monty has health insurance through Lian's job.

- His child care at the YMCA is also a great resource and teaching environment for Monty to learn to play with other children, specifically on the playground.

- Lian belongs to a local church with a strong church community that's willing to work with Monty consistently every week on the family's goal for Monty to participate in group activities during Sunday school activities.

- Marcus's parents live nearby and visit just about every month.

- Lian has a large, supportive family who visit several times each year from Maine.

Do you have any additional concerns that you have not yet shared or that others have shared with you about your child? Is there anything else you would like to tell us that would be helpful in planning supports and services with you to address what is most important to your child and family?

Lian wants to find a support group to help her cope better with Monty's trouble getting along with other kids and going out in the community. Marcus wants to find a baby sitter who Monty likes so he could visit friends occasionally during the week when Lian is traveling.

(continued)

Figure 4.1.   *(continued)*

Child's Present Levels of Development				
Developmental area	Description of skills/status (list child's skills in each developmental area, describe status, include information about sensory needs in each domain)	Developmental level (percentage of delay, standard deviation, age equivalent)	Information source (instrument[s], parent report, observation)	Evaluator's name and evaluation/ assessment date
Adaptive Feeding, eating, dressing, sleeping (e.g., holds a bottle, reaches for toy, helps dress him- or herself)	*Removes pants; lifts arms to help with dressing* *Tries to use a spoon, but still prefers using his fingers* *Goes to sleep well/ sleeps through the night*	*Delay: 1.5 standard deviation*	*Battelle Developmental Inventory–Second Edition (BDI-2)* *Parent interview* *Occupational therapist (OT) observation*	*Parents with Madison Self, 4/1/12* *Marcus with Christina Dew, OT, 4/21/12 and 4/25/12*
Cognitive Thinking and learning (e.g., looks for dropped toy, pulls toy on a string, does a simple puzzle)	*Searches for removed toy* *Plays Peekaboo* *Explores new places* *Does a simple puzzle*	*Within typical range*	*BDI-2* *Parent report* *Speech-language pathologist (SLP) observation*	*Parents with Madison Self, 4/1/12* *Marcus with Jennifer Evans, SLP, 4/21/12*
Expressive communication Making sounds, gesturing, talking (e.g., vocalizes vowels, points to objects to express wants, uses two or more words)	*Monty babbles in long sentence-like form* *Has three words (Mama, Da, and no)* *He uses the words routinely and correctly* *No is the word he uses most often* *He points, grunts, or screams to get what he wants*	*Delay: 1.5 standard deviation*	*BDI-2* *Parent report* *SLP observation*	*Parents with Madison Self, 4/1/12* *Marcus with Jennifer Evans, SLP, 4/21/12*
Receptive communication Understanding words and gestures (e.g., looks when hears name, points to body parts and common objects when named, follows simple one- and two-step directions, understands simple words)	*Follows two-step directions (e.g., "please get your shoes and bring them to me")* *Points to named objects* *Knows names of parents and other relatives (Mom, Dad, Gamma, Abuela, Tia Maria, Tia)*	*Within typical range*	*BDI-2* *Parent report* *SLP observation*	*Parents with Madison Self, 4/1/12* *Marcus with Jennifer Evans, SLP, 4/21/12*

(continued)

Developmental area	Description of skills/status (list child's skills in each developmental area, describe status, include information about sensory needs in each domain)	Developmental level (percentage of delay, standard deviation, age equivalent)	Information source (instrument[s], parent report, observation)	Evaluator's name and evaluation/ assessment date
Physical: Fine motor Using hands and fingers (e.g., reaches for and plays with toys, picks up raisin, strings beads)	Opens and closes small train parts Uses pincer grasp to feed himself Is trying to use a spoon	Within typical range	BDI-2 Parent report OT observation	Parents with Madison Self, 4/1/12 Marcus with Christina Dew, OT, 4/21/12 and 4/25/12
Physical: Gross motor Moving and using large muscles (e.g., rolls from tummy to back, sits independently, walks holding on)	Loves to run Walks up and down stairs with one hand held Parents note he can be clumsy Runs into things and people	Within typical range	BDI-2 Parent report OT observation	Parents with Madison Self, 4/1/12 Marcus with Christina Dew, OT, 4/21/12 and 4/25/12
Social-emotional Interacting with others (e.g., smiles and shows joy, makes good eye contact, seeks help from familiar caregivers, takes turns, shares toys)	Beginning to engage in parallel play Does not enjoy playing with other children Beginning to imitate his father during play Explores house independently Smiles/shows joy at seeing parents and familiar adults Pats Mom when she is upset Cries when peers cry	Delay: 1.5 standard deviation	BDI-2 Parent report OT observation	Parents with Madison Self, 4/1/12 Marcus with Christina Dew, OT, 4/21/12 and 4/25/12
Vision (e.g., visually tracks object, attends to faces of familiar people, returns head to starting point when watching slowly disappearing object)	Passed screening Recognizes familiar adults from a distance Tracks objects in all directions Parents report no concerns with his vision		Screening SLP observation Parent report	Parents with Madison Self, 4/1/12 Marcus with Jennifer Evans, SLP, 4/21/12
Hearing (e.g., turns head, smiles, or acts in response to voices and sounds; responds to name)	Turns head to loud and soft sounds Responds to name Passed screening		Screening SLP observation Parent report	Parents with Madison Self, 4/1/12 Marcus with Jennifer Evans, SLP, 4/21/12

(continued)

Figure 4.1. *(continued)*

Initial Eligibility for Part C Services

Evaluating and assessing each child and determining the child's initial eligibility for Part C early intervention services must include using informed clinical opinion. Eligibility determination is a team decision.

☑ Your child is eligible for Part C Services because he or she has (*check one or more below*):

☐ A 1.5 standard deviation or 25% delay in development in one or more areas (*check all that apply*):

☐ Cognitive ☐ Physical: Fine motor ☐ Physical: Gross motor ☑ Adaptive

☑ Social-emotional ☑ Expressive communication ☐ Receptive communication

☐ A diagnosed condition that is likely to result in delay in development (*identify*):

☑ Informed clinical opinion (*check and provide explanation if this is the only method used for determining eligibility, although clinical opinion must be used throughout evaluation and assessment*):

In addition to delays in standardized test scores on the BDI-2, Monty scored in the atypical range on the Infant/Toddler Sensory Profile. Parent report and these scores indicate he is highly sensitive to daily activities with loud or bright environments and has a tendency to avoid activities that are overstimulating to him, such as those with noise, a lot of bright or changing light, and a lot of people. SLP observed Monty to demonstrate substantial frustration related to his inability to be understood by others. The SLP feels his lack of expressive communication contributes to his delays in social-emotional development.

Summary of Functional Performance

Positive social-emotional skills (including social relationships) (*relating with adults, relating with other children, following rules related to groups or interacting with others*):

Summary of child's functioning:

Monty has some age-appropriate functioning, but exhibits more immediate foundational skills and behaviors. He shows affection to both parents and extended relatives, particularly female relatives and adult women who are friends of the family. Monty displays a range of emotion and responds empathically to others' sadness by showing sadness and patting them or trying to give them a comfort object. Monty calls for his Mom and Dad by name when he wants them to help him or when he wants to share something with them. When adults ask him questions, he knows to nod in response, but these types of exchanges are typically limited to quiet settings such as his home. It is harder for Monty to respond to questions from adults in busy or loud settings. Monty has not yet been observed using toys or other objects to engage peers, although he will engage adults with his trains. These exchanges with adults are brief. For example, he will show or give one of his trains to the adult and then continue to play with the toy on his own. Monty jabbers while showing his trains to his parents. The vocalizations are not yet articulated words or fully understandable sounds, so his parents don't usually converse back. When his parents imitate his vocalizations, he continues to vocalize more.

When another child is playing quietly, Monty will sometimes play alongside him or her in his YMCA classroom. Monty typically avoids playing alongside multiple children or playing alongside any children in settings with loud background noises. He often clings to his teacher during his school day and at church child care, particularly when many children are playing loudly inside. Monty frequently seeks out familiar adults for soothing himself when upset at home, in child care, during Sunday school child care, and in community settings. Monty often acts out by hitting or kicking whatever or whoever is around him when in busy environments with a lot of noise or touching from other people if he is not constantly being held by parents or familiar caregivers. Monty is beginning to understand routines at child care and responds to the soft music they play when cleaning up to go outside or to eat lunch. Monty's score in personal-social was 1.5 standard deviations below the mean on the BDI-2.

Outcome descriptor statement (*select one*):

At 20 months, Monty shows occasional use of some age-expected skills, but has more skills that are younger than those that are expected for a child his age in the area of positive social-emotional skills.

(continued)

Summary of Functional Performance (continued)

Acquiring and using knowledge and skills (including early language/communication) (*thinking, reasoning, remembering, and problem solving; understanding symbols; understanding the physical and social worlds*):

Summary of child's functioning:

Monty engages in simple pretend play with his Dad when playing with trains and animals, making the animals eat or fight. He will search for objects that have been taken away, often looking for specific trains, but is not able to tell others which item he is looking for with words. Monty can turn toys on and off independently and make the toys function in a variety of ways. He has taken apart several of his trains recently and has tried putting them back together, often fitting a piece or two before starting a different activity. Monty also puts together puzzles appropriate for children his age and takes apart and puts together train tracks. He likes to turn the remote control on and off and likes to explore the drawers in his dresser. When asked to put away toys, Monty will put different toys in the appropriate place when asked.

Monty can say three words; however, these can be difficult for others outside the family to understand and are rarely heard other than during quiet times with his parents at home and during play with Dad, with the exception of the word no. He does not yet use words other than no, Mama, and Da regularly across settings and situations. He points to items that he wants and understands familiar, recurring two-step directions such as going to get his shoes and bringing them to his Mom when he is getting ready for school. Monty uses gestures effectively to communicate when calm, but often gets over-whelmed in social situations with peers or in loud settings and may cry, scream, hit, or kick when he is frustrated, rather than using gestures or words.

He will listen to a short story, but usually loses interest after about 2 minutes. He can point to pictures in a book and sometimes jabbers along with the adult reading the book, imitating the adult's voice and some of the sounds in the words he or she uses. Monty responds to his own name and recognizes a lot of objects, showing his understanding of named objects by pointing to them from pictures or picking them out of a group. Monty's talking includes a lot of jabbering that sounds like sentences.

Assessment tools indicate that receptive communication and cognitive functioning were within normal limits for children Monty's age. In addition to parental and care provider concerns, Monty demonstrates an expressive communication delay of 1.5 standard deviation on the BDI-2.

Outcome descriptor statement (*select one*):

Monty shows many age-expected skills, relative to same-age peers, but continues to show some functioning that might be described like that of a slightly younger child in the area of acquiring and using knowledge and skills.

(continued)

Figure 4.1.   *(continued)*

Summary of Functional Performance (continued)

Use of appropriate behaviors to meet own needs (*taking care of basic needs [e.g., showing hunger, dressing, feeding, toileting]; contributing to own health and safety [e.g., follows rules, assists with hand washing, avoids inedible objects, if over 24 months]; getting from place to place [mobility] and using tools [e.g., forks, strings attached to objects]*):

Summary of child's functioning:

Monty likes to play outside and can independently climb a slide ladder to slide down with supervision for safety. He runs on grass and uses most playground equipment when the playground is not crowded with other children. Monty also follows safety rules, such as holding hands when walking to the playground with his parents. Monty sometimes climbs into a chair and occasionally uses the chair to reach what he wants on the countertops. He tries to use a spoon with much spilling and usually abandons it after a couple of attempts to get the food in his mouth. He prefers using his fingers when eating. Monty can drink from a regular cup with some spilling. Monty can remove his pants by himself and helps his parents get him dressed by extending his arms and legs. He cooperates with tooth brushing, by holding still and opening his mouth upon request. Sometimes he tries to brush his own teeth, but only rubs back and forth on the front teeth before handing the toothbrush to his parents. Monty falls asleep on his own after his parents finish his bedtime routine. Monty rarely uses his words to communicate what he needs to others and is very difficult for others to understand. He typically fusses when hungry or gestures to show people what he wants or needs. Monty will go get toys himself or gesture to others for help in getting those toys that are out of reach. In particularly loud surroundings or settings with lots of other people, however, Monty rarely seeks out toys or initiates play independently, preferring instead to cling to a familiar caregiver or sometimes hitting or kicking other children if pressured into playing near them in these situations.

Gross and fine motor subdomains on the BDI-2 were within normal limits. Adaptive skills were assessed at 1.5 standard deviations below the mean.

Outcome descriptor statement (*select one*):

At 20 months, Monty shows occasional use of some age-expected skills, but has more skills that are younger than those that are expected for a child his age in the area of using appropriate behavior to meet his needs.

(continued)

Assessment Team

The following individuals participated in the evaluation and assessment.

Printed name and credentials	Role/organization	Assessment activities
Jennifer Evans, CCC-SLP	Speech-language pathologist, CompHealth	☑ Child's present levels of development ☑ Eligibility for Part C services ☑ Contributed information for summary of functional performance ☑ Participated in selecting outcome descriptor statements
Christina Dew, OT	Occupational therapist, CompHealth	☑ Child's present levels of development ☑ Eligibility for Part C services ☑ Contributed information for summary of functional performance ☑ Participated in selecting outcome descriptor statements
Madison Self	Service coordinator	☑ Child's present levels of development ☑ Eligibility for Part C services ☑ Contributed information for summary of functional performance ☑ Participated in selecting outcome descriptor statements
Marcus Finch-Sawyer	Parent	☐ Child's present levels of development ☐ Eligibility for Part C services ☑ Contributed information for summary of functional performance ☑ Participated in selecting outcome descriptor statements
Lian Finch-Sawyer	Parent	☐ Child's present levels of development ☐ Eligibility for Part C services ☑ Contributed information for summary of functional performance ☑ Participated in selecting outcome descriptor statements

Family role in child outcomes summary process (*check only one*):

✔ Family was present for the discussion and the selection of the descriptor statements

___ Family was present for the discussion, but not the selection of the descriptor statements

___ Family provided information, but was not present for the discussion

---

Family information on child functioning (*check all that apply*):

✔ Received in team meeting   ___ Collected separately   ✔ Incorporated into assessment

___ Not included (please explain)

Assessment instruments informing child outcomes summary:

BDI-2

Other sources of information (*e.g., practitioner observation, information from child care provider*):

Practitioner observation, parent report, child care provider information

(continued)

Figure 4.1. *(continued)*

Functional IFSP Outcomes for Children and Families

Outcome number: _1_   Start date: _5/1/12_   Target date: _8/1/12_

What would your family like to see happen for your child/family? *(The outcome must be functional, measurable, and in the context of everyday routines and activities.)*

Monty will eat a meal while sitting at the table at a restaurant.

What's happening now related to this outcome? What is your family currently doing that supports achieving this outcome? *(Describe your child and/or family's functioning related to the desired change/outcome.)*

Monty currently walks into a restaurant and sits in a booster seat. He allows his parents to carry him to the buffet and he lets them know what he wants by gesturing or through his other actions. Monty frequently gets under the table at restaurants, leans on his parents, tries to pull them up to leave, and does not eat his food.

Parents currently carry him when he asks to be carried and to get food; his mother brings games and/or gives him her telephone to play games to distract him; and recently, his father tried putting him in a darker booth farther from noises, which he found worked well to keep Monty from going under the table. Monty's parents also take his food to go and encourage him to eat it once they get home.

What are the ways in which your family and team will work toward achieving this outcome? Who will help and what will they do? *(Describe the methods and strategies that will be used to support your child and family to achieve your outcomes within your daily activities and routines. List who will do what, including both early intervention services and informal supports, such as family members, friends, neighbors, church or other community organizations, special health care programs, and parent education programs.)*

Parents will continue to try the following strategies:
- *Sit by a window for natural light or sit in darker areas in the restaurant*
- *Choose a quiet corner at the restaurant*
- *Give Monty sunglasses to wear inside if he chooses*
- *Hold Monty when moving around in crowded spaces*
- *Give Monty a break from the activity by putting on headphones to block out noise, covering him with a coat, or letting him get under the table when he shows signs of discomfort*
- *Help him choose his favorite foods*
- *Bring games and toys for Monty*

OT will use coaching to help the family identify additional strategies to promote Monty's successful participation in going out to eat.

OT will provide occupational therapy services to support Monty and assist the family in implementing strategies.

OT and SLP will work together with Lian and Marcus to identify strategies to support Monty's use of words to express his wants and needs. Mealtimes in restaurants will be the first activity setting to be addressed, but the team will support Monty's successful use of words over time across all daily routines and activity settings.

SLP will provide speech-language pathology services to Monty and his family through joint visits with the OT to identify strategies to help Monty communicate with his family more successfully during restaurant outings.

Marcus and Lian will use strategies when going out to eat, share what is working and not working, help develop additional strategies, and share Monty's progress toward this outcome.

How will we know we've made progress or if revisions are needed to outcomes or services? *(What criteria [i.e., observable action or behavior that shows progress is being made], procedures [i.e., observation, report, chart], and realistic time lines will be used?)*
- *Monty doesn't go under the table at the restaurant as soon as the family sits back down from getting food.*
- *Monty starts eating within 5 minutes of when the family returns to the table from the buffet.*
- *Monty eats his meal while there are mild distractions nearby, such as sounds or bright lights.*

How did we do? *(Review of progress statement/criteria for success)*

Date: _____ Achieved: We did it!

Date: _____ Continue: We are part way there. Let's keep going.

The situation has changed:

Date: _____ Discontinue: It no longer applies.

Date: _____ Revise: Let's try something different.

Date: _____ Explanations/comments:

(continued)

Outcome number: __2__   Start date: __5/1/12__   Target date: __8/1/12__

What would your family like to see happen for your child/family? (*The outcome must be functional, measurable, and in the context of everyday routines and activities.*)

Monty will interact with other children during swimming classes at the YMCA.

What's happening now related to this outcome? What is your family currently doing that supports achieving this outcome? (*Describe your child and/or family's functioning related to the desired change/outcome.*)

Monty loves to play in the water. Monty last took swimming classes 2 months ago. In this class, all the parents and toddlers got into the water together and the teacher provided a mix of parent–toddler activities as well as opportunities for the toddlers to interact with each other. Marcus got in the water with Monty, and Monty was very excited at the beginning of each class. After about 5 minutes, he wanted to leave. When the toddlers were asked to line up along the side of the kids' pool, Monty tried to get as far away from the other kids as possible and would not participate in any toddler group activities.

What are the ways in which your family and team will work toward achieving this outcome? Who will help and what will they do? (*Describe the methods and strategies that will be used to support your child and family to achieve your outcomes within your daily activities and routines. List who will do what, including both early intervention services and informal supports, such as family members, friends, neighbors, church or other community organizations, special health care programs, and parent education programs.*)

OT will meet with Marcus and Monty at the YMCA to observe settings and identify Monty's interests during play in the water and the challenges Monty has in staying engaged in water play when he is at the YMCA pool outside of class.

OT will use coaching to help the family identify additional strategies to promote Monty's successful participation in swimming classes.

OT will provide occupational therapy services to support Monty's successful participation in swimming classes and assist the family in implementing strategies.

OT and SLP will work together with Lian and Marcus to identify strategies to support Monty's use of words to express his wants and needs.

SLP will provide speech-language pathology services to Monty and his family through joint visits with the OT to identify strategies to help Monty communicate with his family and others (especially other children) more successfully.

Marcus will use strategies when taking Monty to play in the pool at the YMCA, share what is working and not working, help develop additional strategies, and share Monty's progress toward this outcome.

When swim classes start, the OT will meet with Marcus and Monty at the YMCA to observe swim class and Monty's participation during class. The OT and Marcus will identify strategies to assist Marcus in promoting Monty's participation.

How will we know we've made progress or if revisions are needed to outcomes or services? (*What criteria [i.e., observable action or behavior that shows progress is being made], procedures [i.e., observation, report, chart], and realistic time lines will be used?*)

- Monty doesn't ask to leave before the parent–child activities that happen during swimming class end.
- Monty and Marcus can stay in swimming class the entire 45-minute period.

How did we do? (*Review of progress statement/criteria for success*)

Date: _____ Achieved: We did it!

Date: _____ Continue: We are part way there. Let's keep going.

The situation has changed:

Date: _____ Discontinue: It no longer applies.

Date: _____ Revise: Let's try something different.

Date: _____ Explanations/comments:

(continued)

Figure 4.1.   *(continued)*

Outcome number: __3__   Start date: __5/1/12__   Target date: __8/1/12__

What do we want to accomplish *(desired outcome)*? *Lian will identify and participate in a parent support group for parents of young children.*

Who will do what? *(strategies/activities)*
- *Madison will use coaching to identify what resources Lian has already considered.*
- *Madison will support Lian in identifying options for specific parent support groups within an acceptable driving distance from her office and home.*
- *Lian will attend parent support group options and evaluate which best meets her needs with Madison's support.*

Review date: _____

Progress code (circle one):   Achieved   Continue   Discontinue   Revise

Comments:

Outcome number: __4__   Start date: __5/1/12__   Target date: __8/1/12__

What do we want to accomplish *(desired outcome)*? *Marcus and Lian will agree on and obtain babysitting services for Monty for Marcus to gain access to while Lian travels.*

Who will do what? *(strategies/activities)*
- *Madison will use coaching to identify what resources Marcus and Lian have already considered.*
- *Madison will support Marcus and Lian in establishing criteria for agreed-on babysitting services.*
- *Madison will support Marcus and Lian in identifying options for babysitting services.*
- *Marcus will use the agreed-on babysitting services and evaluate the experience with Madison's support.*

Review date: _____

Progress code *(circle one)*:   Achieved   Continue   Discontinue   Revise

Comments:

Summary of Services

Early intervention services	Outcome number (list all that apply)	Frequency/ intensity	Methods	Setting	Natural environment (Y/N)	Start date	End date	Agency(ies) responsible
OT	1, 2	twelve, 1-hour visits in 3 months	Direct service Teaming Joint visits	Home Community	Y	5/1/12	8/1/12	CompHealth
SLP	1, 2	six, 1-hour visits in 3 months	Direct service Teaming Joint visits	Home Community	Y	5/1/12	8/1/12	CompHealth
Service coordinator	3, 4	5 visits in 3 months	Direct service Teaming Joint visits	Home Community	Y	5/1/12	8/1/12	Anywhere Early Intervention Program

Checklists for Developing Participation-Based Individualized Family Service Plan (IFSP) Outcome Statements

Child: _____ Monty Finch-Sawyer _____ Date: __ 5/1/12 __

Service coordinator: ____ Madison Self ____ Primary service provider: ____ Christina Dew, OT ____

Reviewer: _____ Shelden/Rush _____ Date of review: __ 5/31/12 __

Instructions

These checklists include practice indicators of the key characteristics for writing participation-based individualized family service plan (IFSP) outcomes in early childhood intervention.

The three checklists describe the steps for developing family- and child-focused, participation-based IFSP outcome statements by 1) gathering information by identifying family and care provider priorities as they relate to child participation in everyday activity settings; 2) observing families and their children engaged in real-life, everyday activities across settings and with important people in their lives; and 3) documenting family- and/or child-focused, participation-based outcome statements on the IFSP. Each section contains indicators of a specific area of writing participation-based IFSP outcomes. For each indicator, determine whether the program is adhering to the aspect of the practice described. Space is also available for notes or examples of adherence.

	Are practices characterized by the following?	Yes	No	Examples/notes
Gathering information	1. Information is gathered about child and family activity settings, routines, interests, current participation, and desired participation in real-life situations and settings.	Y	N	*Detailed information included about child interests, family activity settings, and priorities.*
	2. Service coordinator listens for possible IFSP outcome statements during conversations with family members and care providers as they share their priorities, questions, and ideas.	Y	N	*Context is included in both child-focused outcomes (mealtimes at restaurant and swimming lessons at the YMCA).*
	3. When met with statements from parents or care providers about delayed skills, service coordinator probes further into how the delay influences child participation in existing or desired activity settings or routines.	Y	N	
	4. Service coordinator specifically does not ask parents about their concerns or goals for the child because this information came out of the conversation about family priorities.	Y	N	
	5. Context is used as the benchmark for how the child's participation will be enhanced and/or developed within and across activity settings.	Y	N	*(continued)*

Figure 4.2. Monty Finch-Sawyer's Checklist for Developing Participation-Based Individualized Family Service Plan (IFSP) Outcome Statements.

Figure 4.2.　*(continued)*

	Are practices characterized by the following?	Yes	No	Examples/notes
Observe families and children	1.　Observations of the child, family, and other care providers take place within the context of multiple real-life activity settings in the home and community that are both successful and challenging prior to developing the IFSP.	Ⓨ	N	*Observations included the family home and local restaurant.* *Both parents were involved in the assessment process.*
	2.　Parents and other care providers are involved in the observations by participating as they typically would during the real-life activity or routine.	Ⓨ	N	

	Are practices characterized by the following?	Yes	No	Examples/notes
Document IFSP outcome statements	1.　Child, family member, or other care provider is the actor or learner in the outcome.	Ⓨ	N	*IFSP includes both child- and family-focused outcome statements.* *Activity settings of mealtime at restaurant and YMCA swimming lessons are the contexts listed on the IFSP.* *IFSP outcome statements are clearly understandable by all team members.* *Third word phrase is 1) eat a meal at a restaurant and 2) interact with the other children at swimming lessons.*
	2.　Outcome is based on a family priority.	Ⓨ	N	
	3.　Outcome is based on child participation in everyday activity settings and child interests or a parenting support.	Ⓨ	N	
	4.　An activity setting (i.e., context) is listed in the outcome statement.	Ⓨ	N	
	5.　Outcome statements are discipline free (i.e., separate goals are not written for each discipline).	Ⓨ	N	
	6.　Outcome statements are written in words that all team members can understand.	Ⓨ	N	
	7.　Outcome statements are stated as close to how the parent or care provider actually stated the outcome as possible.	Ⓨ	N	
	8.　The third word in the outcome statement is a functional concept rather than a specific skill.	Ⓨ	N	
	9.　Special occasions or life events meaningful to the family are used as time lines.	Y	Ⓝ	
	10.　The family measures progress of the outcome.	Ⓨ	N	
	11.　Outcome statements include active rather than passive words (e.g., *tolerate, receive, increase, decrease, improve, maintain*).	Ⓨ	N	

Primary Service Provider Teaming Process—Initial Referral to Individualized Family Service Plan (IFSP) Process

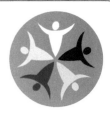

Child referred to early intervention program

Early intervention program assigns child to geographic team based on child's address
Team leader assigns referral to service coordinator

Service coordinator contacts family to schedule face-to-face visit

Possible first team meeting

Service coordinator initiates Welcome to the Program at team meeting

Visit 1

Service coordinator conducts initial face-to-face visit with family
Service coordinator explains program to family
Service coordinator explains rights, procedural safeguards, consents, and financial information
Service coordinator gathers information and identifies activity setting/context for functional assessment
Service coordinator explains next step in the early intervention process to the family
If needed, team identifies two members (including most likely primary service provider [PSP]) to conduct evaluation

Second team meeting

Service coordinator continues Welcome to the Program by sharing information gathered in Visit 1
Team identifies most likely PSP

Visit 2 if automatically eligible

Functional assessment completed by most likely PSP
If service coordinator is present, service coordinator and most likely PSP complete individualized family service plan (IFSP)
If service coordinator is not present, IFSP completed at next visit

Visit 2 if eligibility to be determined

Documentation of child's eligibility using existing documentation
If testing is necessary, two team members conduct evaluation in home (one evaluator is most likely PSP)
Inform family of results unless need more information
If service coordinator is present, inform family of eligibility

Team meeting—ongoing

Third team meeting

Service coordinator continues Welcome to the Program at team meeting

Visit 3

Most likely PSP and another team member conduct functional assessment in identified activity setting
Service coordinator joins most likely PSP (and other team member) to complete IFSP Joint plan developed for next visit

Team meeting—ongoing

Checklists for Developing Participation-Based Individualized Family Service Plan (IFSP) Outcome Statements

Child: _____ Date: _____

Service coordinator: _____ Primary service provider: _____

Reviewer: _____ Date of review: _____

Instructions

These checklists include practice indicators of the key characteristics for writing participation-based individualized family service plan (IFSP) outcomes in early childhood intervention.

The three checklists describe the steps for developing family- and child-focused, participation-based IFSP outcome statements by 1) gathering information by identifying family and care provider priorities as they relate to child participation in everyday activity settings; 2) observing families and their children engaged in real-life, everyday activities across settings and with important people in their lives; and 3) documenting family- and/or child-focused, participation-based outcome statements on the IFSP. Each section contains indicators of a specific area of writing participation-based IFSP outcomes. For each indicator, determine whether the program is adhering to the aspect of the practice described. Space is also available for notes or examples of adherence.

	Are practices characterized by the following?	Yes	No	Examples/notes
Gathering information	1. Information is gathered about child and family activity settings, routines, interests, current participation, and desired participation in real-life situations and settings.	Y	N	
	2. Service coordinator listens for possible IFSP outcome statements during conversations with family members and care providers as they share their priorities, questions, and ideas.	Y	N	
	3. When met with statements from parents or care providers about delayed skills, service coordinator probes further into how the delay influences child participation in existing or desired activity settings or routines.	Y	N	
	4. Service coordinator specifically does not ask parents about their concerns or goals for the child because this information came out of the conversation about family priorities.	Y	N	
	5. Context is used as the benchmark for how the child's participation will be enhanced and/or developed within and across activity settings.	Y	N	

(continued)

Observe families and children	Are practices characterized by the following?	Yes	No	Examples/notes
	1. Observations of the child, family, and other care providers take place within the context of multiple real-life activity settings in the home and community that are both successful and challenging prior to developing the IFSP.	Y	N	
	2. Parents and other care providers are involved in the observations by participating as they typically would during the real-life activity or routine.	Y	N	

Document IFSP outcome statements	Are practices characterized by the following?	Yes	No	Examples/notes
	1. Child, family member, or other care provider is the actor or learner in the outcome.	Y	N	
	2. Outcome is based on a family priority.	Y	N	
	3. Outcome is based on child participation in everyday activity settings and child interests or a parenting support.	Y	N	
	4. An activity setting (i.e., context) is listed in the outcome statement.	Y	N	
	5. Outcome statements are discipline free (i.e., separate goals are not written for each discipline).	Y	N	
	6. Outcome statements are written in words that all team members can understand.	Y	N	
	7. Outcome statements are stated as close to how the parent or care provider actually stated the outcome as possible.	Y	N	
	8. The third word in the outcome statement is a functional concept rather than a specific skill.	Y	N	
	9. Special occasions or life events meaningful to the family are used as time lines.	Y	N	
	10. The family measures progress of the outcome.	Y	N	
	11. Outcome statements include active rather than passive words (e.g., *tolerate, receive, increase, decrease, improve, maintain*).	Y	N	

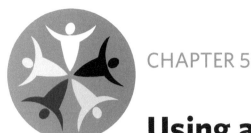

CHAPTER 5

Using a Primary Service Provider

Putting the Approach Into Action

Implementing a PSP approach to teaming depends on using natural learning environment practices and an adult interaction style (coaching) that builds the capacity of parents and other care providers to support the growth and development of the children in their care. More specifically, the information gathered (i.e., child and family priorities, interests, activity settings) between the initial contact with the family and the development of the IFSP is the foundation for the interaction and involvement of the team. In addition to the characteristics and implementation conditions described in Chapter 2, the early intervention program should consider the following recommendations for the IFSP process, beginning at initial intake to intervention to accomplish the intended outcomes resulting from using the PSP approach to teaming practices.

- All initial visits, evaluations, assessments, and intervention visits should occur in the family's natural environment.

- The service coordinator begins to gather information from the family about activity settings and child interests at the initial visit to ensure that their activity settings are the contexts for assessment and intervention.

- Evaluation is used to determine eligibility and is conducted by members of the core team rather than a separate evaluation team with members who only perform evaluations and never serve as a PSP. Results of the evaluation should be provided to the family during this visit, unless extenuating circumstances exist.

- Assessment is differentiated from evaluation and is conducted at a separate visit by the most likely PSP and another team member, if necessary, and within the context of everyday activities to assist in developing participation-based IFSP outcome statements. Assessing and developing the IFSP are conducted during the same visit.

- The final decision of who will serve as the PSP and SSP, as well as the frequency and intensity of the services being delivered, occurs at the IFSP meeting.

The focus of this chapter is to provide detailed information on how to describe the role of the PSP with individual children and families, explain the role of other team members in supporting the PSP, identify the PSP, determine frequency and intensity of services, identify the need for role

 Remember

Who will serve as the primary service provider and secondary service providers, as well as the frequency and intensity of the services being delivered, is decided at the IFSP meeting.

assistance, and delineate any reasons, if any, that might exist to change the PSP for a specific child and family.

EXPLAINING THE PRIMARY SERVICE PROVIDER APPROACH TO TEAMING

All programs need an easily understandable and synchronized explanation of how early intervention services are provided. Every team member is responsible for accurately explaining the program, including contract providers. The content should include an explanation of how the services are delivered in a manner consistent with the *Mission and Key Principles of Providing Early Intervention Services in Natural Environments* (Workgroup on Principles and Practices in Natural Environments, 2007b), which includes the use of a PSP (Key Principle 6). Any variance to the synchronized message should be based on the audiences' prior experience with early intervention, knowledge of the existing program, and expectations of early intervention services. Appendixes 5A and 5B contain tools to use when explaining or sharing information about a PSP approach to teaming. The first tool is a fact sheet providing key points succinctly describing the teaming practices. The second tool is a sample brochure for families and referral sources. Program brochures should be in color as opposed to the black and white sample provided in the appendix.

Reflect

How does your program currently ensure that program staff and contractors share a synchronized description of your program with families and referral sources?

Talking With Families, Teachers, and Other Care Providers

The basic script content when talking with care providers should include a general description of the team members, their roles, and use of a PSP approach to teaming. The script should also include using natural learning environment practices and the caregiver's role during and between schedule visits. The explanation should refer to research in an understandable way as the basis for why the services are provided in this manner. The practitioner providing the explanation should be succinct and encourage questions. Some parents, teachers, and other care providers will be able to clearly identify what they want from the early intervention program, whereas others will need more support in determining the type of assistance that will best meet their needs. The initial conversation takes time, so practitioners should plan accordingly in order to ensure that the visit is as relaxed and informal as possible. The information shared at the initial visit will likely need to be repeated by the service coordinator and PSP over time.

Take Action

The following points can be used to remember the script for explaining the program to new families, teachers, and other care providers.

- Our team
- Use of a primary service provider (PSP) approach to teaming
- Opportunities for role assistance
- Research supporting use of a PSP
- Time and location of visits
- Natural learning environment practices

Sample Script

Following is a sample script for use by early intervention practitioners when introducing the program. The early intervention practitioner should begin the conversation by asking the individual what they already know about the program. The practitioner should then tailor the script to current understanding and need for additional information.

I work with a team of specialists who have a variety of backgrounds and qualifications, such as special education, early childhood education, occupational therapy, physical therapy, and speech-language pathology. We also work with social workers, psychologists, and nurses, so if we need to talk with them or get additional information, then we can pull them in easily. You will have one person from our team whom you will see most often. This person, whom we will call a primary service provider, or PSP, is a member of the much larger team of highly experienced and skilled professionals. The team supports you and your PSP, who works most closely with you. If you and/or your PSP have questions or need some specific assistance, then your primary provider will ask for help from the team. When you and your primary provider need support, your provider will go back and talk with all of the team members during our weekly team meeting. Your PSP may talk with one or two of them and share what you have tried or talked about and get some ideas, or another member of the team may come with your primary provider to visit you.

You may be wondering or others may ask you why we just have one person from our program who comes to see you on a regular basis. The latest research tells us, and families report, that it is more beneficial to have just one person supported by a team of people than it is to have a number of people working directly with you and your child. When a lot of different people ask you to do things, that is time taken away from the typical activities that you and your child enjoy doing or need to do together, or worse, it may even mess up your routine and activities.

Research in child learning and development has helped us see the value of everyday activities that occur in your home (classroom) or in the community as sources for children's learning opportunities. Our approach, which is consistent with national recommendations for how early intervention services should be provided, supports you in finding the best opportunities for promoting child growth and development. These opportunities center on the child's interests and everyday activities. Research has shown that children are more likely to pay attention to and learn during activities that they find fun and interesting. Because you and other caregivers are such an important part of this process, our time together will be spent identifying the things you do or want to do in order to provide your child increased opportunities to take part in interest-based activities.

You and your primary provider will decide together when and where to meet based on what you are focusing on at the time. Because we know children are learning all the time in their everyday activities, we try to meet you in those places and during those activities you identify as learning opportunities. We will vary our days and times for visits based on your priorities and the day of the week and time of day that the activity typically occurs. For example, depending upon what we all decide, your primary provider may meet you at your home, the park, McDonalds, or in the child's classroom setting.

You know your child best, so you and your provider will be working closely together to figure out what opportunities your child has to take part in daily activities, what they like to do, and what you and other members of your family (preschool program) are doing and can do to help them take part in these activities. So when you meet with your primary provider you will be talking about what you have been doing since your last visit and how, or if, it has helped your child do the things that they like and need to do. During your visits, you and your primary provider will try some things together to help with mealtime, morning routines, bath time, or other activities that are important for your child and family. By participating in these everyday activities, you and your primary provider will be helping your child learn new skills to improve development. Your primary provider can also talk with you and share information about child development, parenting ideas, supporting positive behavior, and resources in the community that can help child learning or support you in addressing other identified priorities. Before your primary provider leaves, the two of you will always come up with a plan for what you are going to do until the next time you get back together as well as what you will do at the next visit. What questions do you have about our program or the early intervention practices we use?

This script provides general information to the parent, teacher, and other care providers about the practices used by the early intervention program, refers to current research to support the intervention practices, and describes their roles during visits. In addition to the content in this script, the early intervention service coordinator must also share other information required by Part C during the initial visit (e.g., procedural safeguards, eligibility requirements).

Explaining the Practices to New Families, Teachers, and Other Care Providers

Practitioners should be mindful that the entire process may be unfamiliar to individuals who are new to early intervention. Although practitioners move through the process on a daily basis, families new to early intervention are likely in the midst of an experience that is very personal, emotional, and uncharted territory for them. The procedures, terminology, steps in the process, intervention practices, and the people now involved in their lives are just being introduced and will require repeated explanations. Key Principle 4 of the *Mission and Key Principles for Providing Early Intervention Services in Natural Environments* stated that the early intervention process "must be dynamic and individualized to reflect the child's and family members' preferences, learning styles, and cultural beliefs" (Workgroup on Principles and Practices in Natural Environments, 2007b, p. 2). The first conversation with the family should account for the families' desires, expectations, and current knowledge while simultaneously being sensitive to the family's response to the possibility of needing early intervention services. Because this is a new experience for families, programs should emphasize how the program can assist them in meeting the priorities they have for their child and family. It is often tempting for programs implementing a new approach to describe current practices in comparison with previous program implementation or contrast the program's practices to services provided by other agencies and programs. Families and other care providers new to early intervention need to know what the program does do and why, not what the program used to do or does not do. For example, some practitioners feel compelled to explain early intervention in terms of an educational model versus a medical model or explain how services were different prior to implementing a primary provider approach to teaming (Adams, Tapia, & The Council on Disabilities, 2013). These types of comments serve only to confuse families without prior experience with early intervention or other formal resources.

 Remember

New families, teachers, and other care providers need to know what the program does do and why, not what the program used to do or does not do.

Explaining the Practices to Families, Teachers, and Other Care Providers With Prior Experience With a Multidisciplinary Teaming Approach

When practitioners are explaining current early intervention practices to people with previous experience with programs using a multidisciplinary model of team interaction (e.g., a therapy clinic, hospital, early intervention program), the practitioner should ask the person to describe past services and perceptions of the effectiveness of those services. Practitioners should be listening closely for similarities and differences related to the current program's practices. For example, a parent might describe previous service delivery as having an SLP, OT, and PT who each came to their home at different times to work with the child on a regular basis. When asked about the effectiveness, the parent could positively describe the previous services as well as comment on the child's progress despite the challenge of planning around multiple visits from different providers. In this scenario, the practitioner could take the opportunity to ensure the child and family that they would have access to the needed disciplines as well as address the complications of dealing with many people and interaction styles on a regular basis. The practitioner should also ask questions to obtain an in-depth understanding of what the individual expects from the early intervention program. The practitioner should be listening for information that matches the description and purpose of Part C early intervention.

Unfortunately, some care providers may expect services that are no longer considered recommended practice or supported by current research due to the variance in implementing services for infants and toddlers with disabilities across programs, agencies, and settings. Using specific examples that the person provides, practitioners should then share alternative examples of how the program's practices differ and why. For example, a parent perceives a child needs physical therapy services to provide specialized handling techniques or a specific exercise protocol based on the child's diagnosis or developmental delays and has prior experience with an agency or provider that delivered this type of service. In this case, the practitioner should explain that early intervention does provide therapy services with the purpose of promoting the child's participation in real-life activities while supporting the parent/care providers' ability to improve the child's development of new skills and strengthen current abilities throughout daily routines and activities, not just when the early intervention practitioner is present. The practitioner should be prepared to talk about the existence (or nonexistence) of current evidence to substantiate specific intervention strategies as well as share the evidence supporting the use of parent-mediated practices that promote natural learning within and across everyday contexts. Instead of the PT being limited on visits to handle the child or implement an exercise protocol, the family members and the therapist would work together to use child interests to build on existing opportunities to maximize the child's participation during everyday activities and identify new strategies and techniques to achieve the desired outcomes. If the exercises or handling techniques are evidence based, then they would certainly be included as possible options for supporting the child and family as part of their regular activities (e.g., parent holding a child with torticollis in a position for bottle feeding that requires the child to look away from the side of the contracture). Skills other than motor will naturally occur as part of the activity because interest-based, everyday routines are the venue for early intervention (e.g., getting a bath involves not only the motor aspect of sitting and moving, but also includes opportunities for communication, social-emotional interaction, thinking and problem solving, and self-care). Considering the long-term perspective related to a child's development during their tenure in the early intervention program, the PT might or might not be the best option to serve as the PSP. This decision would be made by the team, which always includes the family.

Take Action

The following points can be used to remember the script for explaining the program to families, teachers, and other care providers with prior experience.

- Use ordinary life situations as natural learning opportunities.

- Use child interests.

- Discuss the important role parents, teachers, and other care providers play in the child's learning.

- Use a primary service provider approach to teaming.

Families, teachers, and other care providers with prior experience receiving services from a program using 1) a multidisciplinary teaming model; 2) decontextualized, deficit-based, practitioner-implemented intervention; and 3) homework for carryover may need explanations of practices that include comparisons. See the sample script provided in the following section.

You may notice several differences between the therapy or intervention you receive from our program and what you might get or might have received from other professionals. First, our intervention uses real-life situations (e.g., eating meals, riding in the car, getting dressed, going out on the playground) and the natural opportunities for children to learn within those situations as early intervention. Other approaches attempt to teach skills or behaviors in isolation or separate from how children will use them in real life. For a child to practice going up and down stairs on the way to play outside is much more meaningful than for a child to practice stair climbing in a therapy room or even in the home when this is not part of a real-life situation for the child.

A second difference is that our interventions use not only real-life situations, but also those that children prefer and that keep their interest for longer periods of time. The longer the child stays involved in an activity, the more the child has an opportunity to learn increasingly complex behaviors. The provider in other types of therapy and intervention decides the activity the child should do and spends a lot of time and energy trying to get the child to do those things. The result is that the child is often bored and frustrated with the activity, which limits learning opportunities.

The role that caring adults play in the child's learning is the third important difference between our approach and others. Caregivers are provided guidance and support on how to use everyday activities to promote learning so the child is learning all the time. Our staff members do not have to be present for the child to be learning and developing. In other approaches, the therapy happens only to the child with or without the important people in the child's life involved. The child gets far less intervention with little impact on development.

The final difference between our program and others is that we understand the value of participating in activities that are fun and meaningful to you and the child; therefore, we want to reduce the number of people coming into the home or classroom on a regular basis by having one person on our team as your primary contact. This notion of a primary person is based on research that points out how conflicting ideas brought in by multiple people can be confusing and unhelpful to families. Although you will have one person as your primary contact, you will also have a team of professionals for support. The team will be available when you and your primary provider have questions, and, when necessary, the team will work with you and your PSP to identify the information needed for ongoing support. This may occur as part of the regular team meeting or by having another team member attend a visit with you and your primary provider to give needed support and plan future joint visits as necessary.

Talking With Physicians and Other Referral Sources

Early intervention programs depend on other professionals within the community, agencies, and programs to assist with identifying potentially eligible children for screening, evaluation, and services. Maintaining communication is essential. Referral sources need to be assured that the early intervention program will be responsive to the identified needs of the child and family. Community partners differ in their expectations when making a referral to early intervention. Some physicians, for example, may expect a direct order to be followed (e.g., child needs speech services twice weekly), whereas others may expect the early intervention program to identify needs and develop treatment plans (e.g., an order from a physician to evaluate and treat). In Part C, the outcomes and needed services are decided by the IFSP team and cannot be directed by a single team member. Input from physicians regarding needed services is important and becomes part of the information considered when developing the plan. Open communication between physicians as well as other referral sources and the early intervention program is necessary to maintain a common understanding of the role of early intervention, evidence-based practices in early childhood intervention, and the mandates of Part C. The desires of the physician, other referral sources, families, and the early intervention program can generally be met when there is respect and understanding among all parties.

The sample script used for explaining the practices to families, teachers, and other care providers may be adapted when talking with physicians and other referral sources. The following key points may be helpful to include as part of the explanation as well as to respond to specific questions the physician or representative from another program may ask.

- Similar to evidence-based medicine, early intervention programs are required to use evidence-based practices in early childhood and family support, which has resulted in changes in approaches to services and supports for individual children and their families (Adams, Tapia, & The Council on Disabilities, 2013).

- Similar to the concept of a medical home, early intervention programs use a teaming approach in which a PSP is identified as the key contact between the program and family to provide direct services as well as identify, obtain, and coordinate additional services needed from other team members.

- Part C requires that early intervention occur within the context of everyday child and family routines. As a result, the role of the PSP is to ensure that families and care providers know how to support and challenge the child within their care throughout their daily activities, thus promoting desired or needed skill development. Intervention, therefore, is not limited to only when the early intervention practitioner is present to work with the child. Refer physicians to Adams, Tapia, and The Council on Children with Disabilities (2013) for more information about the use of coaching and natural learning environment practices in early intervention.

- Using a PSP does not limit access to services but provides each child and family with a designated team of professionals, which minimally includes ECSE, occupational therapy, physical therapy, service coordination, and speech-language pathology. The end result of this team approach yields more coordinated, comprehensive, efficient, effective, individualized, and timely service delivery.

- Using a PSP approach to teaming does not mean less service. This teaming approach does not prescribe a particular frequency and intensity of service; therefore, the PSP, family, other care providers, and other team members plan together to delineate the amount of service necessary to achieve the IFSP outcomes in the shortest amount of time. The frequency and intensity of service delivery is not solely based on the child's diagnosis and impairments, but instead is determined by the parents' and other care providers' need for support in helping to achieve the identified outcomes.

- The frequency, intensity, and type of service for a particular child and family cannot be dictated by any one team member. The IFSP team is responsible for this decision. The parent has right of refusal of services, but they cannot dictate the final decision. The most helpful prescriptions from physicians are those that leave the decisions of type and amount of service delivery to the expertise of the early intervention team. Prescriptions that state "evaluate and treat" assist the team in maintaining a more individualized approach based on all of the information gathered throughout the evaluation and assessment process. More restrictive physician prescriptions such as "physical therapy services twice weekly" may actually limit the type of service the child and family receives and may lead the parent to believe that the child is not receiving appropriate services because the IFSP team's decision may not actually match that of the prescribing physician. The physician prescription may serve as a gatekeeping function in a multidisciplinary or interdisciplinary model of teaming to prohibit maximizing services based on billability. Selecting a PSP and SSP, however, holds the team accountable for appropriate service delivery decisions.

- The PSP will send regular (no less than quarterly) summary reports that specify the level of participation in services, updates on progress, and the plan for the next quarter in order to maintain open communication and keep physicians and other referral sources informed about child and family progress (see examples of a blank and filled-in version of the Early Childhood Intervention Physician Progress Report in Appendices 5C and 5D).

- In addition to therapy for children, Part C provides for a holistic approach to support for the child and family. As a result, families have access to parent supports, service coordination, and other community resources as needed. Early intervention is much more comprehensive than only a venue for obtaining occupational therapy, physical therapy, and speech-language therapy.

- Participation in early intervention is voluntary. Although some judicial systems and social services agencies may mandate enrollment, early intervention programs cannot require parent participation under Part C.

An approach similar to academic detailing used by pharmaceutical sales representatives has been the most effective means for interacting with physicians and other referring agencies (Clow et al., 2005). Academic detailing involves maintaining a professional presence (i.e., attire and demeanor) in physicians' offices and building a relationship (i.e., frequent visits by the same person) based on trust and respect that will foster credibility of the early intervention program, resulting in ongoing referrals. The role of the early intervention program is to assure community partners that children and families will receive the most up-to-date and appropriate services possible, rather than trying to convince them that a primary provider teaming approach or any other specific type of early intervention practice is better or more appropriate than what the referral source may be recommending.

 Take Action

Develop a script for how your program can explain using a primary service provider approach to teaming to physicians and other referral sources.

IDENTIFYING THE PRIMARY SERVICE PROVIDER

Role expectation in a PSP approach to teaming requires that all team members be competent and confident in their own discipline, child development, parenting supports, natural learning environment practices, and coaching. All core team members must be available to potentially serve as a possible PSP, with the exception of the service coordinator, in systems that use a dedicated service coordination model. Although a dedicated service coordinator may use a coaching style of interaction and provide parenting and family supports, they do not serve as the primary provider. The person selected to be the PSP is the member of the team who is the best possible match for a family. It is important for team members to look at long-term goals and outcomes when considering who should be the primary provider, including all outcomes the family has prioritized and what is known about certain conditions, diagnoses, and specific developmental disabilities. The long-term trajectory assists the team in choosing the best person available for the duration of the family's involvement with the program and decreases the likelihood of needing to change the PSP as priorities and outcomes change. The team will then provide role assistance to the PSP, child, and family through joint visits, team meetings, and coaching with other team members.

When the Selection Process Begins

The team should consider the fewest number of people needed to provide high-quality supports and services on a regular basis for an individual child and family because of the negative effect of having multiple providers involved in families' lives. When the referral is first made to the early intervention program, the team immediately begins thinking about the best possible match for the family. The team is not deciding who the primary provider will be at this point, but rather is considering the best person to match the child and family with the information known at the present time. As the IFSP process continues (assessment, evaluation, and multiple conversations with the family), the team learns more about possible options for the role of PSP and begins to discuss their thoughts with the family, asking them their opinions and ideas along the way. The team members will put forth their ideas and suggestions about who would make a great PSP, and the family is involved in the discussions. This person is referred to as the most likely PSP. The final decision for who will be selected as the PSP occurs at the IFSP meeting after developing all of the outcome statements.

How to Choose the Most Likely Primary Service Provider

The most likely PSP is identified based on four categories or types of factors that are considered in a specific sequence and have multiple levels of complexity: 1) parent/family, 2) child, 3) environmental, and 4) practitioner.

 Remember

The four types of factors used to select the most likely primary service provider are

1. Parent/family

2. Child

3. Environmental

4. Practitioner

Parent/family factors are the family's priorities and requests for services to support their child's learning and development. This would also include a prescription from a physician for a specific therapy that a family might present to the early intervention program. Other parent/family factors include the family dynamics (e.g., how the family defines itself, how the family members interact with one another) as well as characteristics of individual family members (e.g., primary culture, language, diagnosis or condition) and availability of the family to participate in early intervention services.

Child factors include specific characteristics that are unique to each child deemed eligible for the program. These factors are the child's diagnosis or condition as well as any needs identified by the family or other team members during the evaluation and assessment process. Other child factors include child-specific interests (e.g., toy trains, new puppy, favorite blanket) and activity settings (e.g., snuggling with grandma, eating snack at child care, playing on the slide at the park) in which the child currently participates and/or needs to be involved. The team must also consider the child's availability as a factor (e.g., avoiding naptime, hospitalizations, illness).

Environmental factors are the third type of factor to consider when identifying the most likely PSP and include the child's and family's natural learning environments, such as the child's home, locations within the community (e.g., church, park, grocery store), or the preschool or child care setting if applicable. Safety considerations such as presence of animals, health risks (e.g., second-hand smoke), and locations that could present potential risks or harm to the early intervention practitioner are also included as environmental factors. The distance of the child and family's natural learning environments from the early intervention program is another environmental factor. The distance factor should be discussed prior to final selection of the PSP because the driving distance may affect the practitioner's ability to schedule visits. Availability is also a factor that may affect opportunities for scheduling visits across environments and activities. For example, visiting during naptime or the teacher's planning time at child care would be times when the child and teacher are not available to participate in a real-life activity.

Practitioner factors include, first and foremost, the knowledge and expertise of each individual practitioner as it relates to the parent/family and child factors. Both professional and personal expertise should be taken into account during this discussion. For example, if a particular child has feeding issues, then the person(s) on the team with specialized skills related to feeding should be considered as most likely PSP. Personal knowledge and expertise may be matched with a family's interests, activity settings, and lifestyle (e.g., outdoor activities, farm life, sports activities). Practitioner factors also include the primary provider's assigned area of service within a geographic region. For example, if a team has multiple SLPs, then they may be assigned to a specific area within a county or school district to decrease drive time. The SLP serving the area in which the child resides would be considered as the most likely PSP. The billability of the service being provided is also a practitioner factor. Billing is a required consideration for those programs required to obtain third party payment.

In special circumstances, a practitioner factor could also be a prior relationship with a family. For example, if a family has an older child who participated in the early intervention program, then the person who worked most closely with the parent or care provider at that time may be the best choice to become the PSP. The relationship may already be established, and the primary provider and family already know how to work with one another; therefore, the primary provider will also know the family's interests, routines, and activity settings. The team member with a preexisting relationship may be the best choice because they are competent and confident in child development, parenting supports, and coaching and also know when to seek support from other members of the team. Similarly, all other factors being equal, a practitioner may have developed a special rapport with the family during the early steps in the IFSP process. Because of this bond, the family may feel more comfortable with this team member fulfilling the role of the PSP.

Availability is a final practitioner factor for identifying the most likely PSP. If a team member's schedule is essentially full and they cannot take another family onto their workload, then they may not be available to be the primary provider. If, however, they are the best and only person who should be the PSP for the family, then the team will have to determine if some adjustments can be made to enable them to provide support to the new child and family. If the best person on the team cannot be made available and no other team member has the knowledge and skills necessary to support the family, then the team may have to identify a resource outside the team. Rarely does a team have to seek outside resources because adjustments can usually be made within the team for the family to have the best possible PSP.

The Selection Process

The Worksheet for Selecting the Most Likely Primary Service Provider (see Appendix 5E; also see Figure 5.1) may be used to assist a core, geographically based early intervention team using a PSP approach to teaming with the selection of who will serve as the most likely PSP.

The term *most likely* is used in the worksheet because the final decision of the PSP is not made until the IFSP meeting when the team members are discussing the service delivery options (i.e., who, how often). The worksheet may be used at the initial visit through all steps in the early intervention process up to and including the IFSP meeting. The worksheet can be used early in the process and can assist in selecting evaluation team members and the person(s) most appropriate for conducting the functional assessment. The items listed on the worksheet are intended to be 1) information gathered throughout the early intervention process up to and including the IFSP

Worksheet for Selecting the Most Likely Primary Service Provider

Core team as options for primary service provider (PSP)

Early childhood (EC) _____ Occupational therapist (OT) _____

Physical therapist (PT) _____ Speech-language pathologist (SLP) _____ Other _____

		Most likely PSP(s) identified based on			Most likely PSP options selected (list)	Secondary service provider (SSP) options selected (list)
	Parent/family factors	Child factors	Environmental factors	Practitioner factors		
Tier 1	List priorities with contexts	List diagnosis/condition/ needs (long-term view)	Circle natural learning environments • Home • Community • Preschool • Child care • Other	List knowledge/expertise (personal/professional)		Role overlap
	List parent/physician request	List interests/activity settings				
Tier 2	Family dynamics Individual parent/caregiver characteristics • Language/culture • Knowledge/expertise • Diagnosis/condition • Other		Safety Distance from program office	Primary service area in geographic region Billability Prior relationship Rapport		Role overlap
Tier 3	Availability	Availability	Availability	Availability		Role overlap

Most likely PSP is:	Role gap? If so, explain:	Role assist (SSP):

Notes:

Figure 5.1. Worksheet for Selecting the Most Likely Primary Service Provider.

meeting as well as 2) discussion points for the team as part of the conversation about who on the team would most likely be the best PSP.

The first step in the process is to list all of the members of the core team at the top of the worksheet because all core team members are always potential PSPs. The box does not include the service coordinators because they do not serve as a PSP in a program with dedicated service coordination. Individuals who are a part of a program in which service coordination is also a role of a service provider would be represented by their discipline at the top of the worksheet.

The worksheet can be conceived as a funnel. At its widest point, all team members with the exception of dedicated service coordinators are eligible to be a PSP. The decision-making process consists of the four sets of factors previously described now further divided into three tiers. These tiers are used as filters to determine the most likely PSP(s) at each tier until the best, most likely PSP emerges as well as any supports the PSP might need from an SSP through joint visits.

Beginning at Tier 1 and parent/family factors, the team lists and discusses the parents' priorities for the child. Rather than a list of skills the parents would like for the child to learn, the priorities are written and discussed as participation-based IFSP outcomes that include the most helpful context for the child to participate. Context is critical because it assists in determining the PSP. The team also considers any specific parent/physician requests with equal weight of other team members. For example, if the family or physician believes the child needs occupational therapy, then an OT should remain as an option for most likely PSP unless another factor in Tier 1 or possibly Tier 2 would indicate that another team member would be a better, most likely PSP. Factors on the worksheet are then used to explain to the family how the options for the most likely PSP were identified. The team then moves to child factors in Tier 1 and shares the child's diagnosis or condition, if applicable, as well as any of the child's needs gathered up to this point. The team keeps the long-term perspective in mind rather than only what the child might need right now and discusses the child's interests and activity settings identified thus far. Next, the team moves to the environmental factors in Tier 1 and circles the natural learning environments identified to date during conversations with the family. Finally, the team moves to the practitioner factors in Tier 1. Of the original core team members listed at the top of the worksheet, the team determines who has the professional knowledge and expertise based on their discipline perspective and experience as well as perhaps personal experiences to assist the parents in achieving their priorities for the child based on the child's diagnosis, condition, and/or needs as well as the current natural learning environments.

Most often, more than one team member could be the most likely PSP at this point. The team lists the names of the most likely PSP(s) in the shaded section on the worksheet. Based on the long-term perspective, if a team member has been excluded as the best, most likely PSP, but will still be needed to support the PSP and family at this point, then the team lists their name as an SSP option on the worksheet. If only one team member is listed as the most likely PSP in Tier 1, then the team has successfully identified the most likely PSP. The team then writes this person's name in the darker shaded box at the bottom of the worksheet labeled "Most Likely PSP." The team now determines if any role gaps exist. That is, the team ascertains what additional knowledge and skills will perhaps be necessary to help support the PSP and family related to the parent priorities as well as the child's diagnosis/condition and needs. The team lists the role gaps in the box identified as such on the worksheet. Next, the team decides who may be needed to serve as an SSP to support the PSP during one or more joint visits and lists this person's name in the last box on the last row of the worksheet. If more than one team member is listed in the most likely PSP area at the end of Tier 1, then the team has role overlap. This means that more than one person currently has the ability to serve as the most likely PSP; therefore, the discussion continues as the team proceeds to Tier 2.

Tier 2 begins with the team considering the parent/family factors of family dynamics and individual parent or care provider characteristics. Examples of family dynamics include, but are not limited to, multigenerational households, parents who are divorced and have joint custody, foster families, reunification efforts with a child's biological family, or parents with differing opinions about child rearing and/or intervention. If a team member has more experience working with families in similar situations, then they would continue to move forward as a possible most likely PSP.

The team also considers individual parent or care provider characteristics in Tier 2. The primary language of the parent/family is the first characteristic the team considers. If the primary language (other than English) is spoken by one or more of the most likely PSPs listed in the gray box on Tier 1, then those team members are still considered as the most likely PSP and proceed through Tier 2. If none of the identified most likely PSPs from Tier 1 speak the family's primary language, then an interpreter will be needed, and all of the potential PSPs will continue through Tier 2. Parent knowledge/expertise is the next parent characteristic considered. For example, if the parent is a grandparent raising the child, a foster parent, or a teenage parent, then these could be factors to assist with deciding the most likely PSP. If a parent has prior knowledge or experiences, then this could rule in or rule out certain team members who were still considered most likely PSP. A parent diagnosis or condition is the final parent characteristic that could potentially affect the most likely PSP through Tier 2. For example, if the team knows the parent has a mental health issue, then perhaps a member of the team still in consideration has experience working with parents who have a similar diagnosis. This team member would proceed through Tier 2, whereas others could be taken out of consideration at this point.

Next, the team considers the environmental factors in Tier 2. Personal safety may be an issue and, if so, should be discussed. No individual team member should feel that their personal safety is at risk. By the same token, the entire team should ensure that individual values, biases, or preferences do not result in misinterpretation of an environmental situation as a threat to personal safety. If an individual continues to have unrealistic personal safety concerns, then the team leader or supervisor will need to support that team member in moving forward. At this point, if multiple team members are still considered as the most likely PSP, then perhaps gender could be a factor in determining the most likely PSP or the availability of another team member to go with the most likely PSP would need to be considered. The team also considers the distance between the family's home, child care, or other natural environment in which the parent would want direct supports from the program office. For example, if one of the remaining most likely PSPs has very few hours available for a new family who lives 1-hour away, then other most likely PSPs should remain in consideration as a result of the discussion in Tier 2.

Practitioner factors are the final set of factors to consider in Tier 2. Sometimes individuals who are part of programs that have more than one particular discipline are assigned to specific areas of the geographic region that the core team supports. For other teams, certain team members may go to a specific part of the catchment area on certain days. In these cases, the primary service area may help determine who should continue to be considered as the most likely PSP. If an early intervention program relies on billing and one team member still in consideration for most likely PSP is able to bill a third party payer for their services, then this would continue to keep them as an option for PSP. In contrast, if someone cannot bill for the service, then the team may decide to no longer consider this person as an option. Finally, the filters of prior relationships and rapport are considered. If a team member is still in consideration and provided supports to this family for a previous child, then that team member may move forward in the selection process. Similarly, if the parent and a team member established strong rapport during the process from initial contact to IFSP meeting, then this should also be considered if all other factors are equal between this individual and other possible PSPs.

At this point, the team lists the names of the remaining most likely PSPs in the shaded section in Tier 2 as well as any other SSP options. If only one most likely PSP remains, then the team has identified the best candidate. The team writes this person's name in the darker shaded box at the bottom of the worksheet labeled "Most Likely PSP" and determines if any role gaps exist. Then the team determines who may be needed to serve as an SSP to support the PSP during one or more joint visits and lists this person's name in the last box on the final row of the worksheet. The team continues to have role overlap if more than one person is listed in the most likely PSP area in Tier 2; therefore, discussion will need to continue to Tier 3.

The team continues the discussion in Tier 3 with the parent/family factor of availability. The team considers all the days and times when the parent and/or child care provider is available to meet with the remaining team members who could be the most likely PSP. The team must also consider the child's availability across environments. If these days and times are possibilities for one or more of the remaining team members at this point, then that team member moves forward in Tier 3 as a candidate for the most likely PSP. Next, the team concludes the discussion of most likely PSP and looks at the practitioner factors of availability. If the remaining practitioners are available, then they move forward as the most likely PSPs. Some teams may consider availability as a first factor in determining who on the team could be the most likely PSP. Practitioner availability is the last factor because the goal of the team is to provide the very best PSP the team has to offer to every family. The potential very best person should not be eliminated without considering all of the other factors. Availability can be considered when all factors are equal between team members at the end of Tier 3. If only one most likely team member is remaining and unavailable, then the team's conversation moves to finding a way to enable that team member to be the most likely PSP for the child/family or move back up through the tiers to see if another team member should be reconsidered for the possibility of most likely PSP.

The team lists the names of the most likely PSPs in the shaded section in Tier 3, and if only one most likely PSP remains, then the team has identified the most likely PSP. The team determines if any role gaps exist and decides who will be the best person to serve as SSP. Role assistance can be provided to the PSP through one-to-one conversations, during team meetings, and via joint visits. The team then writes this person's name in the last box on the last row of the worksheet. If more than one team member is listed in the most likely PSP area in Tier 3, then the team continues to have role overlap. At this time, the remaining individuals determine who is willing to poten-

tially serve as the PSP. If for any reason the parent was not present during this discussion, then the team should present the suggestion for the most likely PSP and review the worksheet, sharing the information previously discussed.

The overall process for using the worksheet to select the most likely PSP and possible SSP takes less than 10 minutes in most circumstances. The conversations become faster once teams work together over time, and the worksheet simply serves as an outline for the conversation.

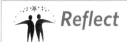

Reflect

How does this process for selecting the most likely primary service provider compare with your current strategy for making this decision?

The Mitchell family case study located in Appendix 5F demonstrates how two different teams use the Worksheet for Selecting the Most Likely Primary Service Provider to discuss the possibilities of who might be the best PSP with the Mitchell family during the IFSP process. The teams are identical in each scenario, with the exception of a few different team members. The teams serve the same geographic catchment area and number of children and families. These examples are provided to show how thoughtful consideration of the practitioner factors on a team can influence the decision of who would be the best team member to serve as the most likely PSP.

FREQUENCY AND INTENSITY OF SERVICES

Once the decision is made regarding who will serve as the PSP, the frequency, intensity, and duration of the supports provided by the PSP and any needed SSP must be specified. Previous methods for determining frequency and intensity of services have been discussed in the literature since the 1980s and determined ineffective. The decision-making criteria have included, but not been limited to, the child's age, severity of the child's disability, family socioeconomic status, mother's education level, availability of time in the practitioners' schedules, child therapy history, practitioner judgment of the parents' ability to follow-through with a home program, third party reimbursement caps, and cognitive referencing (Atwater et al., 1982; Borkowski & Wessman, 1994; Carr, 1989; Cole et al., 1990, 1991; Cole & Mills, 1997; Farley et al., 1991; Krassowski & Plante, 1997; Notari et al., 1992). Hallam et al. (2009) conducted a study in early intervention and reported that child and family factors including age of entry into the program, gestational age, Medicaid eligibility, use of third party insurance, and children's developmental levels influenced the amount of services provided. Other authors described factors such as the teaming approach used, values and philosophy of the early intervention program, and management and delivery of services as highly influential on the type and amount of early intervention services received (Dinnebeil et al., 1999). Palisano and Murr (2009) discussed perspectives on the intensity of occupational and physical therapy services for young children with developmental considerations. This discussion included the concepts of episodes of care, readiness of the child for activity and participation, method of service delivery, and the effect of practice in natural learning environments as options for determining intensity of therapy services. Although multiple variables have been discussed in the literature in terms of making decisions about how much intervention should be provided to individual children, no method emerges as a clear evidence-based strategy for making these types of decisions (Bagnato et al., 2011; Caracci et al., 2018; Gee et al., 2016; Houtrow, Murphy, & The Council on Children with Disabilities, 2019; Kuhn & Marvin, 2016; Zeng et al., 2012).

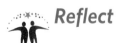

Reflect

What is the basis for your decisions about frequency and intensity of services?

The frequency and intensity of services listed on the IFSP should include the PSP as well as any and all SSPs. A flexible approach to scheduling is necessary in light of the absence of empirical data on frequency and intensity of service and in consideration of the use of natural learning environment practices and the mission of early intervention to support the parents' and care providers' abilities to promote child learning and development. This approach is based on the needs of the parents and care providers (related to the child's strengths and needs) and the priorities chosen as outcomes on the IFSP. This approach is referred to as *FAB scheduling*, which is *f*lexible and *a*ctivity based and involves *b*ursts of support.

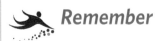

Remember

FAB scheduling is *flexible*, *activity* based, and involves *bursts* of support.

Scheduling That Is Flexible

Intervention is traditionally scheduled in blocks. For example, an early intervention practitioner identifies time slots during their week for visits with individual children and families. Once a child is placed in a time slot, regular visits occur on the same day and at the same time unless the practitioner or family needs to reschedule the appointment for a specific reason. The advantages to a blocked scheduling approach are that it is easy for the parent and practitioner to remember (e.g., Ramon on Tuesdays at 2:00 p.m.) and it is easy for the practitioner to manage their schedule (e.g., practitioner can plan ahead; knows when they have an available opening). In contrast, flexible scheduling has many advantages and provides availability of the practitioner based on the immediate needs and priorities of the child and family. Each future visit is scheduled at the end of the prior visit based on the joint plan developed between the care provider and the PSP. For example, the PSP asks the parent when they should return for the next visit based on what the parent will be doing between visits. For urgent situations, the PSP can meet more frequently with the parent while allowing for needed time for practice and implementation between visits. The time between visits may increase as the parent's competence and confidence in supporting the child's learning and development increases. Flexible scheduling is more consistent with using natural learning environment practices specifically related to contexts in which children's skills and behaviors typically occur throughout the day. Joint visiting is an implementation condition of a PSP approach to teaming (see Chapter 6) and requires team members to be available to accompany one another when needed, often with short notification. A flexible approach to scheduling also allows more and varied options for joint visits.

Scheduling That Is Activity Based

Many practitioners plan visits with children and families based on open time slots in their weekly schedules. Another reason a practitioner might schedule at the same day and time is to capitalize on the absence of other siblings or important people in the child's life to eliminate potential distractions for the child or perceived chaos by the practitioner. This type of scheduling interferes with implementing natural learning environment practices. The child's environment, regardless of possible distractions, is the context in which the child must learn, and the parents need to be supported in fostering child participation and development. Furthermore, if a practitioner schedules a visit at the same time each week, then they are either limited to intervention within the activity setting that would naturally occur during that time or forced to create activities that would not usually occur during their typical day. For example, if a child tends to avoid sensory experiences such as hearing loud noises, playing with other children, being hugged and cuddled, or eating foods with varying textures and the practitioner visits Wednesdays at 4:00 p.m. when the children are engaged in watching television while their mother prepares dinner, then the practitioner is always limited to the activity settings of meal preparation and/or television watching. Once the child's participation improves in these activity settings, if blocked scheduling continues, then the practitioner may be inclined to create games for the young children to play to address the child's sensory issues, such as ring-around-the-rosy, duck-duck-goose, or red rover. With the parent in the kitchen cooking dinner, these additional activities are limited to when the practitioner or another willing adult is present to facilitate and supervise the interaction. The practitioner may also feel the need to create the games or other learning opportunities because they devalue the activity occurring at the time (i.e., children watching television).

Alternatively, if a practitioner is using activity-based scheduling, then each visit will be planned around the priorities of the parents or child care providers within the context of the activities that typically occur on that day and time. For instance, the child previously described would most likely need support during mealtime, bath time, tooth brushing, and bedtime routines. The practitioner would plan to go at the time of day when these activities occur so that the natural consequences and real-life circumstances are present. Consider a situation in which bath time is problematic for a child and family. The family bathes the child in the evening, which can be a challenging time to schedule a home visit. If, however, the practitioner requests the family to bathe the child at a different time of day for their convenience, then the family may be willing to do so, but the energy level of the child and family will be different, the amount of time allocated to the activity could vary, the possibility of confusing the child and causing other negative outcomes increases due to changing the schedule, and the challenge of generalizing the strategies and skills to the real-time context will have to be overcome. Practitioners may voice concerns regarding their availability to participate in activity settings or routines that occur outside of an 8:00 a.m. to 5:00 p.m. workday due to personal commitments, family issues, or limitations on the number of available visits after 5:00 p.m. (i.e., a practitioner willing or available to provide evening services one night each week).

The nature of early intervention services requires practitioners to be open to alternative scheduling because the lives of children and families do not stop at 5:00 p.m. Learning opportunities exist throughout the child and family's day, evenings, and even weekends. Practitioners are not expected to be present for every bath time or evening meal, but they should be available for initial and occasional visits to support the family's ability to promote the child's participation during the identified activity settings. Practitioners are often challenged by shifting to this type of scheduling as they begin to implement natural learning environment practices. As a result, they have limited flexible times available because they may have some families blocked at times in which the activity of another family typically occurs. Until the practitioner shifts all children and families on their workload to activity-based scheduling, they will continue to have limited options for meeting individual child and family needs.

Scheduling That Includes Bursts of Support

Episodes (or bursts) of care have been discussed as a viable strategy for supporting children with developmental disabilities and their families in order to match the immediate and ongoing needs with appropriate levels of service (Palisano & Murr, 2009). Scheduling using a burst of support is done at the beginning of intervention with a newly enrolled child and family (i.e., frontloading)

Remember

Use frontloading

- With new children and families

- To address a pressing need

- For a child with multiple environments

- When initial and immediate expertise or another team member is needed or required

or due to changes in family, child, environmental, and practitioner factors. Frontloading is a scheduling strategy that enables the practitioner and care providers to address pressing needs faster than implementing a less frequent approach. For example, a child with severe feeding challenges (e.g., losing weight, vomiting, swallowing issues, making the transition to oral feeding) should be seen frequently, especially initially, to address support for all critical people feeding the child and during all meals. A practitioner can use frontloading for a child in multiple environments (e.g., home and child care, grandma's house and home) to more quickly observe and support the child's participation across environments, people, and times of day. The practitioner might schedule several visits with the family within the first week or 2 weeks following enrollment instead of starting out with weekly visits.

Teams must consider the long-term view of the child and family when selecting the PSP. In some instances, however, the expertise of a team member other than that PSP may initially and immediately be required in the short term. For example, children with a diagnosis of cerebral palsy with quadriplegia often have many assistive technology needs that require the knowledge and expertise of multiple team members. The team member selected as the PSP may need intensive support from other team members as specialized equipment needs are identified and the effectiveness of using the equipment is assessed across environments. The PSP and SSP would implement high-frequency joint visits (i.e., burst of support) in this situation to ensure that an initial plan is being implemented that meets the needs of the PSP, SSP, parents and other care providers, and child.

Scheduling a burst of support can also occur when there are changes in family, child, environmental, and practitioner factors. The burst of support is used to help the child and family through substantial changes that could disrupt the achievement of child and family outcomes and ameliorate the possible negative effects of life-changing events. For example, family factors to consider for which a burst of support might be appropriate include, but are not limited to, the birth or adoption of a new infant, parental divorce, family illness or death, recent parental diagnosis of a mental health issue, parental unavailability (e.g., death, incarceration, abandonment, alcohol or drug abuse), or parental job change or loss. Child factor changes for consideration include, but are not limited to, developmental growth spurt, regression of skills, new health issue or condition (e.g., diagnosis, surgery), or disruption of a routine due to a family or environmental change. Changes in environmental factors will affect the entire family unit and should be considered for a burst of support. Environmental factors include the family moving to a new location, transitions in child care, the family moving in with an extended family member or vice versa, homelessness, or the family's community experiencing a natural disaster. Practitioner factor changes can also be a good time for a burst of support. For example, if a practitioner serving as PSP leaves the team, then the new PSP and family should consider a burst of support to quickly get to know one another and decrease any possible negative effect the change in provider might have on

Remember

Other times for a burst of support include

- Life-changing events

- Developmental growth spurt

- Regression of skills

- New health issue

- Family moving to new location

- Transition in child care

- Homelessness

- Natural disaster

- Change in the primary service provider

the child and family. Depending on the circumstance or issue, a joint visit may be part of the burst of support because of the need for specialized expertise and knowledge.

Appendices 5G and 5H are two documents that depict an example of the workload of an OT working full time in an early intervention program and the current month's calendar of her schedule. These documents are provided to share an example of FAB scheduling. The workload list provides the total number of children and families on the practitioner's ongoing workload and delineates her other responsibilities, which include evaluations, IFSP meetings, joint visits (for children on her workload as well as not on her workload), and team meetings. The numeral in parentheses next to each child's name on the list indicates the number of visits scheduled for each child that particular month. The calendar shows the variations in the time of day of the visits as well as when visits are scheduled in the child care center (CCC) in order for the OT to participate in previously identified activity settings that occur at that time for the child and family/child care provider. Joint visits (JV) are also noted on the calendar as well as the discipline of the other team member participating in the joint visit. The calendar also indicates the visits that require an interpreter's participation (Interp), which may affect FAB scheduling. The calendar indicates 11 visits for the Donovan family as part of frontloading as a burst of support following the child's IFSP meeting that occurred at the end of the previous month.

Making the transition to FAB scheduling can be one of the most challenging aspects of implementing a PSP approach to teaming. This approach to scheduling vastly differs from more traditional block scheduling, and practitioners' unfamiliarity with the strategies and perceived ambiguity with visit-to-visit scheduling can create anxiety and an initial feeling of loss of control over one's own schedule. Administrators may find new challenges for tracking workload numbers because practitioners' schedules may no longer reveal obvious openings, which is why workload maximums are determined by team rather than individual (see Chapter 3). Although new to many practitioners, FAB scheduling offers maximum flexibility and alignment with natural learning environment practices. Once all team members have shifted their entire workloads to this type of scheduling, the practitioners and families find it more helpful and flexible, and a different type of sense of control of the schedule develops over time.

Take Action

Look at how you currently schedule visits with families. How could you move to FAB scheduling?

ROLE OF THE PRIMARY SERVICE PROVIDER WITH INDIVIDUAL CHILDREN AND FAMILIES

Practitioners who work in early intervention have different roles when working with families under Part C than in other settings within their professions. Early intervention visits in natural environments can be more complex than visits in health care or school settings. Not only is the focus of an early intervention visit broader in scope than other types of therapy or education, but the early intervention practitioner also has to be prepared to provide supports in many new and varied environments with adults who are important to the child. Practitioners should plan visits to occur at the time, place, and with the typical materials present where family or child care activities that will be the focus of the visit occur. Practitioners are supporting families and other care providers in their abilities to enhance their child's development. This includes knowing and using evidence-based intervention practices from the fields of early childhood (general and special education), infant mental health, occupational therapy, physical therapy, speech-language pathology, and so forth to promote parent-mediated child participation in everyday activity settings. Building the capacity of the adults in the child's life requires that practitioners use an interaction style with adults that supports their learning. Reflective and informative conversations with parents and other caregivers help practitioners establish child progress toward IFSP outcomes and global early intervention child outcomes.

The PSP uses coaching as the adult learning strategy with the parents and other care providers to build their capacity to promote the child's learning and development. Interactions between the coach and care provider minimally include an opportunity for the parent or other care provider to reflect on what they are doing to support the child in accomplishing the desired priorities and for the coach and care provider to generate other strategies or ideas to try within the context of child interest-based activities (Rush & Shelden, 2020). For example, consider a scenario in which the SLP is the PSP for a child and the family's priority is for the child to play with his brother and sister in the backyard. The parents and siblings of the child need support around how to use the child's interests to maximize playing happily and safely together outside. Some of the strategies used by the family will be targeting their responsiveness regarding the child's communication. Other strategies involve the parents' use of behavioral supports during playtime and techniques for assisting the child to keep up with the siblings as they move about the backyard. The SLP observes the family's use of jointly identified strategies to promote the child's participation in backyard play. The SLP also provides feedback on the family's implementation of the plan, demonstrates alternative uses of particular strategies, observes return demonstration by the family to check for understanding, and jointly plans next steps that will happen in between visits.

Three Components of a Visit

Early intervention visits in natural environments can contain three essential components, regardless of the teaming approach. First, practitioners begin by revisiting previous plans, whether developed at an IFSP meeting or during a previous visit. Second, practitioners engage with parents or other caregivers in one or more of three types of interactions—engaging in naturally occurring child learning opportunities, discussing and practicing parenting strategies, and/or providing resource-based parent support. Third, an effective early intervention visit concludes with practitioners and family members developing a two-part joint plan for the future.

Component 1: Revisiting the Previous Joint Plan

The IFSP results in developing desired family and/or child outcomes as well as shared understanding of child and family strengths, abilities, and needs (see Chapter 4). IFSP team members form plans to help the child and family reach these outcomes. Whether these are long- or short-term plans, each visit should start with a conversation about how the previously developed plans are going. Sometimes plans will have worked and are moving along well; other times, intervention methods will need to be adjusted or family time and priorities may have changed. Reviewing previous plans allows for checking in on progress toward child and family outcomes and provides an opportunity to make any changes needed for the day's visit or in the strategies or activities families are pursuing to reach their outcomes.

Component 2: Promoting Child Learning, Parenting, and/or Parent Support

Children spend more time with their parents and caregivers than they can possibly spend with early interventionists. Visits in natural environments focus on the parents'/care providers' abilities to promote child engagement and successful participation in ways that support learning and development through naturally occurring activities. Interventions in natural environments focus on each family's or child care setting's typical routines and activity settings and, therefore, include more than just play. Everyday activities may be child specific, such as dressing or eating meals, or family activities in which the child participates, such as gardening, doing laundry, or cleaning the house.

Practitioners do not need to take toy bags as the content/context for intervention because intervention occurs within a routine or activity, which may or may not be associated with particular toys or materials. If the focus of the intervention is on promoting parent mediation of child participation in a particular activity, then the family would use whatever items they have that would typically be part of the activity. Practitioners may use assistive technology (e.g., specialized spoons, augmentative and alternative communication devices, walkers, positioning devices) and assess the effectiveness of the assistive technology to enable the child to participate within and across their everyday activities. If the purpose of bringing the assistive technology is to assess the child's need for purchase of the item by a third party, then bringing in the equipment is consistent with natural learning environment practices. If, however,

 Remember

The three components of a visit include

1. Revisiting the previous joint plan

2. Promoting child learning, parenting, and/or parent support

3. Developing the two-part joint plan

the intent of bringing the item is the context for the visit (e.g., an iPad is used to promote joint attention while playing a fun game), then bringing the equipment would not be consistent with evidence-based practices in natural environments.

Families are also in the community where their infant or toddler is expected to participate in some manner. For example, parents may ask for support in order to successfully take their infant or young child to the grocery store or enjoy the park while older siblings play. Families may ask for assistance in supporting child care providers where infants and young children spend time.

Practitioners assist parents and other caregivers during the second component of the home visit by affirming the interactions and responsive strategies that parents and other caregivers are using to support child development and child learning. Practitioners use results of observations to reflect with parents about what is going well and those parts of activities and routines that are challenging. Practitioners must first understand the activity and the specific surrounding context before they can identify effective strategies, methods, and modifications that might work within that context. Practitioners share and model evidence-based intervention strategies as well as provide additional information adults can use to support infants and toddlers. Parents and other caregivers can try out the strategies within the context of a naturally occurring interest-based activity with the child. Practitioners promote parent/caregiver reflection and provide feedback following discussion, observation, and practice of specific strategies and techniques.

The second component of the visit is when the PSP would model and teach parents and other care providers specific evidence-based techniques that would promote the child's participation during the activity settings selected as the focus of intervention based on the parent's priorities. A few examples of specific evidence-based intervention techniques that might be used by a PSP include using sign language or giving choices to promote a child's communication, using social stories or picture schedules to assist a child needing support making the transition from one activity to another, using splints or a standing frame to support a child's ability to stand, using swaddling to help an infant sleep, and using adapted feeding utensils to support a child's ability to eat.

The decision for choosing specific teaching strategies and therapeutic techniques in early intervention must be based on several factors. The first and most important factor is that the practice is founded on available research for children under the age of 3 years, or, minimally, derived from research that indicates the practices are promising for children receiving early intervention. Several authors provided guidelines for assisting early intervention practitioners in determining whether a practice has credible evidence to support its use (Adams & Snyder, 1998; Golden, 1980; Harris, 1996; McWilliam, 1999; Nickel, 1996; Rosenbaum & Stewart, 2002; Silver, 1995). Harris outlined specific evaluation criteria that examined the scientific merit of an intervention that 1) has underlying theories supported by valid anatomical and physiological evidence, 2) is designed for a specific population, 3) includes potential side effects, 4) has studies documented in peer-reviewed journals to support efficacy, 5) is supported by well-designed experimental studies, and 6) has proponents who are open and willing to discuss its limitations. In addition, McWilliam delineated the five characteristics of controversial practices for therapists and educators to consider when making decisions about intervention strategies and techniques: 1) claims to cure a disability that theoretically cannot be cured, 2) requires people who are already specialists to undergo even more specialized training or certification, 3) has no published studies that demonstrate the effectiveness of the intervention over others, 4) is described as needing to occur for a certain amount of time (e.g., every 90 minutes), and 5) is debated in court (i.e., legal proceedings to initiate or halt the intervention). These recommendations, taken into consideration with the requirements of Part C that practices used in early intervention must be based on valid scientific evidence, place the burden of responsibility on early intervention practitioners to use a decision-making process beyond personal preference, what they have found to work in the past, or parent request when selecting strategies or techniques to use with a specific child and family.

The second factor stipulates that the parent or care provider is able to implement the technique or strategy when the practitioner is not present. Another factor requires that the strategies fit appropriately as part of everyday routines and activities within a child's natural environment. Using the toys and materials that are available within the child's home or other natural setting,

Remember

Specialized techniques, strategies, and knowledge of the primary service provider (PSP) fit in early intervention when

- Research exists to support the practice for children under the age of 3 years

- Parents and other care providers can continue to use the practice when the PSP is not present

- The practice can be used as part of an everyday routine or activity

- The practice involves using toys and materials already found in the child's environment unless assistive technology is needed

Reflect

How do you currently make decisions about the specific practices you use as part of your intervention to support children and families?

unless the specific situation requires the use of assistive technology, is the final factor when determining if a specific intervention strategy can be used in early intervention. Therapy balls, mats, wedges, bolsters, flash cards, surgical brushes, special food items, surgical tubing, whistles, pinwheels, bubbles, therapeutic music, earphones, cue cards, paper, and crayons are not assistive technology and should not be brought into family's homes or child care settings.

Practitioners may also provide parenting supports during an early intervention visit. Dunst (2005) described parenting supports as "the information, advice, guidance, etc. that both strengthen existing parenting knowledge and skills and promote acquisition of new competencies necessary for parents to carry out childrearing responsibilities and provide their child(ren) development-enhancing learning opportunities" (p. 4). Just as children develop at different rates, parents have different styles of interaction. Some parents are developing or refining their parenting style during early intervention supports, whereas others may have questions about modifications to their parenting practices for an infant or young child with disabilities. Parenting topics include everything from when to introduce toileting, infants' nutritional needs, and independence in daily routines, such as taking a cup to the sink when finished drinking. Other questions such as how to smooth bedtime routines or address challenging behaviors also fall into this category. Parenting information shared with families should also be based on current research as opposed to a practitioner's preferences or own experiences.

Parent support may also be a regular topic during a visit. Early intervention practitioners assist families in identifying and making use of formal and informal resources to address their needs and priorities. The use of informal resources includes those that exist within a specific family's network, such as extended family members, churches, friends, and neighbors. Formal resources are those that are provided by federal, state, and local agencies to support specific needs of families within a specific demographic (e.g., county health departments, social services, food banks, early intervention). For example, practitioners can help families identify formal and informal resources for child care. Formal child care resources might include Early Head Start or Head Start, a child care program that accepts subsidies or vouchers, or a tuition-based center that the family can afford. Informal resources for child care could include a friend, extended family member, or neighbor. The practitioner will have conversations to support the parent in identifying, gaining access to, and evaluating a needed resource as a means to build the parent's capacity to address the need in this current situation as well as in the future. Serving as the resource (e.g., giving the family money, groceries, books, baby furniture, toys, rides to the physician's office) creates dependence on the practitioner instead of operationalizing sustainable resources and strategies that the family can use when the practitioner or program is no longer available. Early intervention practitioners may feel that other family needs and priorities take precedence over child learning and development, especially for families with ongoing complex circumstances. Early intervention is intended to encompass these types of supports that have a direct or indirect effect on the child. Families would naturally focus on basic needs such as housing, food, employment, transportation, utilities, and medical care before prioritizing child learning as a topic of early intervention support.

Component 3: Developing the Two-Part Joint Plan

The two-part plan must be developed at the end of each visit so that interventions will support the child and parent in achieving the IFSP outcomes. Determining what parents and/or caregivers agree to do between visits is the first part of the plan (i.e., Between-Visit Plan). This is typically developed based on the activities and discussion during this or previous visits and may also include activities the practitioner will do, such as identify a resource for a parent or child or find an answer to a parenting or medical question. Discussing the focus of the next visit and determining the activity setting/context, focus, time, and location is the second part of this two-part plan (i.e., Next-Visit Plan). Opportunities exist within each of these components for the parent and the practitioner to actively participate.

Following is an example of the three components of a visit using a PSP approach to teaming and a dedicated service coordination model.

Cindy and her three daughters, Ellie, age 4, Maggie, age 2, and Wendy, age 4 months and eligible for early intervention, live in a mobile home community in a suburb outside of a large metropolitan area. Wendy's physician referred her to early intervention because she has a diagnosis of lissencephaly (smooth brain surface) and needs therapy. Wendy's physician is also concerned with her weight gain and the risk of aspiration pneumonia related to her diagnosis.

INDIVIDUALIZED FAMILY SERVICE PLAN OUTCOMES

- Cindy will know that she is comfortable taking all three girls together to the playground at their mobile home park.

- Cindy will care for Wendy to keep her from becoming sick.

- Cindy will pursue her GED.

PRIMARY SERVICE PROVIDER

The team identified Paula, a PT, as the PSP for Wendy and her family because Paula's expertise and knowledge was the best match to the priorities identified by the family. Paula also has previous experience working with children with a diagnosis of lissencephaly.

ROLE ASSISTANCE

Paula and Cindy identified the need for support from Daniel, an SLP, to ensure Wendy is eating in a way that prevents aspiration pneumonia. Paula also requested support from Joanie, a service coordinator, to help identify resources to support Cindy's goal of obtaining her GED.

FREQUENCY OF SERVICE DELIVERY

Joanie (service coordinator) will visit the family home for 4, 1-hour visits between April 1, 2021, and July 1, 2021.

Paula (PT) will visit the family home for 16, 1-hour visits between April 1, 2021 and July 1, 2021.

Daniel (SLP) will visit the family home (with Paula) for 6, 1-hour visits between April 1, 2021 and July 1, 2021.

Joanie, Paula, Daniel, Maria, an OT, and Cecile, an early childhood special educator, will attend weekly, 1-hour PSP team meetings to support the children on their workloads.

Paula will begin obtaining an understanding of Cindy's current capabilities/understanding regarding the care of Wendy. Paula and Daniel will support Cindy in learning how to position Wendy, feed her, bathe her, watch for ear infections, and so forth. This will require assessing for and assisting in obtaining special equipment for Wendy. Paula and Daniel will also support Cindy in trips to the playground. They will go to the playground, observe Cindy's current approach, and support her in developing new skills and more confidence. This would most likely involve demonstration, ongoing assessment, equipment adaptation, and direct interaction by all of the adults as they discover the best way for Cindy to do this on her own. Joanie and Paula will also work together in supporting Cindy to identify and obtain resources needed for her to pursue her GED.

One to two months later, Paula is well into her visits with the family, and Cindy is ready to take a family trip to the playground. The Between-Visit Plan was for Cindy to get the items she would need to take to the playground and talk up the event with all three girls. Cindy was also writing down any questions or "what ifs" she could think of about the event. They would head to the playground during Paula's next visit, weather permitting.

COMPONENT 1

Cindy was packed and ready to go when Paula arrived. Wendy was in her stroller and was wearing her jacket, hat, and mittens. Maggie and Ellie were in the process of zipping up their coats. Cindy had packed a backpack with a small blanket and snacks for the girls. Cindy was obviously excited about the event and commented that the weather was perfect. Cindy had written down only one question about the trip. She was worried about what to do in case Wendy wet her diaper. She knew that it was not good for Wendy to be out in a wet diaper but felt it might be worse to change her while outside. Paula and Cindy talked this through and Cindy decided she would check on Wendy frequently while at the playground and, if and when she did wet her diaper, they would just return home.

COMPONENT 2

Cindy reminded Maggie and Ellie of the rules for walking outside, and the girls immediately clasped hands and headed out the front door. They problem-solved through several options but decided that having Ellie hold the front door was the best option for assisting Cindy to maneuver the stroller. Once out the door, following direct instruction from Paula regarding safe body mechanics, Cindy could easily carry the stroller down the four steps from their home. Paula noted Wendy's slumped position in her stroller as they walked to the playground. Paula and Cindy brainstormed ways to better position Wendy while in her stroller. Paula demonstrated how to position Wendy's pelvis and buckle the stroller belt for better support. Cindy then gave it a try and they both felt comfortable with Wendy's position and continued their walk to the park. Cindy was able to maneuver the stroller and keep track of the girls. Paula commented on Cindy's ability to keep the girls engaged by the questions she asked the girls while also keeping them focused on being safe. Ellie and Maggie ran toward the swings when they arrived at the playground. The playground swing set did not have an infant/toddler swing available. Cindy looked at Paula and asked what to do. Cindy could figure out how to swing Ellie and Maggie safely, but then Wendy would just be sitting in the stroller. Paula talked with Cindy about Cindy's vision of a successful fun time for all the girls. They discussed multiple possibilities. After Maggie and Ellie were tired of swinging, they moved toward the small slide. Maggie and Ellie were able to go up and down the slide on their own, so Cindy saw this as a great opportunity to get Wendy out of her stroller. Cindy asked several questions and tried several ways of holding Wendy on the slide, but she was not pleased with the results. Paula offered some suggestions and demonstrated some alternatives for Cindy to try. Cindy was able to successfully hold Wendy while being able to see her face and talk to her as she helped her slide down the few bottom feet of the slide. By this time, Wendy did have a wet diaper so the group decided to return home.

COMPONENT 3

After returning from the trip to the playground, Paula and Cindy discussed what went well and what additional supports/ideas she would like to pursue. The Between-Visit Plan that follows is a result of that conversation.

- Cindy will talk with the mobile home community manager about infant/toddler swings for the playground.

- Cindy will place a flyer in the community office to see if other mothers of young children are interested in meeting at the playground.

The Next-Visit Plan includes the following:

- Paula will bring some catalogs of playground equipment (infant/toddler swings) to the next visit.

- Cindy is not ready to go to the playground alone with the girls in between Paula's visits, but would like to go again on Paula's next visit in 2 days.

- Cindy will use the new position and stroller belt during all community outings.

Paula demonstrated the three components as a PSP in this scenario. She used her expertise and evidence-based knowledge related to body mechanics, positioning, child development, parent–child interaction, assistive technology, and parenting strategies for safely including an infant in the slide activity. This particular visit addressed two of the family's three IFSP outcomes. Paula's direct involvement with this family during the visit promoted child development and parenting support.

ROLE ASSISTANCE FOR THE PRIMARY SERVICE PROVIDER

Role assistance is necessary if the PSP or any other team member identifies a need for additional support in their role as the primary liaison between the family and the rest of the team. Role assistance can occur between the PSP and one or more team members as part of colleague-to-colleague coaching conversations outside of the team meeting, joint visits, and coaching during team meetings. Role assistance can also take the form of additional in-depth training for the PSP or any team member for an identified role gap situation.

A PSP can benefit from role assistance in several ways. The first opportunity is when the most likely PSP is selected (see Appendix 5E for the Worksheet for Selecting the Most Likely Primary Service Provider). Needs for role assistance are clearly identified by the time the team moves through the worksheet. Another need for role assistance could occur when a parent or care provider asks the PSP a question and they cannot answer or asks for direct access to another team member representing a discipline different from that of the PSP. For example, after talking with another family member, a parent asks her PSP, who happens to be an early childhood special educator, if the PT could come out to the home for a visit to observe her son's new preference for walking on his toes. The PSP schedules a time with the PT for a joint visit to address the parent's request.

Role assistance could be necessary when a PSP is supporting a child and family and feels stuck regarding additional ideas for helping the parent promote the child's participation during a specific activity setting (e.g., riding in the shopping cart safely at the grocery store). Sometimes when a child makes substantial progress or plateaus and a lack of progress is observed, the PSP may seek role assistance to ensure that they and the parents are doing everything possible to support the child's continued learning and development. Under limited circumstances, teams or programs may experience a situation in which no team member possesses a specific area of knowledge or expertise that is needed by the family, child, or PSP. For programs with more than one team, gaining access to the expertise from another team may be a short-term option. If no other internal option exists, then the team or program may gain access to a community or regional resource as a short-term solution. Long-term answers may include continuing education for one or more team members, contracting with new team members with specific expertise, and establishing a formal mentoring relationship between team members and an identified local, regional, or national resource.

REASONS TO CHANGE THE PRIMARY SERVICE PROVIDER FOR AN INDIVIDUAL CHILD AND FAMILY

One of the purposes for using a PSP approach to teaming is for the family to establish and maintain an ongoing working relationship with a liaison from the team to minimize any negative consequences of having multiple and/or changing practitioners while maximizing the positive benefits. The team considers many factors as they move through the process of selecting the most likely PSP, including the long-term view (up to 3 years) of the child and family in order to make the best possible initial, and perhaps only, decision regarding who will serve as the PSP. As a result, the

PSP rarely changes. The PSP does not necessarily change when IFSP outcomes change; important people, activity settings, or locations in the child's life change; or the PSP may need role assistance from other team members. The PSP should change if the family is uncomfortable with the manner or competence of the PSP or the PSP continually needs role assistance from another team member in the form of joint visits because of lack of knowledge, skill, or confidence. Programs may also be faced with decisions regarding billability of the PSP that may affect long-term sustainability of a particular discipline as the PSP for a specific child and family.

Following is an example of a primary coaching opportunity in a team meeting in which the current PSP, Haley (an OT and service coordinator), is requesting that she be replaced by Kelly, an SLP. Haley feels that she can no longer adequately support the child's needs. The purpose of this scenario is to depict a situation in which the team uses role assistance as a viable alternative to changing the PSP. The team meeting is currently in progress.

Haley:	I've put the Biddle family on the agenda. I have a big request. I feel like I need Kelly's help all of the time with Yolanda's needs. She's made so much progress with all of her other priorities. It's really just the communication aspect that her family is focused on at this time. I think Kelly should be the PSP for Yolanda and her family.
Shannon (EIC):	Haley, thanks for bringing this to the team. Let's think this through. What questions do the rest of you have for Haley?
Geoffrey (PT):	How long have you been supporting Yolanda and her family?
Haley:	Well, it's been over a year. Remember the Biddles adopted Yolanda from the Ukraine when she was 6 months old. She is now 23 months old, so I've been with them for almost a year and a half. We have been through a lot together. She's made so much progress. When she first arrived, they had so many challenges helping her adjust to her new life.
Misty Lynn:	(early childhood special educator) You really think it's best to change the PSP?
Kelly:	I was thinking the same thing. Haley, what's up? How can I support you?
Haley:	Basically I feel stuck. Yolanda is showing no progress in her language development. She just uses gestures or grunts. We've only heard about five words. I know that part of this situation is due to Yolanda learning English, but I'm just not sure I can be helpful.
Shannon:	Haley, what has made a difference when this has happened in the past?
Haley:	I can only think of one time that we actually changed the PSP. Do you remember Virginia and her situation? Remember that. Her grandmother just didn't feel comfortable with me. I can't think of another time that we've switched roles. I just feel like Yolanda's circumstances are different. I'm just not sure how to move forward.
Kelly:	What do you need from me?
Haley:	I'll first tell you that I'm doing everything I know to do. The mother, father, and grandmother are very responsive with Yolanda. They use labeling, waiting, making choices, and narrating, and they are playful and fun. Our focus has been playing outside and community outings, specifically going grocery shopping. We've been trying to use Yolanda's interest in helping her mother to support her communication.
Kelly:	Those activity settings and strategies all sound great. I can also talk with you and the Biddles about how learning English as a second language can affect communication development. How would you like to proceed?
Misty Lynn:	What do you want to do?

Haley: I'd like to do some joint visits with Kelly. I'll need to call Mrs. Biddle to see if that's okay. Kelly, what does your schedule look like late in the morning? I know she tries to run her errands in the mornings before Yolanda's nap, and that time of day would probably work great for a trip to the grocery store.

Kelly: It's pretty packed, but I could fit something in next Monday or Tuesday late in the morning. Would that work?

Haley: Let's hold Monday and I'll confirm with Mrs. Biddle.

Geoffrey: What do you want Kelly to be prepared for on the visit?

Haley: Well, I'd like her to watch us really closely. See what I'm missing and think of any ideas to share. Kelly, I want you to feel free to jump in if necessary.

Misty Lynn: Haley, what would you think of Kelly doing some videotaping? We could all watch the videotape at our next team meeting. That way we could all learn.

Haley: Hmmm. What do you think, Kelly?

Kelly: I'm game if you are. How will Mrs. Biddle react?

Haley: I'll check with her, but we've used video a lot in the past, so I think it will be fine.

Kelly: Okay, sounds good. What about meeting at the grocery store around 10:30 a.m.?

Haley: That should be fine. I'll double check with Yolanda's mom. Now, here's what I'm worried about. Kelly will go on a visit with me, tell me I'm doing a good job, and give me a few new ideas. I'll try the ideas and then in a few weeks I'll be back to feeling stuck—sort of like I'm not really doing anything. Does that make sense?

Shannon: We hear you, Haley. What are some options for preventing this from happening?

Geoffrey: I know it was helpful when I first started when Misty Lynn came with me for several consecutive visits. We then held off for a few weeks and then she came back in the burst of support strategy. I felt like we accomplished a great deal in a very short amount of time.

Haley: That's a good idea, Geoffrey. Kelly, what do you think? Could we pull this off over the next few months?

Kelly: I'm sure we can. We'll just need to be really specific with our scheduling so that I can block my calendar. I also like the videotaping idea. I'd like to brainstorm with you how this could be helpful.

Haley: Great. How about we talk a bit after our meeting today?

Kelly: Okay with me.

Shannon: So what's the plan regarding who will serve as PSP?

Haley: I'm going to continue, with Kelly supporting me as SSP for a burst of support over the next few months. We're also going to get permission from Mrs. Biddle to use the video camera across activity settings to see what we can learn. We will share the videotape at team meeting.

Geoffrey: Haley, how can we make sure that you stay comfortable in your role as PSP?

Haley: With the videorecording and the burst of support through joint visits, I'm feeling better already. I will update you all when we share the videotape at the team meeting. Thanks for your support.

The team was able to consider alternatives when the PSP was feeling inadequate in her ability to support the child and family. Through coaching support, the team identified role assistance strategies of using videotaping and a burst of support from the SLP through a series of carefully planned joint visits. The team was also looking forward to reviewing the videotape during team meetings to assist in supporting the PSP.

ROLE OF THE SERVICE COORDINATOR WHEN USING A PRIMARY SERVICE PROVIDER APPROACH

Case management for eligible children and families was included as a required service in the original authorization of early intervention in 1986 under The Education of the Handicapped Act Amendments (PL 99-457). *Service coordination* was introduced as the new term for case management in the Individuals with Disabilities Education Act (IDEA) of 1990 (PL 101-476). Federal legislation allows individual states to determine the model of service coordination used. Individual programs within some states are allowed to choose the service coordination model and may have a mixed approach within a given program. Dunst and Bruder (2006) identified three major approaches to service coordination in early intervention in a study of state models. First, the dedicated model involves an individual serving in the role of service coordinator only and is employed by an agency that is independent of service provision. Second, the intra-agency model uses a service coordinator only role, but the individual is employed by the same agency providing early intervention services. Third, the blended model provides service coordination through an early intervention practitioner. The study identified that dedicated models of service coordination were less effective than intra-agency and blended models regarding the implementation of evidence-based practices associated with service coordination in early intervention (Dunst & Bruder, 2006).

The type of service coordination model used by a state or program has direct implications on teaming, particularly when using a PSP approach. Using a PSP is based on research that indicates the fewest number of professionals involved in a family's life increases the likelihood of positive child and family outcomes (see Chapter 2; Dunst et al., 2007; Garcia-Grau et al., 2019; Greco & Sloper, 2004; Hughes-Scholes et al., 2015; Law et al., 1998; Shonkoff et al., 1992; Sloper, 2004). A blended model not only ensures better adherence to evidence-based service coordination practices, but it also inherently decreases the number of people involved with the child and family because the service coordinator and PSP are one and the same. Many of the issues related to access and availability of the service coordinators for team meetings and joint visits are minimized with blended and intra-agency models because they are employed by the same agency and should share the same philosophy, technical assistance opportunities, team culture, and so forth. The service coordinators' attendance at team meetings, availability for joint visits, and ability to support children and families as well as the PSP may be limited in a dedicated model. These limitations are typically due to the hiring agencies' provision of case management services for a variety of programs in the community (e.g., at-risk programs, health departments), method of payment for the service coordinator's time, and perceived value of team meeting time.

The roles of primary provider and service coordinator are combined on a team using a PSP approach with a blended model of service coordination. Logistically, using a blended model creates the need to use the Worksheet for Selecting the Most Likely Primary Service Provider from the point of initial contact in order to identify the service coordination role in conjunction with the possible PSP. The decision for who will serve as the primary provider occurs at the IFSP meeting. If the team determines that a person different from the individual who has been providing service coordination to this point would better meet the child and family's needs as primary provider, then the role of service coordinator can shift to the selected PSP. In this situation, the initial provision of service coordination is similar to using interim service coordination, which is not ideal but sometimes unavoidable. An added benefit of using a blended model of service coordination is the ability to bill for service coordination when the topic might not be otherwise billable by the discipline serving in the role of PSP (e.g., OT, PT, SLP). Regardless of the service coordination model, the individual fulfilling this role is responsible for all of the required duties, activities, and documentation. Training is necessary to understand the responsibilities, requirements, and evidence-based practices in fulfillment of service coordination as outlined in the federal regulations as well as how to balance the dual role.

The roles must complement one another in states and programs using dedicated and intra-agency models of service coordination and a PSP approach. The individuals serving in these roles must work closely together to define parameters of responsibility for when the PSP will address parent support issues that arise as part of the conversation during a regular visit. The PSP should address the issue if they have the knowledge, skills, and experience to do so, but, if role gap exists, then the service coordinator would provide role assistance in a timely manner. The service coordinator is typically viewed as the expert on the team for special skills and knowledge related to community resources and supports (e.g., waivers, employment resources, medical assistance, transportation). The service coordinator may need to visit the family without the PSP in situations in which parents identify the need for direct assistance that involves personal and/or confidential information, but the primary provider would know that the visit is occurring and why (e.g., parent support of completing Medicaid application, discussion of referral for mental health supports, assistance related to financial matters).

The decision regarding the model of service coordination used by states and programs is complex and can be influenced by funding mechanisms, systems issues (e.g., lead agency designation, interagency collaboration requirements, a centralized or decentralized Part C structure), and politics (Gomm, 2006). A PSP approach to teaming is possible, regardless of the service coordination model used. The degree of effect on using a PSP approach to teaming, however, is mitigated by the way in which service coordination is structured.

IMPLEMENTATION CHALLENGES AND SOLUTIONS

Challenges exist for programs when implementing a PSP approach to teaming. This section identifies some of the common challenges and misperceptions that can interfere with successful implementation of this teaming approach. The identified challenges include solutions that have assisted teams with implementation.

Making the Transition to a Primary Service Provider Approach to Teaming

Programs moving to the PSP approach to teaming often face challenges for the children and families enrolled in the program as well as the staff members assigned to support each child and family. The transition involves a process that begins with initiating the primary provider approach with children newly referred while changing the approach for children currently enrolled in the program at each child's upcoming IFSP review. The process can actually continue up to 6 months for some programs, which is a substantial amount of time to be juggling multiple teaming approaches. Implementing FAB scheduling with families in a primary provider approach while continuing to support other families with a more traditional type of scheduling can be stressful to practitioners because of the constraints of the traditional schedule. For example, the SLP may have a family currently enrolled that has traditionally received visits on Thursdays at 11:00 a.m. Newly enrolled families may have priorities that require visits around mealtime, and the requirement to continue to see the child and family on Thursdays at 11:00 a.m. limits the flexibility of the therapist's schedule to meet the needs of the newly enrolled family. In addition, the practitioners must make time in their schedules for team meetings, joint visits, evaluations, assessments, and IFSP meetings that may have not been a part of their regular week in the past. Making the transition from having multiple providers to a primary provider can feel like loss of services for many families. Some families may even view the change in service delivery as an effort to save money.

Because programs cannot close for a few days or transition all families simultaneously, the process of implementing a PSP approach to teaming must occur over time and does feel stressful to most team members. Newly enrolled families begin with this approach. Children preparing to exit the program within 6 months of the time the new approach was initiated should likely maintain their current IFSP service delivery unless the team members (including parents) feel otherwise. Programs should next identify children for the transition to a PSP approach to teaming in the order in which IFSP reviews are due. Programs should then consider those children with the fewest number of providers and have the option of requesting an early review of the IFSP to implement the new approach with the family's permission. Other solutions programs have used include identifying families that have expressed or demonstrated difficulty with having multiple providers. It may be more efficient for smaller programs to set a target date for transition and conduct IFSP reviews for all children enrolled in the program within the established time frame.

Open communication is the key to effectively support families through the transition from having multiple providers visit routinely to a PSP teaming approach. Families should be involved in the planning process and provided information to address their concerns and misperceptions that a primary provider approach means reducing the frequency and type of service their child receives. Some programs conduct family forums and develop specific brochures (see Appendix 5B for a sample brochure) to provide all families with factual information about the use of evidence-based practices, which includes the use of a primary provider teaming approach. All service coordinators must be prepared to provide information and answer questions to ensure that families understand that using a PSP does not necessarily equate to less service or only seeing one person, but, in fact, the PSP can visit as frequently as necessary and take other team members as needed to meet the ongoing and changing needs of the child and family.

One Discipline Always Serving as Primary Service Provider

Some programs always have one member serve as the primary provider (typically the individual representing the education role, such as early childhood special educator, early childhood educator, early intervention specialist, early interventionist, child development specialist, special instructor), regardless of whether they use a core team. One reason for this practice includes the prevalence of individuals filling these types of roles in combination with the lack of availability of individuals from other disciplines (e.g., OT, PT, SLP). Another reason for using the educator as the PSP is that the cost of hiring or contracting with therapists is typically higher than using an educator in this role. In addition, some programs have adopted the philosophy that educators have a more global view of children and families and can meet the needs of the majority of children enrolled in early intervention. Then, for those children requiring the involvement of therapists, OTs, PTs, and SLPs are contracted with to provide consultation to the educators.

The lack of availability of disciplines to work in early intervention is a tangible challenge. Solutions to meet this challenge are identified in Chapter 3. In situations in which therapists are available but funds are currently being used to support positions for educators, teacher/therapy assistants, and aides, programs have converted positions to create or increase the number of positions for therapy disciplines to equal (or approximate) the number of positions to support educators. For example, a large early intervention program in the Midwest had traditionally hired educators at a ratio of 3:1 (educators to therapists). The program decided to implement a PSP approach to teaming and developed a plan to reclassify educator and teacher assistant positions to therapy positions based on attrition of existing staff to rebalance their team configurations. To address the additional expense of therapists compared with educators, programs reconfigured existing resources to identify funds to hire or contract with therapists to establish core teams and equalize discipline representation. For those programs exclusively adopting the PSP as generalist, several assumptions exist on the part of the program: 1) the educator knows what the child and family need from all disciplines, and 2) the educator will ask for and receive timely support from other disciplines. This approach can also perpetuate the conception of a hierarchy in which therapists direct the educator regarding how to intervene with the child. Therefore, the solution is to develop geographically based, core multidisciplinary teams of approximately equal numbers of educators, OTs, PTs, SLPs, and other disciplines as available (e.g., nurses, nutritionists, psychologists, social workers) that are all available to serve in the capacity of a PSP. All team members are then available to support the PSP through attendance at regular team meetings and on joint visits with children and families.

Lack of Trust in Other Team Members

A lack of trust of one or more individuals regarding the abilities of another team member to serve as a PSP is a challenge for some teams. The absence of trust may be due to many factors, but it often involves deficient understanding of natural learning environment practices and teaming. In limited instances, however, the distrust may be due to a perceived lack of competence within the person's own discipline, child development, family support, parenting, and so forth. A symptom of this situation may involve an individual team member's belief that they should always serve as the PSP. This may occur because the practitioner thinks another team member is incapable of serving the child and family as well as they could. On the contrary, a team member may never volunteer to serve in the role of PSP due to similar beliefs that other team members may be unable to adequately support them in the role, or the practitioner does not trust themself to serve as the PSP. Solutions that support developing trust among team members include, but are not limited to, further development of team member knowledge and skills through professional development opportunities, joint visits, and team meetings; time for team members to work together; opportunities for shared experiences that allow team members to get to know one another personally and professional; and supervisory intervention as necessary for team members who are unable to fulfill the role of PSP.

Children Enrolled in the Early Intervention Program Receiving Outside Services

Families sometimes seek additional therapy services outside the early intervention program, regardless of the type of teaming approach used. Common reasons that families gain access to outside services include, but are not limited to, a family's belief that more services will result in faster progress, desire to ensure they are doing everything possible for their child, ability to pay for additional services, compliance with physician referral, and dissatisfaction with early intervention services. Whatever the reason, families have the right to gain access to services outside of early intervention, and the service coordinator may even be in the position to assist families in making informed decisions and gaining access to the additional services they want for their children. When families gain access to services outside of early intervention, it should not affect the type, frequency, and intensity of services that are provided by the early intervention program.

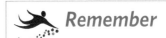 *Remember*

When families gain access to services outside of early intervention, it should not affect the type, frequency, or intensity of services that are provided by the early intervention program.

Teams using a PSP approach are often faced with at least three specific challenges when families seek services outside of the early intervention program. First, teams sometimes believe that the discipline selected to serve as the PSP should not or cannot be the same as the discipline providing service to the child outside of the early intervention program. Teams may be concerned about duplicating services, receiving payment for services, or providing conflicting information or recommendations to the family. Part C requires that early intervention provide the services necessary for the child to accomplish the identified outcomes on the IFSP. The *Mission and Key Principles for Providing Services in Natural Environments* (Workgroup on Principles and Practices in Natural Environments, 2007b) stipulated not only the location of service provision, but also how the services are implemented to support the entire family in promoting the child's growth and development. Services accessed by families outside of early intervention often occur in hospitals, clinics, or developmental centers and are therapist–child focused, which is not consistent with Part C. Services provided outside of early intervention should not factor into the decision of which discipline serves as the PSP and any SSPs identified on the IFSP.

A second challenge is the situation in which a PSP finds themself trying to help family members implement recommendations from the outside therapist(s). For example, a parent is struggling with a recommendation from the clinic-based PT to place dowel rods on the floor in the hallway and require the child to step over the dowels several times daily to improve the quality of the child's gait pattern. The parent purchased the dowel rods and attempted to follow the recommendation, but each time the child approached a dowel, he wanted to bend over and pick it up. The child would then be reprimanded, resulting in frustration for both the parent and child. The parent shared her problem with the PSP from early intervention and asked for help on enticing the child to step over the dowels and walk down the hallway. Some early intervention practitioners might feel compelled to spend time during the home visits to assist the parent in getting the child to comply. Rather than spending time on supporting decontextualized, nonfunctional exercises, the PSP and parent should focus their energies on supporting the child's participation in routines and activities that occur throughout each day. In this situation, the PSP and parent had already identified the child's interest in helping his mother; specifically, laundry time was something that the child really enjoyed. The parent and PSP recognized this as a potential learning opportunity, and the parent decided that she would expand their laundry routine by purposefully dropping articles of clothing down the hallway for the child to bend over, pick up, and carry as he followed his mother back and forth from the laundry room to the bedrooms. The frustration the parent and child experienced during the dowel rod maneuver completely disappeared during their laundry routine because the activity focused on the child's enjoyment of helping his mother with the laundry. Should the parent's requests for assistance with implementing outside therapy exercises continue, the PSP can engage the parent in a reflective conversation about how to approach the clinic-based therapist about the difficulty implementing the home program. Practitioners using this type of approach may encounter parents who attribute child progress to the outside therapy even if the treatment is nonevidence based because it may appear more tangible or real as it focuses on a specific child impairment. Parents may have difficulty in attributing child progress to their own actions within the context of normal routines and activities.

The belief that the child needs more therapy because they only have a PSP is the third, and perhaps the most commonly identified, challenge. The misperception by parents and practitioners is that using a PSP approach to teaming equates to only having access to one team member (i.e., one discipline) and that the frequency and intensity of the service provided is limited to the amount of service typically delivered by that discipline when using a multidisciplinary approach. The child and family have access to any and all team members (i.e., disciplines) in a PSP approach to teaming through joint visits with their PSP and team meetings. Using FAB scheduling does not limit the frequency and intensity of services, but, instead, it promotes flexible scheduling that focuses on prioritized, real-life activities and uses bursts of service as needed by the child and family.

A complicating factor for programs contracting with providers from local group therapy practices is the possibility for self-referral for the child to receive additional therapy outside of early intervention within the contracted therapist's own practice. Although this practice may occur regardless of the teaming approach used, using a PSP approach may exacerbate this practice due to this misperception. A simple solution is to include a provision in all contracts that disallows the contracting practitioner to refer children enrolled in early intervention to the group practice with which they are associated to prevent any real or perceived conflict of interest.

Differences in Teaming Approaches Across Programs

Programs within and across states that use different approaches to teaming are a challenge for families and early intervention practitioners. For instance, a program in the western part of a state uses a multidisciplinary, vendor-based approach to teaming. A family moves across the state and enrolls in a program that uses a PSP approach to teaming. The family may be confused because the program can be implemented so differently within the state's Part C early intervention program. This situation places the responsibility for justifying the use of practices that are consistent with the *Mission and Key Principles of Providing Early Intervention Services in Natural Environments* (Workgroup on Principles and Practices in Natural Environments, 2007b) on the receiving program, and the family and new program begin their relationship under challenging circumstances. Generally, the solution to this situation is for all early intervention programs to implement practices that are supported by Part C federal regulations and the mission and key principles, which include using a primary provider (Principle 6) and

 Take Action

If you are using a primary service provider approach to teaming, how could you and your team members refine your practices (based on this chapter)?

evidence-based practices (Principle 7). Specifically, states that allow programs to implement varying service delivery and teaming approaches should provide materials that support and explain the approved options and examples of the variability that occurs across the state.

CONCLUSION

After reading this chapter, it may be more apparent why implementing a PSP approach to teaming is a process that occurs over time. The process involves each team member developing a deeper understanding of the role of a PSP and how to explain the role to families, physicians, and other referring agencies. The process begins with carefully considering the four factors used to identify the most likely PSP in preparation for final selection at the IFSP meeting. Selecting the PSP is based on role expectation of all potential PSPs' understanding of child development, parenting, and parent support in addition to special skills and knowledge needed. Selecting the primary provider also involves identifying any needs for role assistance based on role gap and role overlap discussed during the process. This deliberate selection process, which includes a long-term perspective, decreases the likelihood that the PSP will need to change. The role of the PSP is to support the achievement of IFSP outcomes by using evidence-based strategies and techniques to promote parent mediation of child participation in prioritized activity settings, which results in development of desired skills and behaviors. The model of service coordination selected by a state and/or program drives how the role is implemented and has direct implications for the teaming process. Although programs and practitioners face challenges to using a PSP approach to teaming, solutions exist to overcome the real and perceived barriers of implementation and can improve the overall quality of early intervention services.

Primary Service Provider Approach to Teaming Fact Sheet

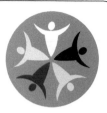

- Every family receives support from a geographically based, multidisciplinary team that minimally consists of an educator, occupational therapist, physical therapist, service coordinator, and speech-language pathologist. Additional disciplines may also be available to serve on the team, depending on the program.

- In a system using dedicated service coordinators, the primary service provider (PSP) and service coordinator work closely together to accomplish the individualized family service plan (IFSP) outcomes.

- All team members (with the exception of the dedicated service coordinator) are available to potentially serve as a PSP.

- All team members are expected to have basic knowledge of child development across all domains and how to promote child learning and participation within the context of everyday life activities in the home, community, and early childhood setting and parent supports (e.g., health care, transportation, education, basic needs).

- One team member is selected by the team, which includes the family, to serve as the PSP. This is the team member the family will see on a regular basis to assist them in achieving the IFSP outcomes.

- The PSP is selected to keep the long-term view (potentially up to 3 years of child/family involvement with the early intervention program) in mind and is based on a combination of family, child, environmental, and practitioner factors.

- The final decision of PSP is determined at the IFSP meeting.

- The frequency of the PSP's visits and joint visits with other team members is based on the current needs of the child/family and is flexible, activity based (different days and times), and may include bursts of service as necessary.

- The PSP receives ongoing support from other team members during informal conversations, team meetings, and joint visits.

- Joint visits occur with both team members and the family present and during the activity setting in which the child, family, or PSP need support in promoting the child's participation.

- The PSP uses evidence-based intervention practices to promote parent mediation of child participation within the context of everyday routines and activities using toys and materials existing in the environment and assistive technology introduced by the team as needed.

- All members attend the regular team meeting, which occurs no less than every other week.

- Each child is discussed in the regular team meeting at least quarterly and more frequently if the PSP and/or family have a question and/or need support from another team member.

- Because working with families is relationship based, the PSP rarely changes, but they may do so if the child's/family's situation changes so dramatically that another team member would be the best match for the family. The PSP does not change just because the child's IFSP outcomes change or are accomplished and new outcomes are developed.

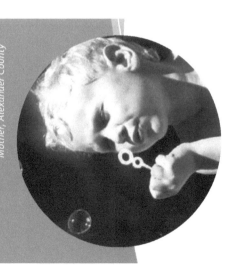

What parents are saying

"We were very happy with all the contact we had with FIPP [and] very pleased with all the services....If it had not been for information from FIPP we would have been lost. No one – schools, teachers, or doctors – had the information or could give us the support we got from FIPP staff."

Father & Mother, Mc Dowell County

"FIPP [has been] a life-changing experience for me...I was equipped by the time I left with excellent parenting strategies that really worked for my child."

Mother, Alexander County

FIPP provides early intervention and family support practices tailored to each family's life circumstances.

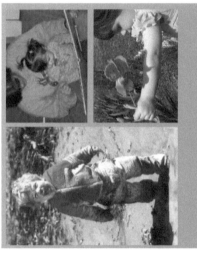

What our research says

95% of parents report that FIPP staff are knowledgeable and helpful about child learning and parenting.

96% of families served by FIPP report that their children made considerable progress in their development as a result of their involvement in FIPP.

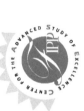

Family, Infant and Preschool Program
300 Enola Road
Morganton, NC 28655

828-433-2661 • 800-822-3477

Family, Infant & Preschool Program Morganton, North Carolina

(continued)

Who we are

The Family, Infant & Preschool Program (FIPP) is a regional early childhood development and family support program serving women who are pregnant as well as infants and toddlers from birth to age five who are at-risk or have developmental disabilities and their families. FIPP provides resources and supports in Alexander, Burke, Caldwell, Catawba, and McDowell Counties in western North Carolina. FIPP has provided services to eligible children and their families since 1972.

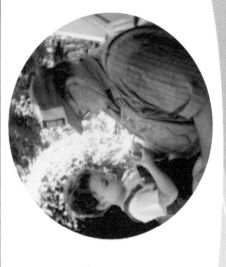

What we do

FIPP is committed to supporting young children and their families using the most effective practices currently available in early intervention.

Teachers, therapists, and family service coordinators at FIPP:

Use evidence-based practices to guide their support.

Use child and family interests as the foundation for intervention.

Focus on enhancing child participation in existing and desired family, community, and early childhood experiences.

Support each family with an identified team of early childhood professionals that includes: early childhood educators, nurses, occupational therapists, physical therapists, psychologists, service coordinators, and speech-language pathologists.

Select one member of the team as the primary service provider to meet with families, child care providers, and teachers in real-life settings (i.e., home, school, child care, preschool, park, store, etc.) with support from other team members as needed.

Partner with parents and other care providers to support them in learning new things and doing what they already do even better to help the child learn and grow.

Help families find answers to tough questions.

Help parents find resources that match what they are looking for.

Believe learning is fun!

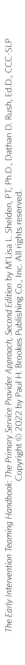

Early Childhood Intervention Physician's Progress Report

Child's name: _____   Date of birth: _____

Physician: _____   Date of report: _____

☐   Family does not want to enroll with our services.

Support or intervention child is receiving	Child progress
☐ Early childhood intervention	Enrolled date:
☐ Evaluation/assessment	
☐ Family support	
☐ Occupational therapy	
☐ Physical therapy	
☐ Speech-language therapy	
☐ Assistive technology	
☐ Other (oral-motor intervention, nutrition, nursing, social work, psychological services)	

If you have any questions regarding this report, please review it with the family or contact the individual below.

(Print) _____   (Signature) _____   _____
          Staff member   Date

From The Family, Infant and Preschool Program (FIPP) Center for the Advanced Study of Excellence (CASE), part of the J. Iverson Riddle Developmental Center (JIRDC) in Morganton, NC; reprinted by permission. Copyright © 2013 Family, Infant and Preschool Program.

The Early Intervention Teaming Handbook: The Primary Service Provider Approach, Second Edition by M'Lisa L. Shelden, PT, Ph.D., Dathan D. Rush, Ed.D., CCC-SLP

Early Childhood Intervention Physician's Progress Report

Child's name: __LaShawn Moore__   Date of birth: __2/08/19__

Physician: __Dr. Christina Campbell__   Date of report: __4/05/20__

☐   Family does not want to enroll with our services.

Support or intervention child is receiving	Child progress
☐ Early childhood intervention	Enrolled date: **06/26/19**
☐ Evaluation/assessment	01/1/20–03/31/20: Visited family's home for 9 of 10 scheduled 1-hour visits. Mrs. Moore cancelled 1 visit due to family illness. The speech-language pathologist was present during 2 visits to support LaShawn and his mother related to communication strategies to use during mealtime.
☐ Family support	Based on our visits this quarter, LaShawn's parents now both feel comfortable placing him in his highchair during family meals. I made a foam seat insert for LaShawn's highchair, which is working well at maintaining him in an upright position. Prior to using the insert, LaShawn was unable to sit in the chair and was fed prior to family meals. LaShawn now joins the family at all mealtimes, is feeding himself finger foods, drinks from a cup with a lid, and only takes a bottle at night. The family is now interested in taking LaShawn out to a restaurant to eat.
☐ Occupational therapy	
☑ Physical therapy	
☑ Speech-language therapy	Prior to our visits this month, bath time was not going well. LaShawn was quickly bathed while screaming and crying. We were able to use a small, inflatable inner tube for LaShawn to sit in during bath time. He immediately liked it, and Mrs. Moore was able to support LaShawn's play during bath time with no crying.
☐ Assistive technology	
☐ Other (oral-motor intervention, nutrition, nursing, social work, psychological services)	LaShawn has shown progress this month related to independent sitting during floor play, getting in and out of sitting on his own while playing with his toys, and pulling up to standing next to the bathtub with minimal assistance.

If you have any questions regarding this report, please review it with the family or contact FIPP.

(Print) _____M'Lisa L. Shelden_____   (Signature) _____M'Lisa L. Shelden, PT_____   ___4/05/20___
          FIPP Staff   Date

Worksheet for Selecting the Most Likely Primary Service Provider

Core team as options for primary service provider (PSP)

Early childhood (EC) _____   Occupational therapist (OT) _____

Physical therapist (PT) _____   Speech-language pathologist (SLP) _____   Other _____

Most likely PSP(s) identified based on

	Parent/family factors	Child factors	Environmental factors	Practitioner factors	Most likely PSP options selected (list)	Secondary service provider (SSP) options selected (list)
Tier 1	List priorities with contexts

List parent/physician request | List diagnosis/condition/needs (long-term view)

List interests/activity settings | Circle natural learning environments
• Home
• Community
• Preschool
• Child care
• Other | List knowledge/expertise (personal/professional) | | Role overlap |
| **Tier 2** | Family dynamics

Individual parent/caregiver characteristics
• Language/culture
• Knowledge/expertise
• Diagnosis/condition
• Other | | Safety
Distance from program office | Primary service area in geographic region
Billability
Prior relationship
Rapport | | Role overlap |
| **Tier 3** | Availability | Availability | Availability | Availability | | Role overlap |

Most likely PSP is:

Role gap? If so, explain:

Role assist (SSP):

Notes:

The Early Intervention Teaming Handbook: The Primary Service Provider Approach, Second Edition by M'Lisa L. Shelden, PT, Ph.D., Dathan D. Rush, Ed.D., CCC-SLP

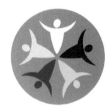

Mitchell Family Case Study

EXAMPLE 1

The early intervention team for the area serving the Mitchell family is responsible for about 100 families. They serve a five county area, and the drive to the Mitchell's house from the office is about 45 minutes (one way). The team uses a blended service coordination model and a primary service provider (PSP) approach to teaming. Their local team currently consists of the following members.

- One full-time early intervention coordinator (EIC) (Greta). Greta has worked for the early intervention program for 20 years. She is the first (and only) EIC for this area. She is from the area and is a well-respected leader in the community. She is divorced and has three grown children, two living close by. She has 12 grandchildren and spends as much time as she can with them. Greta is an avid Seahawks fan.

- One full-time early childhood special educator (Mandi). Mandi has 2 years of experience working in early intervention. She is 30 years old and has a master's degree from an in-state university. She is single and her favorite activities are sewing her own clothes and quilting. Mandi previously worked in a program supporting parents of newborns with disabilities. She prefers indoor activities to outdoor activities.

- One full-time occupational therapist (OT) (Roger). Roger is 42 years old and has lived in this area his entire life. He has a master's degree from a state university and has worked in early intervention for almost 15 years. Roger grew up on a farm. He is married to his high school sweetheart and has nine children. Roger is the team's feeding specialist and has a lot of experience working with children with sensory needs.

- Two physical therapists (PTs) (Ginger works 2 days per week and Martine is full time). Ginger works full time for the regional hospital, and the hospital contracts with the early intervention program for Ginger to work with them 2 days each week. Ginger is 55 years old, has a master's degree in physical therapy, and has worked in pediatrics for about 10 years. Ginger was a PT assistant and went back to school for her physical therapy degree about 15 years ago so she could work with young children. She is divorced, recently moved to the area, and has worked at this hospital for about 9 months. Ginger is very comfortable with all aspects of pediatric physical therapy.

  Martine is 26 years old. This is her first job as a PT. She has a doctorate in physical therapy from an out-of-state university. She had always wanted to move out to the country and accepted this position to do so. She is recently married and has no children. Martine is very athletic and runs marathons to stay in shape. She completed an elective fieldwork experience in her physical therapy program in an orthotics lab.

- Two part-time speech-language pathologists (SLPs) (Tristan works 2 days per week and Stella works 3 days per week).

Tristan is originally from the area and moved back last year. He is 35 years old, married, and has twin boys that are 18 months old. He works 3 days a week for the local school district. Tristan grew up on a farm but currently lives in town near the early intervention office. Tristan has extensive experience in the area of augmentative and alternative communication.

Stella is new to the area. She works for a traveling therapist practice and agreed to accept this position for 2 years. She works 2 days each week for the regional hospital where Ginger works. Stella is single, has no children, and is new to small-town life. She is 28 years of age, is an avid reader, and loves to cook. Stella is very comfortable working with children with feeding issues and does not have much experience with assistive technology.

Greta received the telephone call from Mrs. Mitchell late on Wednesday afternoon. Greta was aware that the Mitchells were moving back to the area. Greta's parents are long-time friends of the Mitchell family, and Greta's younger brother is actually a friend of Mr. Mitchell. Mrs. Mitchell was calling about her youngest son, Ezra. He has a diagnosis of cerebral palsy and had been enrolled in an early intervention program in another part of the state. Greta knew that she needed some basic information from Mrs. Mitchell in order to get the team member who might be the PSP involved with the Mitchells as early in the process as possible. Greta inquired about the family and asked Mrs. Mitchell to share why she had called. Greta also asked generally about the Mitchell family routines as well as what they enjoyed doing together. Greta knew that the team would be meeting on Friday and told Mrs. Mitchell that someone from the team would be in contact with them following the meeting on Friday to begin gathering more information. Based on her telephone call with Mrs. Mitchell, Greta shared the following information with the team.

The Mitchell family lives in a rural, isolated part of the county, and Mrs. Mitchell home-schools all five of her children. Mr. Mitchell is a farmer and has recently moved the family back home to operate his great-grandparents' family farm. The youngest son, Ezra, a 2-year-old, has cerebral palsy and uses a wheelchair, a stander, or just rolls around on the floor, depending on the time of day and what the rest of the family members are doing. Ezra is described as a happy boy by his mom. He has three older brothers and a younger sister; Malakai (15 years old); Isaiah (13 years old); Elijah (10 years old); and Rebekah (4 months old). Ezra was enrolled in an early intervention program in another part of the state prior to the family's recent move. Mrs. Mitchell has Ezra's current individualized family service plan (IFSP) and a copy of all of his paperwork. According to the IFSP, Ezra was receiving weekly visits from the PT and SLP, and the early childhood special educator visited them twice monthly. Mrs. Mitchell shared that Ezra had recently been evaluated by an OT who had planned to start seeing Ezra weekly, but they did not have time to get therapy started prior to the family's move. Mrs. Mitchell explained that Ezra's therapists usually worked with him while she was schooling the older children. When asked to describe Ezra further, Mrs. Mitchell stated that he smiles all the time and says one word, *mom*. She explained that the family can tell what Ezra likes by the degree to which he laughs and smiles. When asked how he participates in family activities, Ezra's mom proudly explained that there is nothing he cannot do with the family. He participates in everything the family is doing by watching. When Greta asked Mrs. Mitchell what they would like to see Ezra doing, she stated that she needed some ideas on how to involve him in homeschool activities and family chores. When Greta asked for more detailed information, Mrs. Mitchell also indicated that the family spent a lot of time outdoors and all of the children had chores, except the infant. She stated that they all struggle with how to include Ezra, especially in the outdoor activities.

Greta shared with the team that she took the opportunity to explain to Mrs. Mitchell that the program in this part of the state was different than where Ezra had previously been enrolled. She described that the approach in this area emphasized evidence-based practices that relied on parent involvement and using natural learning opportunities as the basis for intervention as well as a PSP approach to teaming. She further explained to the team that Mrs. Mitchell particularly liked the notion of the early intervention team helping her find ways to include Ezra in all of the family's activities. She also said, however, that she does not really know how it is possible because Ezra cannot walk, talk, or even sit up without assistance. Greta shared further that Mrs. Mitchell was somewhat skeptical of having a primary provider but was open to the idea. She admitted that the visits from all of the other providers in their previous program were a lot to manage.

Let's listen in on the team as they discuss options for the most likely PSP/family service coordinator:

Greta:	So that's all we know now. I told Mrs. Mitchell that we would pick up the records on our first visit with her. I thought we should take a look at those records before I call the other program.
Martine:	That sounds good, Greta. I'm glad you took the opportunity to talk about our approach. It sounds really different than what the Mitchells have experienced.
Greta:	Thanks, Martine. They will need to hear all of it again. As you stated, we do things very differently than their previous program.
Stella:	Well, I already see Nettie and her family. They live out that way. We've been really busy lately because Nettie has been making so much progress. I've been out there pretty regularly, at least twice a week. I'm not sure that I'm really the best match. Tristan is our go-to guy for augmentative and alternative communication and it sounds like Ezra is most likely a candidate.
Greta:	Hang on, guys. Let's think this through using our new worksheet. This seems like a good opportunity for being systematic about this process. I also think this will assist us as we continue to discuss our teaming approach with the Mitchells.
Tristan:	I was thinking the same thing, Stella. The information that you shared is really about us (the practitioners). How do we shift our thinking to focus first on the Mitchell family and Ezra before we jump in with our availability and expertise?
Martine:	It's tough. I was going to the same place in my head, too. Let's get the worksheet out and really give this a try.
Greta:	Great job, guys. Here is the worksheet. Tier 1, Factor 1, is parent/family factors. This comprises the family's priorities or requests, including anything we might receive from the physician.
Mandi:	Okay, then, we don't know much. How do we proceed?
Greta:	Let's write down what we know. First off, you are all going to be listed up at the top of the worksheet.
Stella:	Even if we don't have time in our schedule?
Greta:	Yes. Everyone is an option as we begin our discussion. We'll talk about individual availability as a final factor in Tier 3.
Tristan:	Okay. We know that Mrs. Mitchell homeschools all of the older children and wants ideas for how to include Ezra. We know that Mr. Mitchell is out working on the farm, but we'll need more detail about all of that. We know that the entire family spends a good deal of time outside and that Mrs. Mitchell said they all have a tough time trying to figure out how to include Ezra.
Greta:	Nice summary, Tristan. What else can we think of related to the parent/family factors in Tier 1?
Roger:	We know that Ezra was receiving ECSE, PT, and SLP services and that the family had just received an order from the physician for OT. So, is this where we take that into consideration?

Greta: Yes. I think that does fit here. What else?

Ginger: I think we're ready to move onto child factors. Let's list all of that equipment that Ezra already has in place. Greta, did you say a wheelchair and a standing frame?

Greta: Yes, and there might be additional items. Mrs. Mitchell just happened to mention these specific items.

Ginger: She also said that he can't walk, talk, or really move very well on his own. The fact that he's 24 months old and already has this type of equipment makes me think that he probably has quadriplegia. We'll have to just go with this for now until we lay our eyes on him.

Tristan: Ginger, I was thinking the same thing. I'm really interested in what approach they're taking with Ezra's communication. If he does have spastic quadriplegia or athetoid-type cerebral palsy, then he will probably have substantial long-term assistive technology needs in this area.

Roger: We'll definitely need to assess, but if we're going with this line of thinking, then his independence related to self-care and all of the issues related to eating are probably going to surface.

Greta: Great discussion. What about Ezra's interests and activity settings? What do we know?

Mandi: Not much. We know that his mom wants to include him in homeschooling, but we don't know anything about what Ezra likes or wants to do.

Roger: Same with outside. We don't even know if he likes going outside, but if his family is always out and about, we'll need to think about ways for Ezra to participate.

Stella: I just feel like we need so much more information.

Greta: We do. Definitely. Remember, this is just to get us started. So, this is a nice segue to environmental factors. What do we know?

Martine: Well, we know he's at home on the farm. We don't know much more.

Greta: The rest of the extended family attends my church. I have a hunch they will too. We'll just need to ask. I think it is important to note that he doesn't attend child care. So we don't have to worry right now about contacting anyone regarding involvement in the IFSP process.

(See Table 5F.1 for the factors just discussed for Ezra.)

Mandi: It sounds like we're ready to talk about where we all fit in. So, let's take a look at our knowledge and expertise—professional and personal. I have to jump in and say that I'm feeling a bit overwhelmed. I just keep thinking about all of those activity settings—the farm, all the kids, all of Ezra's needs. What do you guys think about all of the equipment he has? I would really need a lot of help with all of that. I feel like I wouldn't really know where to start.

Ginger: I feel really comfortable helping address all of the equipment issues, but I am not sure it is the best use of my time to drive all the way out there when I'm only available 2 days a week.

Greta: Ginger, you began with sharing your expertise and knowledge, but it shifted to your availability. We have a lot more to talk about before we get there.

Ginger: Oops! You're right. This is really challenging to separate the two issues. I'm surprised at how much I've been thinking about my schedule.

(The team all comments on the same idea of how pervasive the issue of the practitioners' availability looms as they consider the possibilities of who might serve as primary provider.)

Table 5F.1.   Individualized family service plan factors for the Mitchell family

Tier	Parent/family factors	Child factors	Environmental factors
Tier 1	Ideas for homeschooling Ezra How to include Ezra in chores (feeding the horses, watering/feeding the dogs) Help Ezra to be more independent (eating). Mrs. Mitchell would like time to spend with Rebekah while the boys include Ezra in enjoyable activities (fishing, riding the four-wheeler, riding the horses). Previously received early childhood special education, physical therapy, speech-language therapy, and occupational therapy was soon to begin	Ezra is 2 years old. Ezra has cerebral palsy (quadriplegia). Ezra lights up when his siblings and parents interact with him. Ezra loves to hold Rebekah. Ezra enjoys being outside. Ezra loves the dogs and horses (petting and feeding them).	Ezra spends all of his time at home and with the family at church on Sundays. Parents and Rebekah visit extended family on a neighboring farm once monthly for dinner while Malakai cares for the other children.
Tier 2	Family members include • Mrs. Mitchell (Mary) • Mr. Mitchell (Jeb) • Malakai (brother; 15 years old) • Isaiah (brother; 13 years old) • Elijah (brother; 10 years old) • Rebekah (sister; 4 months old) Mary homeschools all children Family occupation is farming, and the three older boys assist with chores		Live 45 miles from early intervention office on their farm
Tier 3	Mary is available any time Monday through Friday Jeb is available at lunchtime (11:30 a.m.) and evenings (after 6:00 p.m.) Homeschool schedule is • 8:30 a.m.–11:30 a.m. • 12:30 p.m.–2:30 p.m.		

Greta: I agree. The availability consideration is an important one. It's just that we're jumping to it too soon.

Martine: So, I feel comfortable supporting the family, but I'm trying to keep the long-term perspective. Maybe I could go in and help the PSP with all of the equipment needs up front.

Roger: Well, I've been thinking along the same lines. I'd love to step in and serve as the primary for Ezra and his family. You guys know that I'm comfortable with a lot of kids being around (having nine myself), and you also know that my wife homeschools our children. Also, I've lived on a farm all my life, so I would feel right at home. I'm just worried about all the time he might need, and I know that I would need some help from Tristan, early on, related to the communication issues.

Greta: Everyone remember, we're not making the decision without the Mitchells and before we write the IFSP outcomes. We just want to be thinking about the best options from our point of view. Who else feels comfortable addressing the priorities we know about at this time?

Stella: Well, I'm definitely comfortable with the feeding issues, but so is Roger. I'm not the one to help with the augmentative and alternative communication issues that we'll probably face. I also can't say that I'm too excited about tromping around on the farm. I wonder if they have horses?

Mandi: Me neither. I'm nervous about dogs, too.

(The team members all laugh together.)

Greta:	This is good discussion. This is where this all fits together. So, let's write out to the side here who we think we're still considering as most likely PSP.
Roger:	I think I'm in.
Tristan:	Me, too.
Ginger:	I'm not sure how this works, but I think that both Martine and I might be in. But I think we're really better for secondary support. What do you guys think?
Roger:	That makes more sense to me.
Greta:	Then I'll write Roger and Tristan in for PSP and Ginger and Martine in for SSP. Stella and Mandi, does this make sense to you?
Stella and Mandi:	Yes (in unison).
Greta:	Now we're to Tier 2, family dynamics. What do we know here?
Ginger:	I don't think we really know anything here. What do the rest of you think?
Roger:	I agree. Greta, can we just move on?
Greta:	Yes. I think this just emphasizes how much work we have to do to get to know the family. Safety and distance from the office is the next factor to reconsider on Tier 2. We know it is about a 45-minute drive on a clear, no-tractor-on-the-roads day.
	(The team members laugh about the issues they face driving country roads.)
Tristan:	We don't have any safety concerns at this point, but that drive is a big issue for us regarding availability. Can we talk about that now?
Greta:	Not really. We need to consider issues such as prior relationship, rapport with the family, and billing. We can certainly bill for anyone's services. Don't you all agree?
	(The team confirms that billing isn't a complicating factor, initially, but needs to be considered for the future.)
Roger:	This seems premature because we haven't met the family. Do we revisit this once we start the process?
Greta:	Absolutely. We'll keep these factors in mind as we move forward with the family. So, has our list changed regarding Tier 2?
Team:	No.
Greta:	Tier 3 is . . .
Team:	Availability! (The team members laugh, as this is a new way of thinking for them.)
Greta:	Yes. But first, it's about the family's and child's availability. What do we know?
Martine:	Do we know anything?
Roger:	I think we can probably assume this family won't require regular evening visits because of Mrs. Mitchell's request about homeschooling and outside time. We'll need to be open, but it seems that visits during the day will be an option.
Ginger:	What about our availability?
Tristan:	I feel like I have the expertise to support Ezra and his family, but my schedule is really packed. I'm not sure that I can meet all of their needs and expectations at this point and time.

Roger:	I have time in my schedule and I'm already out that way a few times each week. Like I said, Tristan, I know I'm going to need help from you.
Tristan:	I know. I'm going to take a hard look at my schedule to see when I can free up some time. I can definitely find some time for joint visits.
Ginger:	Roger, how comfortable are you checking out all of the assistive technology already in place?
Roger:	I'm very comfortable looking at how it fits and how the family is currently using the different pieces of equipment to support Ezra's participation. I will need some help with the wheelchair. But we don't have to do that right away. I'm really anticipating needing some assistance regarding Ezra's communication. How about I contact Mrs. Mitchell, explain the program again, and schedule to go out on Tuesday morning if she is available? I'll get the paperwork started and really try to move on to the functional assessment. I'll also check out specifically if it's okay for both Tristan and I to come out together. Sometimes, it can be uncomfortable for a mom with two male practitioners. In fact, Greta, what do you think about calling her back to ask about that? That way, if she does have some discomfort, then she won't feel pressure from me and we can move to an alternate plan.
Greta:	I think that's a good idea. I can also check out how much Mr. Mitchell is going to be involved. And I know the older boys will be around, so that should help out too.
	(See Table 5F.2.)
Martine:	It sounds good to me. Roger, what support do you need from Ginger or I?
Roger:	As I said, I'll need some help with the wheelchair, but I feel okay about getting started, unless anything comes up right away.
Martine:	How about I serve as your backup on the equipment because I've got more flexibility in my schedule. Does that sound okay, Ginger?
Ginger:	Sounds excellent to me.
Greta:	Let's summarize. Roger, it appears that based on what we know now, you are our best option for the most likely PSP with support from Tristan and Martine. Is this correct?
Team:	Yes, all good.
Greta:	Okay, then I'll call Mrs. Mitchell and then contact you, Roger. Will you be around this afternoon?
Roger:	Yes, I'll be back by about 2:30.
	(See Figure 5F.1)

Worksheet for Selecting the Most Likely Primary Service Provider

Core team as options for primary service provider (PSP)

Early childhood (EC) __Mandi__ Occupational therapist (OT) __Roger__

Physical therapist (PT) __Martine, Ginger__ Speech-language pathologist (SLP) __Tristan, Stella__ Other _____

	Most likely PSP(s) identified based on			Most likely PSP options selected (list)	Role gap? If so, explain:	Secondary service provider (SSP) options selected (list)
	Parent/family factors	Child factors	Environmental factors	Practitioner factors		
Tier 1	List priorities with contexts *How to include Ezra in family activities* List parent/physician request *Received early childhood special education, physical therapy, speech-language therapy, and referred for occupational therapy*	List diagnosis/condition/needs (long-term view) *Diagnosis of cerebral palsy* *Has wheelchair and standing frame* List interests/activity settings *Homeschool activities*	Circle natural learning environments • (Home) • Community • Preschool • Child care • Other	List knowledge/expertise (personal/professional) *Martine/Ginger: Equipment* *Roger: Large family, homeschooling, lives on a farm, feeding* *Tristan: Augmentative and alternative communication*	*Roger* *Tristan*	Role overlap	*Ginger* *Martine*
Tier 2	Family dynamics Individual parent/caregiver characteristics • Language/culture • Knowledge/expertise • Diagnosis/condition • Other		Safety Distance from program office *Distance from program office is 45 minutes*	Primary service area in geographic region Billability Prior relationship Rapport	*Roger* *Tristan*	Role overlap	*Ginger* *Martine*
Tier 3	Availability *Family has a flexible schedule*	Availability	Availability	Availability *Tristan: Full caseload* *Roger: Has time available*	*Roger*	Role overlap	*Tristan* *Martine*
Notes:					**Most likely PSP is:** *Roger*	**Role gap?** If so, explain: *N/A*	**Role assist (SSP):** *Tristan* *Martine*

Figure 5F.1. The first team's Worksheet for Selecting the Most Likely Primary Service Provider

Table 5F.2. Environmental and practitioner factors for the first team

Tier	Environmental factors	Practitioner factors
Tier 1	Ezra spends all of his time at home and with the family at church on Sundays. Parents and Rebekah visit extended family on a neighboring farm once monthly for dinner while Malakai cares for the other children.	Greta is the early intervention coordinator and has been an early childhood special educator for 20 years. She is divorced with 3 grown children and 12 grandchildren, has lived in the local area her entire life, and is an avid Seahawks fan. Mandi is a full-time early childhood special educator with 2 years of experience. She is 30 years old with a master's degree from an in-state university, is not married, loves to sew/quilt, is not an outdoor person, is new to the area, and has previous experience working with parents of newborns with disabilities. Roger is a full-time occupational therapist (OT) with 15 years of experience. He is 42 years old, has lived in the local area his entire life (grew up on a farm), has a master's degree from an out-of-state university, is married with 9 children, is a team feeding specialist, and enjoys working with children with sensory needs. Martine is a new, full-time physical therapist (PT). She is 26 years old and this is her first job as a PT. She earned a Doctor of Physical Therapy (DPT) from an in-state university. She is recently married, has no children, is new to the area (first time to live in the country), and has completed an internship in an orthotics lab. Ginger has been a PT for 10 years. She works full time for the regional hospital (about 9 months) and is contracted to the early intervention program 2 days per week. She is 55 years old with a master's degree from an in-state university, has previously worked as a physical therapist's assistant, has recently moved to the area, and is comfortable with all aspects of PT. Tristan has been a speech-language pathologist (SLP) for 8 years. He works 2 days per week with early intervention, and he works 3 days per week for local school district. He is 35 years old with a master's degree from an out-of-state university. He originally is from the area and recently moved back. Tristan is married with twin boys (18 months), lives in town near the early intervention office, grew up on a farm, and has extensive experience with augmentative and alternative communication.
Tier 2	Team covers 5-county rural area Mitchell family lives 45 miles from early intervention office on their farm	Stella has been an SLP for three years, and she works 3 days per week with the early intervention program. She is 28 years old with a master's degree from an out-of-state university, recently accepted this traveling therapist position for 2 years, and works 2 days per week with Ginger at a regional hospital. Stella is new to small-town life, is single, has no children, is an avid reader, loves to cook, is comfortable working with children with feeding issues, and does not have much experience with assistive technology.
Tier 3		Stella is currently in that area of the county two times per week. Mandi has the most openings on her schedule but is worried about being able to support all of Ezra's needs. Ginger feels comfortable with Ezra's needs, but it is a long drive when she's only available 2 days per week. Martine has time available, but is thinking about Ezra's long-term needs. Tristan has the expertise that is needed, but does not have any openings in his schedule. Roger has time, knowledge, and both personal/professional experience, but he will need early support from Tristan.

Table 5F.3. Initial individualized family service plan outcome statements for Ezra Mitchell

Outcome 1: Ezra will help feed the animals each day by holding the feed bucket, pouring feed into bowls/pan, and putting away the food bowls.

Outcome 2: Ezra will choose what he wants to eat for snacks and meals by using his communication board to tell his family members what he wants.

Outcome 3: Ezra will join his brothers and his dad fishing at the pond on the weekends while Mrs. Mitchell and Rebekah have some time together.

Table 5F.4. Early intervention service delivery summary

Early intervention services	Outcome number	Frequency/ intensity	Methods	Setting	Start date	End date
Roger (occupational therapist)	1–3	30, 1-hour visits in 3 months	Direct service; teaming; joint visits	Home	5/1/19	8/1/19
Tristan (speech-language pathologist)	1–3	10, 1-hour visits in 3 months	Direct service; teaming; joint visits	Home	5/1/19	8/1/19
Martine (physical therapist)	1–3	4, 1-hour visits in 3 months	Direct service; teaming; joint visits	Home	5/1/19	8/1/19

EXAMPLE 2

Following further assessment and documentation of eligibility, the IFSP team of Mr. and Mrs. Mitchell, Tristan, and Roger developed the following outcomes and service delivery statements for Ezra's initial IFSP (see Tables 5F.3 and 5F.4). A few of the team members have changed in the second example regarding selecting a PSP for the Mitchell family, but all other information is the same as the first example. The information about the new team members is provided next.

- One full-time EIC (Greta)

- One full-time early childhood special educator (Edna). Edna has 20 years of experience working in early intervention. She is 56 years old and has a master's degree from an out-of-state university. She is married and has four grown daughters and six grandchildren. Edna and her husband Ray recently sold their family farm to move into town. Her favorite pastime is spending time with her grandchildren. Edna has extensive experience working with children with severe disabilities.

- One full-time OT (Roger)

- Two PTs (Ginger and Martine)

- Two part-time SLPs (Georgina works 2 days per week and Juanita works 3 days per week).

Georgina is new to the area. She is married and has two little girls that are 18 months and 5 years of age. Georgina works part time to allow her to spend time with her girls. Georgina is a city girl who moved to the country to raise a family. Georgina has 10 years of experience in early intervention. She is one of the team's feeding specialists and has some experience with assistive technology.

Juanita is new to the area. She works for the local school district 2 days each week. She has worked in early intervention for 2 years. Juanita is bilingual (she speaks English and Spanish), is single, and has no children. She is 28 years of age, lives with her sister, and loves to travel. She is the team's expert on sign language and previously worked in a home visiting program supporting children with hearing impairments.

Example 2 begins where the discussion shifts from the early intervention team in Example 1.

Greta:	So that's all we know now. I told Mrs. Mitchell that we would pick up the records on our first visit with her. I thought we should take a look at those records before I call the other program.
Martine:	That sounds good, Greta. I'm glad you took the opportunity to talk about our approach. It sounds really different than what the Mitchells are accustomed to.
Greta:	Thanks, Martine. They will need to hear all of it again. As you stated, we do things very differently than their previous program.
Georgina:	Well, this is interesting to think about. Typically, we would all turn to Edna in this type of situation, right, guys?
	(Team members indicate the affirmative.)
Ginger:	I was thinking the same thing. How do we shift our thinking to focus first on the Mitchell family and Ezra before we jump in with our availability and expertise?
Martine:	It's tough. I was going to the same place in my head, too. Let's get the worksheet out and really give this a try.
Greta:	Great job, guys. Here is the worksheet. Tier 1, Factor 1 is parent/family factors. This comprises the family's priorities or requests, including anything we might receive from the physician.

Edna: Okay, then, we don't know much. How do we proceed?

Greta: Let's write down what we know. First off, you are all going to be listed up at the top of the worksheet.

Roger: Even if we don't have time in our schedule?

Greta: Yes. Everyone is an option as we begin our discussion. We'll talk about individual availability as a final factor in Tier 3.

Edna: Okay. We know that Mrs. Mitchell homeschools all of the older children and wants ideas for how to include Ezra. We know that Mr. Mitchell is out working on the farm, but we'll need more detail about all of that. We know that the entire family spends a good deal of time outside and that Mrs. Mitchell said they all have a tough time trying to figure out how to include Ezra.

Greta: Nice summary, Edna. What else can anyone think of related to the parent/family factors in Tier 1?

Roger: We know that Ezra was receiving ECSE, PT, and SLP services and that the family had just received an order from the physician for OT. So, is this where we take that into consideration?

Greta: Yes. I think that does fit here. What else?

Ginger: I think we're ready to move onto child factors. Let's list all of that equipment that Ezra already has in place. Greta, did you say a wheelchair and a standing frame?

Greta: Yes, and there might be additional items. Mrs. Mitchell just happened to mention these specific items.

Ginger: She also said that he can't walk, talk, or really move very well on his own. The fact that he's 24 months old and already has this type of equipment makes me think that he probably has quadriplegia. We'll have to just go with this for now until we lay our eyes on him.

Edna: Ginger, I was thinking the same thing. I'm really interested in what approach they're taking to Ezra's communication. If he does have spastic quadriplegia or athetoid-type cerebral palsy, then he will probably have substantial long-term assistive technology needs in this area. I'm also already picking up on some signs regarding learned helplessness. We want the entire family to understand as soon as possible how Ezra can participate.

Roger: We'll definitely need to assess, but if we're going with this line of thinking, then his independence related to self-care and all of the issues related to eating are probably going to surface.

Greta: Great discussion. What about Ezra's interests and activity settings? What do we know?

Juanita: Not much. I was thinking about that. We know that his mom wants to include him in homeschooling and wants him to be more independent, but we don't know anything about what Ezra likes or wants to do.

Roger: Same with outside. We don't even know if he likes going outside, but if his family is always out and about, we'll need to think about ways for Ezra to participate.

Georgina: I just feel like we need so much more information.

Greta: We do. Definitely. Remember, this is just to get us started. So, this is a nice segue to environmental factors. What do we know?

Martine: Well, we know he's at home on the farm. We don't know much more.

Greta: The rest of the extended family attends my church. I have a hunch they will too. We'll just need to ask. I think it is important to note that he doesn't attend child care. So we don't have to worry right now about contacting anyone regarding involvement in the IFSP process.

Edna: It sounds like we're ready to talk about where we all fit in. So, let's take a look at our knowledge and expertise—professional and personal. I have to jump in and say that you guys know this is my very favorite situation. I love working with children who have a lot of challenges. I've lived on a farm all my life, so I probably could jump right in. What do you guys think about all of the equipment he has? I feel fine about getting started with all of that, but I would like some help from Martine or Ginger, especially with the wheelchair.

Ginger: I feel really comfortable helping address all of the equipment issues, but I am not sure it is the best use of my time to drive all the way out there when I'm only available 2 days a week.

Greta: Ginger, hang on. You began with sharing your expertise and knowledge, but it shifted to your availability. We have a lot more to talk about before we get there.

Ginger: Oops! You're right. This is really challenging to separate the two issues. I'm surprised at how much I've been thinking about that.

            (The team all comments on the same idea of how pervasive the issue of the practitioners' availability looms as they consider the possibilities of who might serve as primary provider.)

Greta: I agree. The availability consideration is an important one. It's just that we're jumping to it too soon.

Martine: So, I feel comfortable supporting the family, but I'm trying to keep the long-term perspective. I'm really interested in serving as primary for this family. Would you guys trust me in the role? I could address all of the equipment needs up front but would need long-term support from Edna and Georgina. Roger, I'd also probably need some help from you.

Ginger: You're right Martine. Thinking about all the kids and homeschooling makes me think that Roger would have a lot to offer. To answer your question, I definitely trust you and I also think it would be a great experience for you. We can help out with any questions you have.

Roger: I was thinking the same thing. Edna, what are your thoughts?

Edna: This is a good discussion for us to have. I would have really been the primary choice before, but now I'm hearing we have several good options—Roger, Martine, Georgina, and myself.

Greta: This is where this all fits together. Let's write out to the side here who we think we're still considering as most likely PSP.

Juanita: Roger, Martine, Georgina, and Edna. What about Ginger?

Ginger: Yes, I'd be comfortable. I just keep thinking about the drive and, realistically, my availability. It seems like we could all be considered as secondary support as well, depending on who we select as the primary provider.

Greta: Good point. I'll write that down here under role overlap and SSP options.

Greta:	Now we're to Tier 2, family dynamics. What do we know here?
Ginger:	I don't think we really know anything here. What do the rest of you think?
Roger:	I agree. Greta, can we just move on?
Greta:	Yes. I think this just emphasizes how much work we have to do to get to know the family. Safety and distance from the office is the next factor to reconsider on Tier 2. We know it is about a 45-minute drive on a clear, no-tractor-on-the-roads day.
	(The team members laugh about the issues they face driving country roads.)
Edna:	We don't have any safety concerns at this point, but that drive is a big issue for us regarding availability. Can we talk about that now?
Greta:	Not really. We need to consider issues such as prior relationship, rapport with the family, and billing. We can certainly bill for anyone's services don't you all agree.
	(The team confirms that billing isn't a complicating factor, initially, but needs to be considered for the future.)
Roger:	This seems premature because we haven't met the family. Do we revisit this once we start the process?
Greta:	Absolutely. We'll keep these factors in mind as we move forward with the family. So, has our list changed regarding Tier 2?
Team:	No.
Greta:	Tier 3 is . . .
Team:	Availability! (The team members laugh as this is a new way of thinking for them.)
Greta:	Yes. But first, it's about the family's and child's availability. What do we know?
Martine:	Do we know anything?
Roger:	I think we can probably assume this family won't require regular evening visits because of Mrs. Mitchell's request about homeschooling and outside time. We'll need to be open, but it seems that visits during the day will be an option.
Ginger:	What about our availability?
Edna:	I feel like I have the expertise to support Ezra and his family, but my schedule is really packed. The drive is the real issue. Realistically, this is a family that will take 2–3 hours each visit. I'm not sure that I can meet all of their needs and expectations at this point and time.
Martine:	I have time in my schedule and I'm already out that way a few times each week. Like I said, I'm going to need more assistance than any of the rest of you would. Greta, what are your thoughts? Can we afford the time it will take for the team to support me?
Greta:	Absolutely. I see this as an excellent opportunity to enhance our core knowledge as a team. Edna, this means you're going to be needed. How will that work?
Edna:	I know. I'm going to take a hard look at my schedule to see when I can free up some time. I can definitely find some time for joint visits. We can also make good use of the time on the drive. We'll just need to really plan our time well.
	(See Table 5F.5.)
Edna:	Martine, how comfortable do you feel thinking about his communication needs?
Martine:	Well, I'd certainly need support with that, but I was thinking you or Georgina could support me. Also, what about using sign language? Is that something we should consider?

Table 5F.5. Environmental and practitioner factors for the second team

Tier	Environmental factors	Practitioner factors
Tier 1	Ezra spends all of his time at home and with the family at church on Sundays. Parents and Rebekah visit extended family on a neighboring farm once monthly for dinner while Malakai cares for the other children.	Greta is the early intervention coordinator and has been an early childhood special educator for 20 years. She is divorced with 3 grown children and 12 grandchildren, has lived in the local area her entire life, and is an avid Seahawks fan. Edna has been an early childhood special educator for 20 years and works full time. She is 56 years old and has a master's degree from an in-state university. She is married with 4 grown daughters and 6 grandchildren. She loves to spend time with her grandchildren and recently sold the family farm to move into town near the office. Edna has extensive experience with children with severe challenges. Roger is a full-time occupational therapist (OT) with 15 years of experience. He is 42 years old lived, has lived in the local area his entire life (grew up on a farm), has a master's degree from an out-of-state university, is married with 9 children, is a team feeding specialist, and enjoys working with children with sensory needs. Martine is a new, full-time physical therapist (PT). She is 26 years old and this is her first job as a PT. She earned a Doctor of Physical Therapy (DPT) from an in-state university. She is recently married, has no children, is new to the area (first time to live in the country), and has completed an internship in an orthotics lab. Ginger has been a PT for 10 years. She works full time for the regional hospital (about 9 months) and is contracted to the early intervention program 2 days per week. She is 55 years old with a master's degree from an in-state university, has previously worked as a physical therapist's assistant, has recently moved to the area, and is comfortable with all aspects of PT. Georgina has been a speech-language pathologist (SLP) for 10 years and works 2 days per week. She is 35 years old with a master's degree from an out-of-state university. She is new to the area, married with 2 daughters (18 months and 5 years old), is a self-described city girl who moved to the country to raise her family, is one of the team's feeding specialists, and is comfortable with assistive technology.
Tier 2	Team covers five-county rural area Mitchell family lives 45 miles from early intervention office on their farm	Juanita has been an SLP for 2 years and works 3 days per week. She works for the local school district 2 days per week. Juanita is 28 years old with a master's degree from an out-of-state university. She lives with her sister and loves to travel, is bilingual (English and Spanish), is new to small-town life, is single, has no children, is the team's sign language expert, and previously worked in a home visiting program supporting children with hearing impairments.
Tier 3		Edna has a packed schedule, and the drive would be challenging. Ginger feels comfortable with Ezra's needs, but it is a long drive when she is only available 2 days per week. Martine has time available, but she is thinking about Ezra's long-term needs. Georgina has the expertise needed, but there are no openings in her schedule. Juanita feels comfortable, but she is not not sure if this is best use of all of her expertise and knowledge. Roger has time, knowledge, and both personal/professional experience, but his schedule is busy.

Juanita:	It could be a possibility. It's just too soon for us to know, but I like how you're thinking, Martine.
Martine:	I've already learned so much from you guys!
Ginger:	No offense, Martine, but what about all those kids and the homeschooling? What's your comfort level with all of that?
Martine:	I'm comfortable with the fact that I've got a lot to learn, but Roger is available if I need some additional support, right?
Roger:	(smiling) Right, Martine!
Greta:	Remember, we're not making the decision without the Mitchells and before we write the IFSP outcomes. We just want to be thinking about the best options from our point of view. It does sound like we've got a couple of options. Who do we think is our best option, considering what we know at this time?

(Everyone looks around the room, smiling.)

Worksheet for Selecting the Most Likely Primary Service Provider

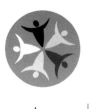

Core team as options for primary service provider (PSP)

Early childhood (EC) ___Edna___   Occupational therapist (OT) ___Roger___

Physical therapist (PT) ___Martine, Ginger___   Speech-language pathologist (SLP) ___Georgina, Juanita___   Other _____

		Most likely PSP(s) identified based on			Most likely PSP options selected (list)	Secondary service provider (SSP) options selected (list)
		Parent/family factors	Child factors	Environmental factors	Practitioner factors	
Tier 1	List priorities with contexts *How to include Ezra in family activities* List parent/physician request *Received early childhood special education, physical therapy, speech-language therapy, and referred for occupational therapy*	List diagnosis/condition/needs (long-term view) *Diagnosis of cerebral palsy* *Has wheelchair and standing frame* List interests/activity settings *Homeschool activities*	Circle natural learning environments • (Home) • Community • Preschool • Child care • Other	List knowledge/expertise (personal/professional) *Martine: Equipment* *Roger: Large family, homeschooling, lives on a farm, feeding* *Georgina: Augmentative and alternative communication* *Edna: Extensive experience with children with severe disabilities, assistive technology*	*Edna* *Roger* *Martine* *Georgina* *Ginger*	*Edna* *Roger* *Martine* *Georgina* *Ginger* Role overlap
Tier 2	Family dynamics Individual parent/caregiver characteristics • Language/culture • Knowledge/expertise • Diagnosis/condition • Other		Safety Distance from program office *Distance from program office is 45 minutes*	Primary service area in geographic region Billability Prior relationship Rapport	*Edna* *Roger* *Martine* *Georgina* *Ginger*	*Edna* *Roger* *Martine* *Georgina* *Ginger* Role overlap
Tier 3	Availability *Family has a flexible schedule*	Availability	Availability	Availability *Edna: Full caseload* *Martine: Has time, wants the PSP role, and is already in location*	*Martine*	*Edna* *Rger* *Georgina* Role overlap
Notes:					Most likely PSP is: *Martine*	Role gap? If so, explain: Role assist (SSP): *Edna* *Roger* *Georgina*

Figure 5F.2. The second team's Worksheet for Selecting the Most Likely Primary Service Provider

The Early Intervention Teaming Handbook: The Primary Service Provider Approach, Second Edition by M'Lisa L. Shelden, PT, Ph.D., Dathan D. Rush, Ed.D., CCC-SLP

Table 5F.6. Early intervention services delivery summary

Early intervention services	Outcome number	Frequency/ intensity	Methods	Setting	Start date	End date
Martine (physical therapist)	1–3	32, 1-hour visits in 3 months	Direct service; teaming; joint visits	Home	5/1/19	8/1/19
Edna (early childhood special educator)	1–3	10, 1-hour visits in 3 months	Direct service; teaming; joint visits	Home	5/1/19	8/1/19
Georgina (speech-language pathologist)	1–3	4, 1-hour visits in 3 months	Direct service; teaming; joint visits	Home	5/1/19	8/1/19
Roger (occupational therapist)	1–3	2, 1-hour visits in in 3 months	Direct service; teaming; joint visits	Home	5/1/19	8/1/19

Ginger: I think we've got three really great options—Martine, Roger, and Edna. It sounds like Martine might have the most to offer at this time because of scheduling. What do you guys think?

(Everyone affirms Ginger's statement.)

Martine: Okay then. I'll give Mrs. Mitchell a call when we finish our meeting.

Edna: What supports do you need from us to get started?

Martine: Thanks, Edna. I know I will need some early support from Georgina or you around Ezra's communication needs, and maybe even Juanita. Roger, I'd like to think about you coming in early as well, just in case I need some specific assistance.

Georgina, Juanita,
Edna, and Roger: Okay, sounds good!

Greta: Let's summarize. Martine, it appears that based on what we know now, you are our best option for the most likely PSP, with formal assistance from Edna, Georgina, and Roger. Is this correct?

Team: Yes, it's all good.

(See Figure 5F.2)

The second team developed the same IFSP outcome statements as the first team for Ezra's initial IFSP (see Table 5F.3). Note the changes in service delivery based on the changes in practitioner factors on the team (see Table 5F.6).

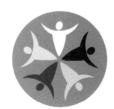

Sample Workload Activity List for Tina, an Occupational Therapist

Tina is an occupational therapist (OT) working in a suburban/rural area in North Carolina. The farthest drive from Tina's office (one way) to any family's home or child care provider is 30 minutes. Her team serves 125 families and consists of the following members.

- Three full-time service coordinators

- One full-time early childhood special educator

- One full-time OT

- One full-time physical therapist

- One full-time speech-language pathologist

Number	Ongoing caseload (number of visits in May)	Evaluations	Individualized family service plan meetings	Joint visits as primary service provider	Joint visits as secondary service provider
1	Smith (4)	Marshall	Marshall	Daniels (1)	Morris (2)
2	Reep (4)	Daniels	Daniels	Short (1)	Reyes (1)
3	Cantrell (2)	Buff	Rodriguez	Smith (2)	
4	Dalton (4)	Dominico	Frank		
5	Jones (4)	Settles			
6	Rodriguez (3)	Scott			
7	Carswell (4)	Tanaka			
8	Roberts (2)				
9	Ramirez (4)				
10	Pasqual (2)				
11	Hess (4)				
12	Perez (4)				
13	Sanchez (4)				
14	Portman (4)				
15	Short (4)				
16	Hernandez (3)				
17	Byrd (6)				
18	Caraway (5)				
19	Daniels (1)				
20	Norman (2)				
21	Frank (1)				
22	Yin (4)				
23	Donovan (11)				

Tina's Schedule *for the Current Month*

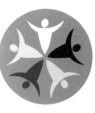

Tina G., OT—May

Monday	Tuesday	Wednesday	Thursday	Friday
3	**4**	**5**	**6**	**7**
9:30 Portman (CCC)	9:00 Byrd (CCC)	8:00 Carswell	8:00 Donovan	8:30 Team meeting
11:00 Smith	10:30 Caraway (CCC)	10:00 Dalton	9:45 Jones	10:15 Smith (JV–SLP)
1:00 Short	11:30 Donovan	11:30 Ramirez (Interp)	11:00 Perez (Interp)	11:30 Donovan
3:00 Evaluate Marshall	2:00 Cantrell	1:00 Sanchez (Interp)	1:00 Hess	2:00 Rodriguez (IFSP)
5:00 Evaluate Daniels	4:00 Roberts	2:30 Reep	3:30 Yin	
10	**11**	**12**	**13**	**14**
9:30 Norman	8:30 Ramirez (Interp)	8:00 Jones	8:00 Donovan	8:30 Team meeting
11:00 Byrd (CCC)	10:00 Perez (Interp)	9:30 Yin	9:45 Dalton	11:30 Donovan
12:00 Donovan	11:30 Donovan	11:30 Portman (CCC)	11:00 Rodriguez	2:00 Frank (IFSP)
3:00 Evaluate Settles	2:00 Reyes (JV–ECSE)	1:00 Sanchez (Interp)	1:30 Caraway (CCC)	4:00 Carswell
5:00 Evaluate Dominico	4:00 Short	3:30 Hess	2:30 Byrd (CCC)	
			4:00 Reep	
17	**18**	**19**	**20**	**21**
9:30 Pasqual	10:00 Short (JV—early childhood special educator)	8:00 Morris (JV–SLP)	9:30 Carswell	8:30 Team meeting
11:00 Smith (JV—early childhood special educator)		10:00 Cantrell	10:45 Short	10:15 Daniels (IFSP)
	11:30 Reep	11:30 Hernandez	12:00 Donovan	11:30 Byrd (CCC)
12:30 Hernandez	1:30 Dalton	1:30 Hess	2:30 Rodriguez	12:15 Caraway (CCC)
3:00 Evaluate Scott	2:45 Ramirez (Interp)	3:00 Jones	4:30 Portman (Home)	2:00 Perez (Interp)
5:00 Evaluate Buff	4:00 Sanchez (Interp)	4:15 Yin	5:30 Byrd (Home)	
	5:30 Donovan			
24	**25**	**26**	**27**	**28**
9:30 Frank	9:00 Portman (CCC)	8:00 Smith	9:45 Carswell	8:30 Team meeting
11:00 Donovan	10:30 Sanchez (Interp)	10:00 Norman	11:00 Perez (Interp)	10:15 Yin
1:00 Reep	11:30 Hernandez	11:30 Morris (JV–SLP)	1:00 Ramirez (Interp)	2:00 Rodriguez
3:00 Evaluate Tanaka	2:00 Hess	1:00 Pasqual	2:15 Dalton	3:30 Byrd (CCC)
5:00 Marshall (IFSP)	4:00 Roberts	2:30 Daniels (JV–PT)	3:30 Jones	4:15 Caraway (CCC)
	5:00 Caraway (Home)		5:00 Donovan	
31				
Holiday				

Key: CCC: child care center; IFSP: individualized family service plan; Interp: requires an interpreter; JV: joint visit; OT: occupational therapist; PT: physical therapist; SLP: speech-language pathologist ECSE: early childhood special education.

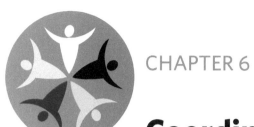

CHAPTER 6

Coordinating Joint Visits

Joint visits are a necessary component when implementing a PSP approach to teaming. A *joint visit* is defined as a type of role assistance in which another team member (i.e., SSP) accompanies the PSP for the purpose of supporting the PSP, the child's care providers, and the child in a timely and effective manner. The role of the SSP is to give role assistance through 1) coaching the PSP and the child's parents and other caregivers by sharing additional expertise and knowledge, 2) conducting further functional assessment, and 3) providing technical support (e.g., construct a seat insert, make a hand splint, teach a child the production of a target speech sound, assist in recommending an appropriate piece of assistive technology, instruct the child how to use a walker, help a mother with breastfeeding) when the PSP feels they need additional ideas, resources, or direct assistance in these areas.

When children have multiple disabilities, teams can mistakenly believe that they need to decide the child's priority area of need and designate that service as the PSP and then add SSPs in the other service areas. Visits by the SSP are not designated solely because a child has multiple needs across developmental domains typically assigned to a discipline other than the primary provider. In other words, joint visits are not provided in order to deliver another type of therapy, but they are implemented because the primary provider, family members, or other caregivers need the assistance of another team member with a particular area of experience, expertise, or knowledge. Similarly, joint visits are not used for the purpose of cotreatment whereby two practitioners are simultaneously providing intervention, but instead are carefully planned visits with the purpose of obtaining support for the PSP and/or care providers.

Three situations exist to indicate that a joint visit may be necessary. First, a PSP may have questions or identify an issue that cannot be addressed within the team meeting and requires that another team member accompany them on a visit to observe the situation and/or provide direct assistance. For example, a PSP believes that a child may need a seat insert in the bathtub in order to have a safe and fun bath time. The team determines that the PT should accompany the primary provider on a joint visit to assess the situation and either adapt a household item or suggest affordable alternatives. Second, another team member may have questions for the PSP during the team meeting that cannot be answered without direct observation of the child within the context of their everyday activities. To illustrate, the PSP who is an SLP described a recent home visit in which the parent used time-out without success when one of her young twins bit the other. The early childhood special educator asked the SLP to explain her response to the mother's use of time-out. The SLP shared that she just waited until the time-out was over and then continued with her support of the twins playing together without fighting. The early childhood special educator probed for the SLP's understanding of using time-out versus using a more positive approach to supporting

Remember

The three reasons for a joint visit are

1. A primary service provider (PSP) may have questions or identify an issue that cannot be addressed within the team meeting.

2. Another team member may have questions for the PSP during the team meeting that cannot be answered without direct observation of the child within the context of their everyday activities.

3. A parent may request access to a team member other than the designated PSP.

Reflect

Think about some examples of when a joint visit by someone from another discipline would have been helpful to you and the family you were supporting.

the child and family. The SLP was interested in learning more, and the early childhood special educator offered to join her on a future visit. Because this type of behavior often occurred during her visits, the SLP decided to talk with the parent and offer the support of the early childhood special educator via a joint visit. Third, the request for a joint visit may come directly from a parent who wants access to a team member other than the designated PSP. For example, following a visit with the child's pediatrician or neonatal follow-up clinic, a parent being supported by a PSP who is a PT requests a meeting with the team's OT. When the PT probes further with the parent, she identifies that the medical provider had expressed concern that the child was not receiving OT services. The parent had described her satisfaction and the child's progress with the team approach being used by the early intervention program to the medical provider; however, he was insistent that the child needed ongoing OT services. As a result, the mother wanted assurance that her child was receiving the needed supports and services from the OT. In this situation, the team should always afford the parent timely access to the desired team member to address the questions and issues. The visit with the OT would occur in conjunction with the PSP.

Joint visits by other team members occur with the PSP at the same place and time whenever possible so that the support needed from the secondary provider is helpful to the family and PSP. The relationship between the PSP and family is not disrupted when a joint visit occurs and the other team member is supporting the PSP. In addition, the opportunity for sharing information between the PSP and the other team member promotes learning opportunities for the PSP, builds trust and respect among team members, and affords the caregivers prioritized and focused opportunities to interact with other team members. The PSP can help the family apply the information in an ongoing and contextualized manner through the role assistance of the accompanying team member.

The frequency and intensity of joint visits is based on the needs of the PSP in light of the child and family outcomes. The SSP should not be needed at every visit but may joint visit with the primary provider for several consecutive visits or periodically over the course of a child's enrollment in a program. The intensity of visits is determined by the primary provider's need for support at a given time to address specific needs of the child, family, or other caregivers. An example might include a situation in which an early childhood special educator is supporting a child and family as the PSP. The child has recently progressed developmentally and is now able to push up into sitting while playing with his toys. The PSP and parents have noticed that the child can only push up with his right arm, not his left, and want the PT on the team to assess the child's progress and provide them with ideas for encouraging the child to get to and play with his toys, regardless of whether the toy is located to his left or right. They all want to make sure that nothing is being missed related to supporting his ongoing development. The PT attends a joint visit with the early childhood special educator during the child's afternoon playtime and affirms the observations of the primary provider and parents. The parents and PSP are supported by the PT in generating new ways to help the child push up with his left arm while playing with his toys. Ideas are also generated during the coaching conversation to support the child to push up into sitting following diaper changes and when being picked up by his parents. The PT asked the primary provider and parents how they would determine if further support was needed, and a plan was developed for the PT to check in with the early childhood special educator at the team meeting in 3 weeks. In this scenario, some people might question why the PT would not need to see the child more regularly or why the PSP did not change from the early childhood special educator to the PT. Based on the needs of the child, family, and skill set of the early childhood special educator, the team members were confident that all needs were being met by the early childhood special educator and family within the context of everyday activities. The early childhood special educator and family can continue to gain access to the PT as needed for further support, as well as any other team member who has needed expertise. The long-term view regarding this child's projected needs and the most appropriate PSP (early childhood special educator) did not change as a result of the child's emerging skill and questions raised by the family and primary provider. If, however, the primary provider felt uncomfortable continuing to support the child and family, then the support provided by the PT could have been increased through additional joint visits. If the additional support was not enough to increase the primary provider's confidence, then a change in PSP from the early childhood special educator to the PT might be warranted.

Consider another situation in which an SLP is the primary provider and the IFSP outcome is related to supporting the child's participation in family mealtimes. The child has cerebral palsy and has recently been able to sit more independently in his highchair and as a result has shown interest in self-feeding. The parent and SLP have tried several spoons but are not having success due to his difficulty holding the spoon and bringing it to his mouth. The SLP explained the new challenge during the team meeting and asked for support from the team. Following discussion, the team determined that the OT would join the SLP on a visit the next week. The joint visit was planned around the noon meal, and the SLP and parent demonstrated the current situation for the OT. The SLP and OT had planned ahead for the OT to take the lead in the conversation and, in anticipation, she brought along some adapted spoons for the self-feeding assessment. As the OT assisted the parent in promoting the child's use of the adapted spoons, all three adults soon realized that the spoons with the larger handles were helpful, but they noticed additional issues with the child's plate slipping as he tried to scoop food. When the plate was stabilized, the child continued to have difficulty with the food falling over the edge of the plate. The OT recognized the need for an adapted bowl and nonslip placemat to enhance the child's success. The mother identified a resource for the placemat and the OT had a bowl that could be tried during a subsequent joint visit prior to the parent making the purchase. The joint visit concluded with a plan for a second joint visit during which the OT will support the parent and SLP in further assessment of the adapted items for self-feeding. The SLP and parent required two consecutive joint visits with the OT and a follow-up visit a few weeks later to ensure continued success.

Conducting a joint visit involves more than just the actual visit including the PSP, SSPs, and the parent. Team members participate in a three-step process in order to implement the most effective and efficient joint visit possible: 1) planning, 2) implementing, and 3) debriefing the visit.

PLANNING THE JOINT VISIT

The PSP is responsible for facilitating two required conversations prior to the joint visit. The first conversation takes place between the PSP and the parent or other care provider. The second conversation occurs between the PSP and SSPs. The Joint Visit Planning Tool (see Appendix 6A) is completed by the PSP prior to and as a part of this conversation. The tool assists the PSP in 1) identifying the specific question or issue to be addressed, 2) reflecting on the relevant background information necessary for the SSP, and 3) developing the plan for the visit.

The PSP and the parent predetermine any questions to ask the SSP, expected outcomes to achieve, and specific actions to take, such as observing the child's participation in a specific activity setting (e.g., mealtime, bath time). This planning conversation is important in order to maximize the efficiency of the time of all parties involved and assist the secondary provider in preparing for the joint visit. For example, the PSP and parent may have specific questions that relate to using a particular type of assistive technology. This conversation with the parent demonstrates the equal partnership among team members; in this case, the parent and PSP. This planning discussion is designed as an opportunity to build the parent's capacity to participate in the upcoming conversation with the SSP as well as engage in future conversations with other professionals related to planning, problem solving, and decision making for their child. Sample questions include, but are not limited to

- "What are our expectations of Roxie, our SLP, during our visit?" "What questions do you have for Roxie?"

- "Who would you be more comfortable taking the lead during the visit, Roxie or me?"

- "We've decided for Roxie to observe playtime when the older children get home from school. What do you need to do to prepare for this?"

- "What day would provide the best opportunity for Roxie's visit?"

The second planning conversation follows the PSP's discussion with the parent or other care providers and involves preparing the SSP for the joint visit. First, the PSP should share relevant background information related to their and the parent's current knowledge and actions taken regarding the specific question or issue. In addition to the child and family activity settings and family priorities, which serve as the focus of the PSP's interactions with the family, knowing and understanding the child's interests is critical to the SSP's preparation. More specifically, the PSP is responsible for planning with the secondary provider about when the visit should occur, what the context will be, and how the SSP can be helpful. This may include sharing specific information so the secondary provider can be prepared to bring possible assistive technology to try with the child and family to support the child's successful participation in a particular activity setting. The secondary provider is at an extreme disadvantage when they are not provided with information from the PSP about child interests and activity settings and only has information related to strategies, techniques, and recommendations to address identified impairments. The PSP and SSP define their roles for the upcoming visit during the planning conversation, including determining who will take the lead in the conversation, model for the parent if necessary, facilitate the parent practicing or applying new information, and take responsibility for developing the joint plan. If the PSP is in the lead, then the secondary provider is there to serve as a resource by observing, supporting, and sharing information with the PSP and parent. If the SSP is in the lead, then the primary provider will function more as a learner alongside the parent. This does not necessarily mean that the PSP is learning from the secondary provider so they can implement a specific technique or strategy, but rather to assist the parent in applying the information over time and within the family's contexts or specific situations.

Example of Planning the Joint Visit

Marileigh, the early childhood special educator on the team, is serving as the PSP in this scenario. Marileigh has been working for the early intervention program since she graduated from college with a degree in early childhood special education 6 months ago. She has been working with Cyd and her son, Roberto, who is 20 months old and has Down syndrome, for the past month. The outcomes on Roberto's IFSP are 1) Roberto will let his mom or teacher know what he wants to eat at meals and when picking a toy at playtime, 2) Roberto's teacher will help him make the transition smoothly from one activity to another at school, and 3) Roberto will be more involved with getting dressed in the morning in order for him and his mother to leave on time. Cyd is a single mother and works full time from 8:00 a.m. to 5:00 or 5:30 p.m. during the week. So far, Marileigh has met with Cyd and Roberto twice at home in the evenings and one time at school with his teachers, Grace and Patrice. Currently, Roberto has two words that he uses most often, *mama* to call for his mother and *dat*, which he uses as a label for everything else. He will frequently point to what he wants and say, "Dat."

As part of the initial visit before the evaluation, Cyd had shared that she and Roberto enjoy looking at books together at bedtime. Their evenings primarily consist of running errands after she picks Roberto up from child care around 5:30 or 6:00 p.m., and then they go home and fix dinner, eat, play for a little while, and bathe Roberto before they snuggle in bed and look at a couple of books together. Roberto loves taking a bath, so they often splash and play in the water.

During the second home visit after the IFSP, Cyd told Marileigh that Roberto has really started to make more sounds when they are playing in the bathtub. Cyd described a little game they play in which Roberto makes a grunting sound and then she grunts back at him. They do this for a few turns until he gets bored and goes back to playing with his bath toys. Marileigh recognizes this as a prime learning opportunity in which Cyd could try to introduce some words for Roberto to imitate. Marileigh and Cyd begin to talk about how they could use this time to expand on the grunting and start using words to label objects and action. Because Marileigh's current visit is coinciding with dinner time, Cyd tries to engage Roberto in the grunting game while he is sitting in his highchair. Roberto plays the game for only a couple of rounds and then starts fussing for his drink. They model the word *milk* and try to get Roberto to repeat it, but he points to the cup in his mother's hand and says, "Dat!" Marileigh asks him, "What do you want?" and Cyd models "milk" while holding the cup of milk just out of Roberto's reach. Roberto protests and shouts, "Dat!" Cyd and Marileigh quickly brainstorm and try a few other ideas with similar lack of success.

As the visit was nearing an end and they began the process of developing their joint plan, Marileigh shared with Cyd that she would like for them to receive some support from Cathy, the SLP on the team, to see if she had other ideas for how they could help Roberto more fully participate at mealtime and bath time by expanding the words that he used during those activities. Cyd agreed, and in the meantime, the two decided that she would continue to introduce the word *milk* during their meals to see if he would try to say it. Marileigh's part of the plan was to bring up the need for Cathy's support during the team meeting, which was going to occur 2 days from the present visit.

As part of the Primary Coaching Opportunity section on the team meeting agenda, Marileigh shared that she and Roberto's mother, Cyd, were experiencing some challenges in supporting his participation in the mealtime routine because he would only grunt or point to what he wants and say, "Dat." Marileigh told the team that the more she and Cyd modeled "milk," the more emphatic Roberto became in pointing and shouting, "Dat!" Marileigh asked the team how she and Cyd could further assist Roberto to participate in mealtime by using his words and what ideas they had to help with this. Cathy, the team's SLP, asked Marileigh to describe or imitate the grunting that he was doing. Marileigh demonstrated how Roberto produced a very harsh "uh, uh" sound, almost in a guttural way. Cathy agreed how great it was that Roberto and his mother enjoyed playing the grunting game together and how his mother was following his lead and imitating him. Cathy expressed some concern about the effect that the repeated harsh onset of production of this sound could have on his vocal folds over time and agreed with Marileigh that using a real word was the next step. Marileigh indicated that she and Cyd feel like they have exhausted their ideas about how to get Roberto to use a word rather than a grunt and another word besides *dat*. Marileigh asked Cathy if she would be willing to accompany her on a joint visit to observe and help Cyd and her with this issue. The team agreed that a joint visit was in order, so Marileigh and Cathy planned to stay a few minutes after the meeting to plan the joint visit.

Cathy: So Marileigh, based on what you shared during the team meeting, it sounds like you need some support helping Roberto's mother support his participation at mealtime by using more of a variety of words instead of just grunting or saying "dat."

Marileigh: That's right, Cathy. As I said in the meeting, I feel like Cyd and I tried a number of things when I was there, but we just didn't have much success. I've already started completing the Joint Visit Planning Tool, so if it's okay with you, I'm going to make notes on it while we talk.

Cathy: Oh sure, that's fine. How can I support you?

Marileigh: We need some more ideas for ways to help him learn to use words.

Cathy: Well, I would normally ask you about the contexts and what you've tried at this point, but you did a nice job of sharing that during the team meeting.

Marileigh: Thanks. I just don't want to miss anything. Like I hadn't thought about the way he is making the grunting could hurt his voice if he does it too much. Because I am still new, I just felt like it would be helpful if you could meet with Cyd and me.

Cathy: No problem. That's why we have a team and members with different areas of expertise. I am happy to share what I know with you and Roberto's mother.

Marileigh: Thanks.

Cathy: Marileigh, I know that you and the mother were focused on mealtime at your last visit as the context for supporting his participation by learning to use words.

Marileigh: Right.

Cathy: What are the other activity settings that happen after they get home, and which one provides the most opportunity for his communication right now?

Marileigh: When I was there the last time, Cyd said that he really seems to be making sounds when they are playing in the bathtub. That's when they started playing the imitation game with the grunting. I was there during mealtime, so we just tried to use some of what she had been doing during the bath. It didn't really go so great. They also enjoy looking at books together and playing before bath time. I probably shouldn't have gone with mealtime to have her show me their little communication game. It kind of flopped.

Cathy: You were still in an everyday activity setting in which he could be communicating. It was just different than how they normally played that game. Based on what you know about the family's activity settings that provide opportunities for communication and build on Roberto's interests, when do you think we should try to schedule our visit?

Marileigh: Well, mealtime was a bust, so do you think we could go around the time he takes his bath, so we could see how she engages him and how he responds?

Cathy: How does that also fit with his interests?

Marileigh: She says that he loves to play in the water and that's where he's starting to vocalize most.

Cathy: His interests at bath time might allow us different ways to keep the activities going.

Marileigh: I can check with Cyd to see if we can go at bath time. She's pretty laid back, so I don't think it will be a problem.

Cathy: When are you going to talk with her about it? Some people may not like the idea of us going into their bathroom.

Marileigh: I am going to call her as soon as we finish meeting and find an evening in your schedule that will work. I mentioned at the last visit that I would like for you to come with me on the next visit. In fact, we didn't schedule a time because we were going to wait and see if you could go out with me in the next few days.

Cathy: Okay, so I think we have a pretty good idea about his interests and an activity that provides opportunities for communication that will be the focus of our visit if the

Marileigh: The way I left it with Cyd was that she was going to continue trying to use some of the strategies we tried during mealtime. Mainly, she was going to keep modeling "milk" and trying to get him to imitate it like they do the grunting in the bathtub. I would like to check in with her about how that is going.

Cathy: Okay. That makes sense and it will give us both an idea about whether that strategy in that context has been effective. If so, we can spend some time building off of that. If not, we can go ahead and make the transition to bath time. Who do you want to take the lead for that part of the visit?

Marileigh: Cyd's not shy, so it won't bother her for you to take the lead. I think it would be most helpful to me if I could watch how you have the conversation and how you might model and share ideas about communication.

Cathy: That'll be fine. So, you will take the lead for revisiting the previous visit, then I will take the lead for the bath time activity. What about the joint planning portion of the visit?

Marileigh: I can pick back up on that and close the visit.

Cathy: Sure, and I want you to jump in and be part of the conversation.

Marileigh: Oh, I will. I see here on the Joint Visit Planning Tool that we also need to talk about when we are going to debrief the visit together. What do you think?

Cathy: Because it's an evening visit, do you think we can meet at the office and ride together? If so, we can debrief in the car on the way back to the office. When will you debrief with the parent?

Marileigh: I would like to give her some time to think about it, but I don't want too much time to pass. So, if possible, I'm going to see if I can call her during her break at work the next day. When can you go with me?

Cathy: I can't go Monday night because I'm going to my son's soccer game. I already have a late visit scheduled for the following night. How about next Thursday night?

Marileigh: I'll call her in a few minutes to see if that might work. Anything else you think you need to know or we need to do to prepare?

Cathy: I can't think of anything. Just let me know if Thursday night works.

Marileigh: Okay, I will. Thanks for doing this with me.

Cathy: I'm glad to do it!

In this scenario, the PSP and parent identified a need for a possible joint visit. The issue was listed as a primary coaching opportunity on the agenda because the team meeting was happening within the next couple of days. Had the meeting been further away and/or had this been a highly critical need, the PSP could have contacted the SLP immediately to talk about the likelihood of a joint visit. During the regular meeting, the rest of the team agreed that the SLP needed to be involved in part because the PSP is relatively new to the team and the field of early intervention and also because both the SLP and PSP believed that seeing the situation was warranted. The PSP initiated the process of completing the Joint Visit Planning Tool to guide their conversation (see Figure 6.1), and both met briefly for the SLP to learn about the child's and family's priorities,

Joint Visit Planning Tool

Primary service provider (PSP): _____Marileigh_____ Family: __Cyd R.__ Child: __Roberto__

Secondary service provider (SSP): __Cathy__ Date of joint visit: __2/06/12__ Time: __6:30 p.m.__

Request for Role Assistance
Question or issue requiring support of another team member
How can we help Roberto use words during mealtime?
What you (PSP) and/or the parent need from the SSP
Strategies to promote using words instead of grunting or saying "dat" at mealtime.

Background Information
Your (PSP) and/or the parent's current knowledge and actions taken regarding the question/issue
Grunting is a game they play at bath time. Have tried modeling "milk." Withheld milk briefly to see if he would produce word. Mother and educator modeled asking question and responding with single word.
Current child interests and activity settings that serve as the context for intervention
Looking at books before bedtime, playing in water during bath, playing at home and school with his favorite toys—trucks and blocks. He doesn't like to stop unless it is his decision.
Current parent priorities
Say something other than "mama" and "dat." Make the transition from one activity to another at school without a fuss.

Plan
a. Conversation that will take place with the family about the joint visit (Questions to consider: When will you have the conversation? What questions need to be answered by the SSP? What does the SSP need to see? What will be the context for the visit? What does the SSP need to know? Who should take the lead—PSP or SSP?) *Talked with Cyd at last visit about having a joint visit with a speech-language pathologist (SLP). We need more ideas. SLP is aware of family priorities and child interests previously listed. We will visit home in the evening after mom gets home from work.*
b. Context for the visit and rationale (date and time) *Family home during bath time because this is the time when parent reports that Roberto is most verbal and where they typically play the grunting game.*
c. Person taking the lead in the visit (SSP or PSP) and rationale *SSP (Cathy—SLP) will take the lead after Marileigh revisits the previous plan. Marileigh will call the mother to see if it is okay to visit during bath time and for Cathy to take the lead in that activity with the mother and Roberto.*
d. Role of the person not taking the lead and the family during the visit *PSP (Marileigh) will observe and help SSP and parent further brainstorm and try ideas during bath time activity.*
e. What is going to happen during the visit *Mother is going to demonstrate how they play the grunting game in the bathtub. The goal will be to introduce some new words during this activity.*
f. Date/time for debrief of the joint visit with the SSP and family *PSP and SSP will debrief visit on the way back to the office on the day of the visit. PSP will call the mother during her break at work on the day after the visit.*

Figure 6.1.   Completed Joint Visit Planning Tool.

interests, and activity settings that serve as the context for intervention as well as specifically how the SLP was going to support the PSP during the visit.

IMPLEMENTING THE JOINT VISIT

The joint visit with the PSP, SSP, and parent occurs after the planning conversations. The visit occurs during the real-life activity setting in which the parent and PSP need support. Plans made between the primary and SSP are implemented in order to address the questions, outcomes, and actions necessary to meet the needs of the parent and primary provider. If for any reason the visit does not go as planned, then the primary and secondary providers are prepared to be flexible and discuss with the parent what would be helpful in light of the unforeseen circumstance. Although one person generally takes the lead during the joint visit, both the primary and SSP will interact with the parent and child as appropriate. The PSP ensures the development of the joint plan prior to the conclusion of the joint visit. This plan may or may not involve additional visits from the secondary provider, but it should always involve follow-up from the SSP via one-to-one conversations and updates during team meeting.

Example of a Joint Visit

Marileigh and Cathy are joining Cyd and Roberto at their home for the joint visit. The visit begins with Marileigh introducing Cathy and revisiting the previous joint plan.

Marileigh: Hi, Cyd! Hi there, Roberto! This is Cathy, our SLP.

Cyd: Hi, Cathy. It's nice to meet you. I have a good friend that I work with and her name is Cathy, too!

Cathy: Oh, wow! It's so nice to meet you. Marileigh has shared with me a little about you and Roberto and what the three of you have been doing together.

Cyd: That's good!

Marileigh: Cyd, thanks for meeting with us today and for agreeing to let us come at bath time.

Cyd: Anything, if it's gonna help this kiddo! He really is more of a chatterbox during his bath. I took off work a little early today, so I've got him fed, we've played awhile, and now he's ready for his bath, even though it's just a little earlier than normal. Do you want to go ahead and get started?

Marileigh: Sure. We can head to the bathroom and you can start getting him ready. We know this is probably a little awkward for the two of you with having us be part of bath time, but this should really give us a picture for how this goes.

Cyd: It's no problem. Neither one of us is shy. He's such a little ham. (Cyd turns to Roberto.) What a silly boy! Aren't you, Roberto? (Roberto smiles really wide and laughs.) It's gonna be a tight squeeze, but there'll be room for a couple of us on the floor by the tub once he gets in and somebody can sit on the toilet lid. (The three exchange glances and all smile.)

Marileigh: While you are running the water and getting the bubbles all fluffed up, tell me about mealtime. When I left last week, you were going to model and prompt him using "milk" to ask for his drink.

Cyd: (laughs) Yeah, right! Everything is still "dat." He's so fun and funny at other times, but he is very serious when it comes to eating, and if he doesn't get what he wants with a "dat," then he starts fussing pretty quickly.

Marileigh:	Well, it's a good thing that we planned for Cathy to join us today. As I mentioned to you on the telephone, she's going to take the lead with you during the bath and I'm going to be more of an observer during this part.
Cyd:	Then, I guess that means you get the toilet seat and we get to splash in the tub. Here, I've got extra towels, Cathy, just in case you get a little wet. We can be pretty crazy in the tub, can't we, Roberto?
Roberto:	Uh, uh!
Cyd:	Oh, you already want to play our game? Are you showing off already, silly man? (Roberto smiles really big as Cyd quickly gets him out of his clothes and into the tub of water and bubbles.)
Cathy:	Is this how your game typically starts?
Cyd:	Yeah, he will usually pull up on the side of the tub and come toward my face and say "uh."

(Just as Cyd says "uh," Roberto pulls himself up and says "uh" very loudly and harshly.) |
Cathy:	Like this?
Cyd:	Exactly. (Cyd leans forward and says "uh" back and the reciprocal vocalizations continue for four to five rounds.)
Cathy:	Wow! He really likes that.
Cyd:	Yeah, he'll keep doing it for a long time.
Cathy:	Why do you think he does it for so long?
Cyd:	He likes it and I keep doing it back. He thinks it's funny.
Cathy:	I'll bet! You are following his lead in an activity he enjoys. You respond just like in a conversation, and he responds back to you. He keeps it up because it's something he has fun doing, which provides him more time to practice getting better at this communication activity.
Cyd:	Yeah.
Cathy:	What do you think he's learning?
Cyd:	That he's got his mama wrapped around his little finger!
Cathy:	Oh, my goodness. Well, maybe so. What else?
Cyd:	It's fun to play in the bath. He's trying some sounds, but I wish he'd use some words and not just grunt. Am I teaching him a bad thing because now he grunts or just says "dat" for what he wants?
Cathy:	Well, you are teaching him that it takes two people to communicate and that when he says something you respond back and that his sounds have some power—they get mom to talk to him and keep her talking.
Cyd:	Yeah, I can see that.
Cathy:	What are some words that we could use here? When he says "uh," what's a word you could say back to him?
Cyd:	Um. (thinking) I'm drawing a blank.

Roberto:	Dat, dat, mama! (Roberto points to a plastic toy boat sitting on the side of the sink just behind his mother's head.)
Cyd:	What? You want the boat?
Roberto:	Dat, dat. (Cyd gives Roberto the boat.)
Marileigh:	Cyd, how does that match what we were trying to do at dinner the other night with the milk?
Cyd:	What? You mean trying to get him to say "milk" before we gave him the cup?
Marileigh:	Yes.
Cyd:	Duh! I could have tried to get him to say "boat," but I bet he would just say "dat."
Cathy:	Would you like to try it?
Cyd:	Sure. (Cyd gets another toy boat from beside the sink and holds it up in front of Roberto.) Boat! Boat!
Roberto:	Dat! Uh!
Cathy:	(quietly to Cyd) Say "boat" again.
Cyd:	Boat!
Roberto:	Uh!
Cyd:	Boat! (Roberto looks away and plays with the other boat he already has in the water. Cyd turns to Cathy and Marileigh.) See what I mean. It's "dat," "uh," or nothing.
Cathy:	Would you like to try something different?
Cyd:	Sure. This isn't working as planned (smiles).
Cathy:	We three adults aren't about to give up yet. (Cyd, Marileigh, and Cathy laugh.) Would you mind if I try something, Cyd?
Cyd:	Go right ahead.
Cathy:	I am going to shift gears here a bit and instead of saying the name of an object that he could refer to as "dat," I am going to try giving him an action word. In this case, I am going to use *pop* because it fits with this activity and we have plenty of bubbles in this bathtub to use. Watch what I do and let's see how he reacts.
Cyd:	Well, that's for sure. Okay. Go for it!
Cathy:	(scoops up a handful of bubbles and then holds her other hand over the bubbles) Roberto, watch! (Cathy quickly presses down on the bubbles until they are gone.) Pop! (Roberto picks up a handful of bubbles and tries to imitate her actions.) Pop! (Cathy repeats the action and word.) Roberto, watch me. Pop! (Roberto repeats her action, but says nothing.)
Cathy:	(to Cyd) What did you see me do?
Cyd:	You showed him how to pop the bubbles and you said "pop," but he didn't say anything.
Cathy:	No, he didn't. Not yet, but he was repeating my actions. What else?
Cyd:	You told him to look at you.

Cathy:	Yes, and I was trying to show on my face that it was his turn to talk just like when the two of you play your "uh" game.
Cyd:	Okay.
Cathy:	I'm going to try it again. (Cathy repeats the activity and models "pop" several more times.) Roberto . . . pop!
Roberto:	Pa!
Cathy:	(nod) POP!
Roberto:	Pa!
	(Cyd, Marileigh, and Cathy clap—more for themselves and their patience than for Roberto, who beams a big, squinty, toothy smile.)
Cathy:	Let's not lose the moment. Cyd, quick, you try it.
	(Cyd follows Cathy's example and Roberto says "pop" three times before losing interest and returning to the toy boats.)
Cyd:	He did it for me!
Cathy:	He sure did! How could you use this?
Cyd:	I can do this every night when we are playing in the bathtub.
Cathy:	What are some other action words that you could gradually try?
Cyd:	Blow? We could blow at the bubbles.
Cathy:	Yes. What else?
Cyd:	We could push the boats across the water and say, "push!"
Marileigh:	What about "go?"
Cathy:	Sure. You could give any of those a try. Just introduce one word at a time. Model the action. Pair it with the word. Wait expectantly for him to take his turn to say it.
Cyd:	I can do that! I think the water's starting to get cold. Come on, big boy. Let's get up and out of the tub.
Marileigh:	Cathy, would that be another word they could try? "Up?"
Cathy:	Sure.
Cyd:	I can hold my hands up to model an action with the word. (Cyd holds her arms up, looks at Roberto, and says "up.")
Marileigh:	Cyd, we'll step out and into the living room while you dry Roberto off.
Cyd:	Okay, we'll be there in just a minute.
	(A couple of minutes later Cyd has Roberto dressed in his pajamas and they join Cathy and Marileigh in the living room.)
Cyd:	Here we are!
Marileigh:	Cyd, we are going to scoot on out of here so you can get Roberto to bed, but before we go, let's talk briefly about our joint plan.
Cyd:	I'm going to try this in the bath every night. I also want to think about words that I could use at mealtime instead of *milk*.

Marileigh:	Okay. Great! When does it make sense for me to come back next?
Cyd:	I know you are going to his child care next week. Could you talk with them about what we did tonight and help them figure out ways to do this at school? I will do the same.
Marileigh:	Sure.
Cyd:	I hate to ask, but I feel like we've turned a big corner. Would you mind stopping by here one night next week so we can keep this going? Maybe we could figure out how to use these ideas at dinnertime.
Marileigh:	That's no problem, Cyd. Actually, I was thinking the same thing.
Cyd:	Great minds think alike! What night is good for you?
Marileigh:	I just need to confirm another appointment on my schedule before I commit. Would you mind if I call you tomorrow to debrief tonight's visit and set the date for our next visit?
Cyd:	That's fine. Can you call me on my lunch break around 12:15?
Marileigh:	I sure can. I'll talk to you then.
Cyd:	Okay. Thanks, Cathy. This was really helpful.
Cathy:	I'm so glad. Marileigh will keep me posted. You two let me know what I can do to continue to help.
Cyd:	Okay, will do! Good night. Roberto, say "bye-bye."
Cathy:	Oh! That's another great word to help him start saying.
Cathy and Marileigh:	Bye-bye, Roberto.
Roberto:	Buh!

Cathy served as the SSP in this scenario and took the lead in the action/practice portion of the visit related to bath time just as she and Marileigh had planned. Marileigh led the conversation about the previous plan and helped to clarify the joint plan for what Cyd will be doing between visits to support Roberto's participation in bath time and mealtimes by using words to communicate his actions. Marileigh and Cyd also planned their next visit. As part of her planned role during the visit, Cathy built on the parent's and child's bathtime play and added to it, based on the parent's priorities. Cathy's support of the parent and PSP included intentional modeling on how to promote communication, which included observation, reflection, modeling, practice by the parent, feedback, and planning. Cathy's actions during the visit serve as the foundation for her debriefing the visit with Marileigh.

DEBRIEFING THE JOINT VISIT

Following implementation of the joint visit, the PSP debriefs with the parent and/or other care providers to evaluate the usefulness of the visit and determine next steps. The primary provider and parent discuss whether the questions were sufficiently addressed, if the intended outcomes of the visit were achieved, and if the actions taken during the visit were helpful. The primary provider and parent also revisit the joint plan that was developed during the visit to implement, update, and/or revise the plan as needed.

The PSP and the SSP debrief in a separate conversation to evaluate the usefulness of the visit, follow up on the joint plan during the joint visit, and determine any next steps. The purpose of this debriefing is for the SSP to ensure that the needs of the primary provider and parent were met. This is also an opportunity for the SSP to engage the primary provider in reflection related to what they learned while observing the SSP in action with the child and parent. Again, the intention of this observation is not for the secondary provider to release all of their discipline-specific expertise, but to support the primary provider in expanding their knowledge base in child development and family support. This would involve knowing what the PSP could share or do immediately without the direct involvement of the secondary provider as well as the when, where, and how the secondary provider will need to be involved to support the PSP with this family and others in the future.

Example of a Debriefing Between the Primary Service Provider and Secondary Service Provider

Marileigh and Cathy debrief the visit they just completed with Cyd and Roberto while driving back to the office. Note the questions the SSP asks the PSP to prompt her reflection as part of the debriefing to examine the extent to which the PSP's capacity was built as part of this role assistance activity.

Marileigh:	Cathy, that was great. It was so helpful. Thank you for going.
Cathy:	You're welcome. How was it helpful?
Marileigh:	First, it was nice to just see you in action. Your interaction with Cyd just seemed so natural and easy.
Cathy:	How so?
Marileigh:	You took what she was doing as part of their bath time play and then you built it into ways they could try to use more words.
Cathy:	What strategies did you see me use?
Marileigh:	You asked her to reflect on what was currently happening and analyze it to determine what she wanted to have happen and try to come up with ways to do that.
Cathy:	You asked her a really nice analysis question there yourself when you had her compare what the two of you had been doing during meals to support his use of words and what she did when she just gave him the boat.
Marileigh:	I guess I did, didn't I!
Cathy:	So, when we first started trying things and I modeled, it didn't work either.
Marileigh:	I know. I have to admit that made me feel kind of good.
Cathy:	Well, gee, thanks. (They laugh.)
Marileigh:	No, that's not what I mean. (Cathy nods and smiles.) It's just that it was nice to see that his mom and I weren't the only ones who experienced the "dat" challenge. Even a person who knows about communication and language development as well as you do may not have success the first time.
Cathy:	Exactly. How else was this helpful?
Marileigh:	I learned some other ways to support use of words, such as moving away from language and using action words. That was a good idea and really worked well in this situation. You also stuck with it and tried several times before he actually tried to say the word. I like how you modeled, but then you had Cyd do it as soon as he said the word.
Cathy:	Yes, a technique that is sometimes helpful is to introduce action words or descriptive words that are meaningful and functional within the context of a particular interest-based activity.

Marileigh: It sure worked in this case.

Cathy: How will you use what I demonstrated tonight?

Marileigh: In terms of communication and language, this gave me some other ideas for supporting communication and helped broaden my knowledge. You also showed me how I can use modeling effectively. You know, one thing that I learned from this whole process was the importance of context.

Cathy: What do you mean?

Marileigh: Cyd had told me how much he likes bath time and how he tries to communicate during that time. But during my previous visit, I went with mealtime, which frustrated him, Cyd, and myself. I should have started with an activity such as the bath that already had higher opportunity for communication.

Cathy: Maybe so. How will you use mealtime now?

Marileigh: Now that we have experienced some success for both Roberto and Cyd, I think we can revisit mealtime and use some of what worked from the bath. We can focus on some action words and descriptive words.

Cathy: Like what?

Marileigh: If she continues to use *up* at bath time, then we can use that word for when it's time to get up in the highchair and he can learn to make that request. We could use *more* to have him request more food or drink.

Cathy: Sure. Don't give up on some of the labels for his food, such as milk, juice, cracker, and so forth. Just don't always ask questions; use labels. Model, wait expectantly, and show him that his words can get him what he wants.

Marileigh: Right. Before I forget, I wanted to ask you about the way he grunts. You had shared some concern that it might be harmful to his voice.

Cathy: Oh, yeah. It was really helpful to actually hear him do that. He does really hit that "uh" hard and forcefully. We do need to give him other ways to play vocally, as well as communicate. I think we made a shift from using that type of communication to words or word approximations, so eliminating the "uh" should alleviate any potential problem.

Marileigh: Okay. That's good.

Cathy: We are almost back to the office. What do you want our plan to be?

Marileigh: I am going to call Cyd tomorrow to debrief tonight's visit and schedule our next visit.

Cathy: How can I be of support to you?

Marileigh: I would like to talk with you after my next visit with her and after I meet with his child care teachers, Patrice and Grace. I think it might be helpful for you to go with me to the child care center at least once to observe and maybe help me explain ways to support his communication during the activities there.

Cathy: I would be happy to do that. How about we get together right after team meeting next week to talk about your next visit with Cyd and Roberto at home? After that, we can determine when it might be good to try a joint visit at child care.

Marileigh: That makes sense to me. I can talk with the child care teachers and ask about you being there with me for a visit.

Cathy: Sounds like we have a plan.

Because the SSP took the lead during bath time, the focus of the debriefing was what the SSP said and did, how it was helpful to the PSP, and how it built her capacity (e.g., confidence, competence) for promoting parent-mediated practices to support child learning within the context of everyday learning opportunities. Cathy wanted to know what was helpful and why in order to assess 1) what Marileigh learned from the visit and how she might use this information to further support the family and 2) how effective the process Cathy used to support the parent and the content was for promoting Marileigh's and the parent's learning. Finally, Cathy needed to develop a joint plan with Marileigh for next steps for support. The two will meet to discuss Marileigh's next visit with Cyd and Roberto as well as possibly schedule another joint visit to occur in the child care setting. Had the follow-up conversation and joint visit not been part of the plan, other options may have included follow-up as part of a quarterly report or primary coaching opportunity during a team meeting.

Example of Debriefing Between the Primary Service Provider and Parent

Following is an example of a debriefing of the joint visit between the parent and the PSP. The debriefing occurs by telephone during the mother's lunch hour. The debriefing could have taken place at the end of the joint visit or during the next face-to-face visit with the parent and primary provider.

Marileigh: Hi, Cyd, it's Marileigh. We had planned for me to call you today at 12:15 to briefly talk about our visit with Cathy last night. Is now still an okay time for you to talk?

Cyd: Sure. I was expecting your call.

Marileigh: Good. I don't want to take up much of your time, but I wanted to get back with you as soon after our visit last night as possible. The reason I wanted us to talk is to find out how the visit with Cathy went from your perspective. How was it helpful to you?

Cyd: I thought we came up with some good ideas last night. I'm glad we can move that playtime beyond just the two of us grunting back and forth. We were beginning to sound like a couple of cavemen. No offense to cavemen or anything. I would never have thought of using some action words. She also kept trying over and over until he finally got it.

Marileigh: How were we able to use his interests?

Cyd: Oh, he loves playing in the tub. It was good to use a time when he is so naturally talkative, even if it started out as just grunting. I can see how it's helpful to find something he likes doing and build it into a learning time.

Marileigh: How can we continue to use what Cathy shared with us?

Cyd: I have been saying "up" a lot. I said "up" when I was trying to put his shirt on this morning, and he held his little arms up. I also said "up" for him to hold his leg up for me to tie his shoe and "up" to pick him up to put him in the car.

Marileigh: Yes, isn't it amazing how much repetition there can be? All those are times for him to hear and possibly begin using that word as part of those activities. I don't want to keep you much longer, but before I let you go, tell me your thoughts about next steps for Cathy's support.

Cyd: What do you mean?

Marileigh: I mean, do you think we have the information and some ideas to move forward for awhile, or do you think we need to have her come back?

Cyd: She was very helpful, but I think we got what we needed for awhile.

Marileigh: I was thinking the same thing, but I wanted to check with you. I am planning to talk with her after our next visit during your dinnertime, and I might find it helpful to have her do a joint visit with me at Roberto's child care. What do you think about that?

Cyd: Sure. I mean if you think it will be useful to you. I didn't have much time this morning, but I started telling Patrice and Grace about what we did last night and how Roberto used some new words. We were all excited.

Marileigh: Okay then. I will talk some more with Cathy and keep you posted. I am scheduled to go see him at child care next Wednesday. Would Tuesday evening work okay for us to meet around your dinnertime?

Cyd: Sure thing. I'll look forward to seeing you then. I can hardly wait to play our little games with the bubbles at bath time tonight!

Marileigh: And I can hardly wait to hear how successful you both are going to be! I'll see you next Tuesday evening.

Cyd: See you then. Bye.

Marileigh: Bye, Cyd!

The PSP and parent take a few minutes following the joint visit to talk about how the visit was or was not helpful and why. This is an opportunity for the PSP to determine what the parent learned and what was useful as well as develop a plan, if needed, for additional joint visits. The information gained from the parent can be useful to share with the SSP about content, interaction style, and the desire for any additional supports by the parent and/or PSP. The debriefings between the PSP and SSP as well as the PSP and parent may happen in any order and may also be a combined conversation between the three individuals.

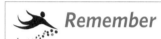 **Remember**

A joint visit has three components:

1. Planning (between primary service provider [PSP] and parent; between PSP and secondary service provider [SSP])

2. Implementing

3. Debriefing (between PSP and parent; between PSP and SSP)

JOINT VISIT CHALLENGES AND SOLUTIONS

Although joint visits are a required condition when implementing a PSP approach to teaming, valid challenges arise. The most commonly occurring challenges are often related to availability factors related to time, expertise, or distance, as well as payment of the services of two practitioners at the same date and time. The following section provides suggestions for addressing typical challenges related to implementing joint visits.

When Joint Visits Are Not "Joint"

On rare occasions when the next available date for the joint visit to occur at the same place and time is too far away, the team may decide to forego a joint visit in these circumstances and schedule a separate visit by the SSP. Planning for and debriefing of the visit are still required when this happens. The PSP and parent discuss the need for the separate visit and plan what activity setting needs to occur during the visit, what questions the parent and primary provider have, and what the secondary provider will be doing during the visit. The primary and SSP must also plan together based on the information the primary provider obtains from planning with the parent. The SSP conducts the visit with the family and debriefs the visit with the family and then

Remember

Separate visits by the primary service provider and secondary service provider are rare and can compromise the efficiency and effectiveness of the intervention process.

Take Action

If you are not already working on a team using a primary service provider approach, coordinate with another service provider seeing the same family and generate ideas for how to have a joint visit with the family.

the primary provider and discusses the information shared, actions taken, and the joint plan. The primary provider also debriefs the parent based on the conversation with the secondary provider, which includes discussing the helpfulness of the visit and the status of the joint plan developed between the parent and SSP. The decision to implement separate visits requires substantial thought and planning and can compromise the efficiency and effectiveness of the intervention process.

Geographic Barriers

The human resources needed for a joint visit are not available or at best difficult to gain access to in some instances due to time or geographic limitations. For example, a PSP needs access to an SLP for a joint visit because she and a child care provider have specific questions regarding speech sound development. In this program area, the SLP only drives to this county 1 day a week and her calendar is booked for the next 3 weeks. Although a joint visit with both the PSP and SLP onsite with the child care provider is preferable, the team opts for having the SLP join the visit via conference call to discuss the questions. The team could have also considered additional options of a web-based platform using webcams, enabling the SLP to see and interact with the child and child care provider. In circumstances in which observation of the child in context is necessary, teams can also use video to record the child in action and then share this video during a team meeting or with the needed team member and then engage in a one-to-one conversation via telephone, e-mail, or web-based technology.

Team Role Gap

A team may not have the necessary expertise to support a particular child and family in certain situations. The team needs to gain access to support from an individual or resource outside of the core team that can provide the information. For instance, a team receives a referral for a child with a diagnosis of cortical blindness and no one on the team has strong expertise in supporting children with this diagnosis. The state, however, has regional specialists available to support infants and toddlers with visual impairments. The service coordinator contacts the regional vision consultant to invite her to participate in developing the child's IFSP and request assistance for supporting this child. The vision specialist participates on the team as an SSP and attends joint visits to support the primary provider when they are scheduled to be in the area. Similarly, other regional specialists for low-incidence disabilities would serve as adjunct members of the core team and participate in joint visits with the assigned PSP when available.

Payment for Joint Visits

Paying two practitioners who provide support to a child on the same date at the same time is another complication related to joint visits. Most third party payers do not provide payment to two providers for simultaneous service delivery. Programs have a few options when this is the case. One option is to use third party reimbursement to pay for one of the visitors and program service delivery funds to pay for the time of the SSP. A second option is to establish fiscal policies that designate a rate for the SSPs. The primary provider most often bills the third party payer in these situations and the secondary provider receives the established rate from the early intervention program. The expectation is that programs determine a means for paying practitioners for their time involved in joint visits in order to effectively support children and families enrolled in the program.

CONCLUSION

Joint visits are a safety net used by programs implementing a PSP approach to teaming to ensure that the child, care providers, and primary provider have timely access to the knowledge and expertise of needed team members to support the achievement of IFSP outcomes. This chapter identified three situations in which joint visits may be necessary when a question or situation arises for the PSP, parent, or another team member and is beyond the scope of what can be accomplished during the team meeting. Joint visits require deliberate planning with the SSP and the parent or care provider. Debriefing of joint visits helps to guarantee that the primary provider received the role assistance necessary to continue supporting the child and family as well as identify next steps for follow-up. A regularly scheduled team meeting is the other safety net to afford timely support for the PSP, child, and family. Chapter 7 focuses on how to structure team meetings that are efficient and effective.

Joint Visit Planning Tool

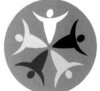

Primary service provider (PSP): _____Family: _____ Child: _____

Secondary service provider (SSP): _____ Date of joint visit: _____ Time: _____

Request for Role Assistance
Question or issue requiring support of another team member
What you (PSP) and/or the parent need from the SSP

Background Information
Your (PSP) and/or the parent's current knowledge and actions taken regarding the question/issue
Current child interests and activity settings that serve as the context for intervention
Current parent priorities

Plan

a. Conversation that will take place with the family about the joint visit
    (Questions to consider: When will you have the conversation? What questions need to be answered by the SSP? What does the SSP need to see? What will be the context for the visit? What does the SSP need to know? Who should take the lead—PSP or SSP?)

b. Context for the visit and rationale (date and time)

c. Person taking the lead in the visit (SSP or PSP) and rationale

d. Role of the person not taking the lead and the family during the visit

e. What is going to happen during the visit

f. Date/time for debrief of the joint visit with the SSP and family

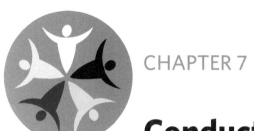

CHAPTER 7

Conducting Team Meetings

A common planning/meeting time is an implementation condition for using PSP teaming practices that is based on literature for effective teams (see Chapter 2; Bell, 2007; Borrill et al., 2001; West, 2012). The team meeting provides participants with a predictable time for role assistance, which may include discussion, idea generation, questioning, and critical thinking. It also contributes to the acculturation and socialization of the team identity and serves as the venue for developing a heightened sense of accountability and commitment for completing the task before the team.

Multidisciplinary, interdisciplinary, transdisciplinary, and a PSP approach to teaming mention the use of a formal team planning time or meeting (Shelden & Rush, 2010; Woodruff & McGonigel, 1988). All team members come together on a regular basis in a formal team meeting, whereas an informal team meeting may consist of only the individuals most actively involved with a specific child and family (Limbrick, 2004, 2005; Limbrick-Spencer, 2001). Formal team meetings are typically scheduled for a particular day and time. Informal team meetings occur as needed by individual team members. This chapter focuses on the formal team meeting.

The purposes of team meetings in multidisciplinary, interdisciplinary, and transdisciplinary models is typically to share information about a child and family based on a specific team member's interactions or interventions with the child or family. Depending on the teaming model, input from other team members may range from none (multidisciplinary) to sharing information and resources (interdisciplinary) to teaching and supporting other team members to use strategies and techniques typically done by another team member (transdisciplinary) (Woodruff & McGonigel, 1988). The purpose of the team meeting in a PSP approach to teaming is threefold: 1) joint accountability among team members for all families served by the team, 2) to share information among team members as families move through the early intervention process, and 3) for role assistance in the form of colleague-to-colleague coaching to support the PSP in building the capacity of the parent or care provider to support the child's participation in everyday activities in the home, community, and early childhood program settings and identify needed or desired parent resources (Shelden & Rush, 2010). The team meeting discussion may be used to determine the status of the current situation, what currently is or is not working, and what the PSP and care provider(s) have already tried or discussed, followed by sharing necessary resources, supports, and information from other team members. This process may include scheduling a joint visit for another team member to accompany the PSP to offer direct supports during a scheduled visit to the PSP, child, and/or care providers (see the Joint Visit Planning Tool in Appendix 6A).

Other literature, especially the business literature, describes how to conduct effective meetings, but research related to the characteristics of successful meetings is relatively nonexistent

Remember

Literature on effective team meetings indicates

- Only necessary participants should attend.

- Attendees should represent diverse perspectives.

- Attendees should have the knowledge and expertise to accomplish the task.

- The meeting should have clear guidelines.

- The meeting should be led by a competent facilitator.

- The meeting should have a prepublished agenda with time limits.

Remember

Research identifies three components to ensure effective team meetings:

1. Logistics

2. Facilitation

3. Participant interaction style

(see Appendix 2B). Literature that describes how to conduct meetings does not include the research-based characteristics of team meetings or even conceptual and theoretical frameworks for this type of meeting. Available literature on effective team meetings indicates that only necessary participants should attend (Daniels, 1993; Kayser, 2011; Pell, 1999), and the attendees should represent diverse perspectives (Doyle & Straus, 1986) and have the knowledge and expertise to accomplish the task (Bell, 2004; Doyle & Straus, 1986; Larsson, 2000). Furthermore, the meeting should have clear guidelines (Holpp, 1999; Rogelberg et al., 2012), be led by a competent facilitator (Doyle & Straus, 1986; Holpp, 1999; Kayser, 2011; Weaver & Farrell, 1997), and follow a prepublished meeting agenda (Daniels, 1993) with time limits (Holpp, 1999; Kayser, 2011; Pell, 1999), which assists in clarifying the purpose of the meeting (Rogelberg et al., 2012; Weaver & Farrell, 1997).

GUIDELINES FOR EFFECTIVE TEAM MEETINGS

The following guidelines for PSP team meetings were developed using existing literature on effective teaming characteristics (Bell, 2007; Daniels, 1990; Doyle & Straus, 1986; Holpp, 1999; Kayser, 2011; Larsson, 2000; Rogelberg et al., 2012; Weaver & Farrell, 1997) as well as through interviews and surveys completed by members of a multidisciplinary early childhood intervention team that had been working together and using a PSP approach to teaming. The literature and data identified three components to ensure effective team meetings—logistics, facilitation, and participant interaction style.

Logistics

Meetings for teams serving 100 children and families or more should be scheduled weekly at a time when all members can attend to guarantee multidisciplinary representation and a diverse perspective (Doyle & Straus, 1986) as well as ensure that the team has the necessary knowledge and expertise to accomplish the task (Bell, 2007; Doyle & Straus, 1986; Larsson, 2000). A weekly formal meeting time is necessary in order for teams to routinely meet time lines, effectively assist families through the IFSP process, and learn how to develop and maintain the ability to work collaboratively as a team. Team meetings may occur every other week for teams with relatively small caseloads or as team members become more comfortable and knowledgeable about working together, thereby becoming more efficient in their use of time. In our experience, teams that meet less than every other week are unable to maintain fidelity to the characteristics and implementation conditions of a PSP approach to teaming.

The average length of the formal meeting for most teams is 60–90 minutes. This amount of time allows team members to feel comfortable discussing issues and questions while ensuring that all agenda items are appropriately addressed. Not every child and family supported by the team is discussed at every team meeting, but every child and family should be discussed over a 3-month period to ensure that necessary supports are provided and outcomes are met. More detailed information about how time is allocated is discussed later in this chapter.

The day and time of the team meeting must consider the availability of part-time and contracted team members. As a result, the team meeting will be scheduled at the time convenient for the team members who give the program the least amount of their time. This is one of the reasons that program management should hire or contract with the fewest number of team members who give the most amount of time to the program. For example, consider a team that contracts with the local school district for an SLP's time. She is available every weekday after 2:30 p.m. This team's meeting time must occur during her available working hours, which means sometime after 2:30 p.m. Another example might be a situation in which a PT contracts with the team for 4 hours per week. At least 1 of those hours must now be spent in the team meeting, so the most hours this PT would have available to fulfill the role of a PSP and conduct joint visits is 3 hours each week.

All team members must be present for the entire team meeting. Unlike traditional team meetings in which participants provide status reports on the children and families they serve, members in this type of team meeting are available to provide role assistance to others serving as primary provider and receive information, ideas, and strategies from members of other disciplines. If a discipline is missing or leaves the meeting after they have shared information about the families on their caseload, then the other team members would be denied access to the knowledge and expertise that would have been provided by that person.

Meeting ground rules should be established early in a team's development and as new members join and revisited on a regular basis. Ground rules are the operating principles that define how team members work together during the meeting in order to be efficient, effective, and respectful of one another and the families they serve. Once ground rules are established and agreed on by all team members, it is the responsibility of each individual team member to abide by and enforce them. The ground rules provide a basis for conversations if and when team members fail to uphold what was agreed on by the team. Sample ground rules include, but are not limited to

- Start and stop the meeting on time

- Share the air time

- Arrive to the meeting on time and stay for the entire meeting

- Prepare for the meeting in advance

- Share information about families only in ways that members would if the family members were present

- Use everyday language that all team members will understand

- Give undivided attention to the team meeting (e.g., no cell phones, texting, e-mails, note writing)

- Team meeting attendance is required (e.g., no scheduling of other meetings, home visits, evaluations during this time)

Parents should be informed of the team meeting and invited to attend in person or via conference call or other technology if they so desire. Families should know that team meetings are different than IFSP meetings; therefore, they will be invited to attend only the portion of the meeting that directly relates to their family and discussions are generally very brief. In most instances, families want to be informed when information about their family is going to be shared at the team meeting in order for them to submit questions or

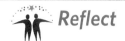 **Reflect**

How does your team ensure that parents are aware of and invited to participate in team meetings in which their child is going to be discussed?

requests for specific information if they do not plan to attend. If parents choose not to attend, then the PSP should ask them to send questions or updates to the rest of the team and provide timely feedback to the parents following the team meeting.

Because team members are required to participate in the meetings, program administrators must have mechanisms in place to compensate them for their time spent in the meetings. Payment for team meeting time is most commonly an issue for programs with contracted providers because it is not typically reimbursed by third party payers. Many state and local programs have identified procedures to ensure that practitioners are compensated for team meeting time, including developing fiscal policies that establish rates for team meeting participation, paying regular hourly rates, and using bundled rates that include time spent in team meetings.

Facilitation

Team meetings should be led by a skilled facilitator (Doyle & Straus, 1986; Holpp, 1999; Kayser, 2011; Weaver & Farrell, 1997) who follows an agenda (Holpp, 1999; Kayser, 2011) that has been developed prior to the team meeting (Daniels, 1990). The team meeting facilitator is a team member and may or may not be someone other than the formal team leader. Facilitation should not rotate among team members, but rather be the same person for each team meeting. The person responsible for facilitating the team meeting must be someone who either currently has or can develop the skills necessary for ensuring that the guidelines for meeting facilitation (see Appendix 7A) and interaction among participants (see Appendices 7B and 7C) are closely followed. Appendix 7D provides a checklist for program administrators or teams to select a competent and effective team meeting facilitator.

The role of the team facilitator is to establish and maintain the structure of the meeting, make certain that the meeting ground rules are followed, and ensure the agenda and all team meeting processes are implemented efficiently (Appendices 7E and 7F). Following each agenda item, the team facilitator asks the PSP to state an action plan and confirm receipt of the information and support needed. The facilitator recognizes that team meeting time is useful for networking, obtaining informal supports, and experiencing the team culture for all members. The facilitator's responsibility is that team meeting time is used for its intended purpose, however, due to the limited amount of time available, the costs of bringing all team members together, and the critical need to address all items on the team agenda.

Ensuring that each meeting has a prepublished agenda is another responsibility of the facilitator. Prepublishing the agenda may be accomplished by posting it to a location on a program's intranet in order for individual meeting participants to add agenda items prior to the meeting (see Appendix 7G). Another option might be for team members to call in agenda items to the facilitator or support staff prior to the meeting. Prepublishing the agenda allows the meeting facilitator to assign times to each item on the agenda prior to the designated meeting time, thereby increasing the efficient use of time during the meeting (Holpp, 1999; Kayser, 2011; Rogelberg et al., 2012).

🏃 *Remember*

The following are five types of team meeting agenda items.

1. Primary coaching opportunities—approximately 10 minutes per family

2. Quarterly updates—approximately 5 minutes per family

3. Welcome to the program—under 5 minutes per family

4. Transitions—approximately 2 minutes per family (if discussed)

5. Closures—approximately 2 minutes per family (if discussed)

The following are optional agenda items.

1. Announcements

2. Scheduling

Team Meeting Agenda

The team meeting agenda may consist of five types of items: primary coaching opportunities, quarterly updates, welcome to the program, transitions, and closures (see Appendix 7H). Announcements and scheduling are optional items that may be added to the agenda. The primary purpose of the team meeting is to provide opportunities for individuals serving as PSPs to receive support related to their work with individual families as well as provide support to other team members based on their experiences and area of expertise. The primary coaching opportunities item on the agenda allows PSPs to ask questions and pose issues as a mechanism for receiving role assistance from other team members. The time allocated for primary coaching opportunities typically ranges from 10 to 15 minutes per family, depending on the needs of the primary provider. Quarterly updates is the second agenda item. Every family should be reviewed by the team at least quarterly to remain current regarding each family's status in the program. Quarterly updates consist of a 5-minute overview of the current plan for supporting the family, status of the plan, and next steps. New children and families recently assigned to the team, along with their status in the program (e.g., intake, evaluation, assessment, program planning), are introduced to the team as part of the welcome to the program item on the agenda, which usually takes no longer than 5 minutes. Transitions of families to other programs and closures (e.g., graduation, disenrollment) are shared as part of the remaining two agenda items. Rather than discuss all transitions and closures during the meeting, these two agenda items may be considered as discussion items at the discretion of the person who added the item to the agenda and if time permits.

Announcements and scheduling are optional agenda items. Announcements should be either pre-printed on the agenda or included as an additional handout or part of an electronic message to team members, rather than shared verbally, because team meeting time is limited and costly to programs. Similarly, because scheduling usually involves only a few team members, all scheduling should be held until the end of the meeting at which time team members can coordinate their schedules. In order to ensure that all team members have their scheduling needs met, the facilitator should allow enough time at the end of the meeting for scheduling to occur while all team members are still present.

Participant Interaction Style

The interaction style of participants affects how team members serving as PSPs may receive information from other team members and the usefulness of the information. Implementing written participant guidelines for team members can help them prepare (Holpp, 1999; Rogelberg et al., 2012; Weaver & Farrell, 1997) to present information in the team meeting (see Appendix 7B) as well as provide support to other team members by using a capacity-building interaction style during the meeting (see Appendix 7C). The meeting facilitator is responsible for ensuring that all participants adhere to the written guidelines.

Presenting Information in Team Meetings

The person presenting information during the team meeting is also responsible for being prepared and organized in order to maximize efficient use of the team meeting time. Team members present information for the following agenda items: 1) welcome to the program, 2) quarterly updates, and 3) primary coaching opportunities (see Appendix 7H). The Individual Family Staffing Report (see Appendix 7I) is a tool to assist the person presenting information prepare for the team meeting and document a plan developed as part of the discussion at the meeting.

Welcome to the Program

The purpose of this agenda item is to ensure that all team members have knowledge of new children and families being served by the team. Prior to the meeting, the team member conducting the initial visit should have a clear understanding of the family's reason(s) for seeking program supports and a preliminary notion of the family's priorities. During the meeting, the team member shares the reason for the referral, any information already learned about the family's priorities, and the supports needed from the team. This could be a point at which the discussion of most likely PSP is initiated.

Consider a situation in which the service coordinator has just completed an initial visit with a family referred by a local pediatrician. The service coordinator shares that the pediatrician referred this 6-month-old child to early intervention because of her concerns about the child's weight and difficulty feeding from her bottle. The parents' priorities at this point are for the child to eat more during a shorter period of time and gain weight. The family is also struggling with the child's sleep schedules and fear she has flipped her days and nights, sleeping most of the day and staying awake most of the night. The service coordinator also shares that the family does not really have a set routine for her mealtimes, naps, or bedtime. They enjoy playing with her, but reported that she seems irritable and fussy most of the time. She does have a favorite pacifier and blanket that she snuggles. The service coordinator mentions that she needs to schedule the child's evaluation at the end of today's meeting.

Primary Coaching Opportunities

The purpose of primary coaching opportunities is for the PSP to obtain resources and/or supports (i.e., role assistance) from other team members to ensure that they are effectively addressing the family's priorities and child's needs. The PSP should use the Individual Family Staffing Report (see Appendix 7I) prior to the team meeting to identify their need for role assistance from other team members and determine how to present the situation to the rest of the team in a concise manner. The PSP should state the need for role assistance in the form of a question or an issue during the team meeting and share their and the parents' current knowledge/actions taken regarding the topic or issue. If the topic is related to child learning, then the PSP should also share the child's interests and activity settings that serve as the context for intervention as well as current parent priorities. If the topic is about parenting or parent support, then the primary provider should inform the rest of the team what resources they and the parents have already gained access to or considered. For example, if a primary provider needs additional ideas or resources for supporting a family around identifying a new child care provider, then the primary provider might ask the team members, "What child care providers on the north side of town provide care for parents who work second shift at the mill?" The primary provider should then share what they and the parents had already explored and could further clarify what the parents' criteria might include prior to sharing possible child care resources. Following this discussion, the PSP is responsible for providing feedback to the other team members regarding whether they are giving the support and role assistance needed. The PSP restates or clarifies question(s) or issue(s) as needed and ensures that they have a concrete and specific action plan, which might include a joint visit with another team member, before the facilitator moves to the next item on the agenda.

Example of How the Primary Service Provider Gains Access to Support Through the Team Meeting

The purpose of the following scenario is to illustrate how the PSP gains access to support from the team as part of a primary coaching opportunity listed on the agenda of the team meeting. Steve, the OT on the team, has a need for role assistance related to one of the families he serves regarding housing resources. His other team members include Bev, the EIC, who also serves as team meeting facilitator; Debbie, an early childhood special educator; Beth, a PT; Dee Dee, a psychologist; Molly and Lois, service coordinators; and Kirra, an SLP.

Bev:	The next item we have on our agenda is a primary coaching opportunity for Steve. Steve, what's the issue or question you are bringing to the team today?
Steve:	I have been working with the Beam family for the past 7 months. You may remember they have four children ranging in age from 6 months to 8 years of age. Renatta is a little more than 2 and she is the child in the family who has an IFSP. Mr. Beam has been out of work for more than a year, and Mrs. Beam does not work outside the home. They have used what little savings they had and relied on family and friends to help them stay in their apartment, but the money has run out, so they will no longer have a place to live at the end of the month. I need some resources to share with this family for housing.
Dee Dee:	Steve, what informal and formal resources have you and the family already pursued?
Steve:	Sorry. I meant to share that and forgot.
Bev:	That's okay. Go ahead and share that with us now.
Steve:	The family has talked with their extended family, but most of them are in similar circumstances and just don't have any more money to give them. It's not easy to move a family of six with such little children in with another family member, so they have ruled that out as a possibility. The dad just got into a job retraining program that starts next month, but it will take him 3 months to finish the program. They live over in Miller County, so I am just not familiar with the resources over there for this sort of thing.
Molly:	I work with a lot of families in Miller County and, frankly, there aren't many resources there.

Steve: They just have 2 weeks to find something.

Lois: What about the homeless shelter here in this county?

Steve: Transportation is a problem. They have one car that Mr. Beam works on all the time to keep running, but the job retraining program is in Miller County, so I don't think the car could make it back and forth every day.

Debbie: The homeless shelter might be an option for the mother and children, but they don't have facilities for men. The only men's shelter is across town.

Steve: They wouldn't want to split up. I know that for sure. They are really close, and Mr. Beam helps out a lot with the children.

Lois: What about the churches there in Miller County? Have they checked with them? Sometimes they know of temporary housing.

Steve: I could ask them about that.

Molly: Oh, yeah. The churches in that area have formed a group called the Miller County Ministries. Most of them have combined their efforts related to food pantries, funds to help pay utility bills, and so forth.

Bev: Steve, what do you think the family would think about checking with them as a plan?

Lois: Do they pay rent or have a place where they all could stay?

Molly: I don't know, but it might be a place to start. Maybe if they can't help with the rent, they could assist with food and help with their utility bills. Then the family could put whatever resources they have left toward the rent. I can give you the contact number, Steve.

Steve: That would be great. Thanks.

Bev: So, what's your plan, Steve?

Steve: I am going to get the contact number of the Miller County Ministries from Molly, and then I'll share it with the family during my visit tomorrow because they don't have a telephone. I feel better prepared to brainstorm options with them now and can help them evaluate the pros and cons of what we've talked about today.

Bev: What's your back-up plan if that doesn't work?

Steve: I guess I can share the information with them about the homeless shelter in this county or maybe we could figure out options for transportation and then we can look into other resources here in town.

Bev: All right. Anything else you need from the team about this today, Steve?

Steve: No, I'm good for now. Thanks.

This scenario illustrated how a team member brings a question or issue to the team in the form of a primary coaching opportunity. In this situation, Steve asked about resources for housing. Rather than starting to list resources, the team ensured they had knowledge of what Steve and the family had already considered and asked about both formal and informal resources. Once they understood this information, they began asking him about other options and shared information. Although Steve looked to the service coordinators on his team for this type of expertise, other members contributed as well. Not all team members had information or ideas to provide. Team members were respectful of one another and built on one another's ideas. As the conversation neared an end, the facilitator checked with Steve to ensure that he had a plan as well as back-up ideas to discuss with the family. See Figure 7.1 for a completed Individual Family Staffing Report for the Beam family.

Individual Family Staffing Report

Family name: _____ *Beam* _____   Team meeting date: _____ *2/14/21* _____

Child's name: _____ *Renatta* _____   Last review in team meeting: _____ *12/08/21* _____

Primary service provider: _____ *Steve* _____

Secondary service provider(s): _____ *N/A* _____

Type of staffing (check one)	Discussion/outcome
☐ **Welcome to the program** (before the individualized family service plan) Information needed by other team members • Reason for referral • Information gathered about child interests, activity settings, and family priorities • Steps in the early intervention process that have been completed • Supports needed from other team members	Plan:
☑ **Primary coaching opportunity** Information needed by other team members • Question/issue you are bringing to the team for support • Your or the parent's current knowledge/actions taken regarding this topic/issue • If child learning, then current interests and activity settings that serve as the context for intervention • Current parent priorities • Video share	**Role assistance** 1. Response to the question/issue discussed during team meeting Plan: *Get telephone number of Miller County Ministries from Molly.* *Talk with family at visit tomorrow about contacting resource and evaluate pros/cons.* *Consider transportation options in order to use a housing resource in town.* *And/or* 2. Joint visit with _____ on _____ at _____ Plan for joint visit: • Conversation to occur with parent: • Context for joint visit and why: • Person taking lead in joint visit and why: • When to debrief joint visit: *(continued)*

Figure 7.1. Completed Individual Family Staffing Report for the Beam family.

Figure 7.1. *(continued)*

☐ **Quarterly update** Information needed by other team members *Child learning* • Child's current interests and activity settings • Ways in which you and parent are promoting child's participation • How your actions and/or interactions relate to the parent priorities *Parenting support (e.g., sleep, behavior, nutrition, toileting)* • Topics, questions, or issues currently being addressed • Ways in which previous supports are being addressed *Parent support (e.g., housing, transportation, employment, medical)* • Topics, questions, or issues currently being addressed • Ways in which previous supports are being addressed • Informal and formal resources to meet identified needs	Plan:
☐ **Transition** Information needed by other team members • Transition plan	Transition plan:
☐ **Closure** Information needed by other team members • Reason for closure	Follow-up:

Team members present (signature and discipline):

_____*Steve, occupational therapist*_____   _____*Bev, early intervention coordinator*_____

_____*Molly, service coordinator*_____   _____*Kirra, speech-language pathologist*_____

*Debbie, early childhood special educator*   _____*Lois, service coordinator*_____

_____*Dee Dee, psychologist*_____   _____*Beth, physical therapist*_____

Quarterly Updates

The purpose of the quarterly updates is to make sure that all children and families are brought to the attention of the full team on at least a quarterly basis. If a family is brought to the team during the primary coaching opportunities section of the agenda, then this may also serve as the quarterly update. For quarterly updates, prior to the meeting, the PSP should determine what progress has been made or changes in status have occurred with the child and family since the last update. During the meeting, the PSP should share information related to interactions with the child and family regarding child learning, parenting support, and/or parent support. The PSP should document the current plan for the child and family and any next steps on the Individual Family Staffing Report (see Appendix 7I).

Providing Support to Other Team Members During the Team Meeting

The role of other team members when not presenting information about a particular child and family is to provide support and serve as a resource to the presenting team member. Rather than immediately moving to making suggestions or recommendations, team members should use an interaction style that builds the capacity of the presenter for both the current and possible future situations. Team members should use the same principles used to coach parents when supporting other team members in the context of the meeting (Rush & Shelden, 2020). Team members must be certain that they clearly understand the presenter's question or issue. If the question or issue is unclear, then members of the team should seek clarification of the question or issue. Understanding what the presenter already knows, has done, or is thinking in relation to the issue or question before providing additional information or ideas is important in order to avoid making suggestions that the primary provider has already tried or considered.

Team members should be respectful of each other's lines of questioning and must allow others to finish their questions, comments, or thoughts prior to jumping in with another question or before sharing additional information. Team members who are not actively asking questions should be listening to what is being asked to avoid duplication of questions and information and avoid needlessly jumping into the conversation. Only one person should talk at a time during primary coaching opportunities. The questions or information should be directed to the presenter, rather than another team member (i.e., sidebar conversations are distracting). The focus of the discussion should be on the PSP to ensure their needs are being met. All team members should be sensitive to sharing the air time with other team members. When a team member asks questions, they are open to varied possibilities as answers because having a predetermined answer that they are trying to get the presenter to say is coaxing rather than coaching.

Information, strategies, and ideas are shared only after the question or issue has been adequately defined and the presenter has been given the opportunity to reflect on their actions, intentions, ideas, and possible solutions/actions. All team members need to avoid giving advice (e.g., statements that include the following words: *should, ought to, need to*) and actively ensure that the presenter is getting the type of support they would find most helpful. Team members are responsible for checking the presenter's understanding of any information that is being shared and listening to the presenter and reading their body language as feedback regarding whether the information received is the type of support the PSP needs. The team must ensure that the presenter has a concrete and specific plan to implement prior to ending the coaching conversation and that the plan includes a mechanism for sharing the outcomes of plan implementation either with the entire team or key individuals during a follow-up meeting/conversation. As a reminder, the team meeting facilitator has ultimate control of the meeting and their requests to close a conversation are to be respected.

Example of a Challenging Meeting for the Team Facilitator

Challenging meeting situations for the team facilitator may include, but are not limited to, formation of new teams, new member joining an existing team, team members with strong personalities, and lack of clear ground rules. The following scenario provides an example of a situation in which the facilitator has to provide redirection and support team members in using effective team meeting practices. In this example, Beth, the PT and PSP on the team, needs support related to a child's behavior.

Bev: Beth, I see you are on the agenda with a primary coaching opportunity for Jason Raines. What is your issue or question for the team?

Beth: Thanks, Bev. I have been working with Jason and his family for about a year now. He is really a cute kid, but he sure has a mind of his own. His mother is really good, but she is just about at her wits' end. I mean, his behavior has really gotten out of control. She has tried everything. It's a really good family. The dad is involved, and I've met the grandparents.

Bev: Beth...

Beth: They don't live too far from me, so I see them out in the community a lot. His behavior seems fine when I see him out, but it must really be another story when they are at home.

Bev: Excuse me, Beth, but please share your question or issue with us, which is the reason you put this on the agenda as a primary coaching opportunity.

Beth: Oh, sorry. The mother needs some help with his behavior, and I'm just at a loss for what to do.

Kirra: What happens?

Dee Dee: I could go out on a joint visit with you.

Steve: Shouldn't we know what you've already tried? The Individual Family Staffing Report says to tell us what you've already tried.

Dee Dee: What does she want or expect his behavior to look like?

Beth: She uses time-out. She has to drag him over to the naughty spot and he hits, kicks, and screams all the way there. I'm telling you, when he kicks you with those AFO [ankle foot orthosis] on his legs, you know you've been kicked. He kicks with the heel of his foot, and I've seen the bruises on his mom's legs to prove it. I mean, ouch!

Dee Dee: Oh my gosh! Not another time-out mom!

Bev: Whoa, guys! Hold up a minute! How does what is happening right now match our team ground rules and guidelines for participating in team meetings?

Lois: Not!

Bev: Beth, we need you to be specific and follow the outline on the Individual Family Staffing Form under Primary Coaching Opportunity. In response, we need to ask you only one question at a time. Dee Dee, we don't have enough information yet to determine if a joint visit is necessary, and remember our ground rule of only talking about parents within the team meeting as we would if they were sitting right here.

Dee Dee: You're right, Bev. I'm sorry.

Bev: Beth, what I've heard you say is that you and the mother need some support around Jason's behavior. She's tried time-out, but that hasn't been successful in the current situation. So, we have a general idea of what support you need and we know what the mother has tried, but we are missing the context. Tell us when the behavior seems to be happening.

Beth: At bedtime. I've been working with the parents to make the transition from the crib to his own bed so he can be more independent at getting in and out of the bed by himself. The problem is that he does not want to go to bed. When they try to make him go to bed, he starts hitting and kicking. The mom is a big believer in time-out. She's seen it on television, she uses it, but it's not working for bedtime. They just have to let him fall asleep wherever, and then they carry him to bed.

Kirra: I'm wondering if this could be communication based. Does he understand what his mother wants him to do? Can he follow simple instructions?

Beth: Yes, I think so. He . . .

Debbie: You could use picture cards to help him with the transitions.

Steve: I was thinking that, too, or maybe let him have more control over the bedtime routine, like the mom could allow him to pick out his own pajamas?

Dee Dee: We need to focus on child interests instead of on a punishment such as time-out. I'm telling you, time's up for time-out! We've got to help parents understand that!

Molly: Do we need to refer to a behavior specialist?

Bev: Hold on. Let me interrupt, please. Beth, how is this helpful?

Beth: Well, I have to be honest. I'm getting a little overwhelmed here. I think you all have some good ideas, but you're kind of firing them away at me like there's no tomorrow.

Kirra: Sorry, Beth.

Steve: Me, too.

Dee Dee: I'm trying, but you guys know time-out is my soap box issue.

Bev: So to recap, the issue that you are bringing to the team is the child's behavior at bedtime. He is hitting and kicking to keep from having to go to bed. The mother has tried time-out, but it does not work in this situation. We've heard a lot of ideas thrown out, but how can we better coordinate our supports to ensure that Beth gets what she needs from this discussion?

Steve: Because Dee Dee is so passionate about time-out, why don't you (turns to Dee Dee) start?

Bev: Beth, how does that sound to you?

Beth: I would like to know more about what Dee Dee is thinking about time-out.

Dee Dee: Beth, what do you know about the evidence to support time-out versus options for positive behavior supports?

Beth: I know that we should focus on his interests and use those in situations such as this as well as give him opportunities for what he wants to do, but the hitting came up so fast. Jason's mom has used time-out in the past. I'm not sure how successful it was for her. She seemed to act like it was always a struggle.

Dee Dee: We really don't have research to support the use of time-out for children under 3 years of age. They don't understand why they are being put in time-out and what that has to do with what they were previously doing. Maybe she would be open to some other options to support his behavior because time-out is not always working. What are things he likes that could be associated with the bedtime routine?

Beth: He likes Spiderman, so they had talked about getting him some Spiderman pajamas—kind of like what you were thinking, Steve. He also has a couple of favorite snuggly toys. Oh, and he really likes for his dad to read books to him.

Steve:	All of those could be calming activities to help him wind down and prepare for bedtime.
Dee Dee:	Beth, what supports do you need from us to be able to talk to Jason's mom about time-out and ways to support positive behavior around bedtime?
Beth:	This has been helpful. Like I said, I don't think she really found time-out that helpful, but she didn't know of any other options. Then when the hitting and kicking started, she went right for a punishment technique other than spanking. I believe I can talk with her about this and we can even brainstorm other ideas to support him around bedtime that will prevent it from escalating to hitting and kicking.
Bev:	Then, Beth, your plan is to take this information back to discuss with Mrs. Raines and possibly generate some other ideas of positive behavior supports?
Beth:	Yes, and I can talk more with Dee Dee if I need any other ideas about positive behavior support options and ideas.

Although team members often have the best of intentions and a desire to provide help quickly, firing questions and/or suggestions at the person needing assistance can lead to confusion, conflicting priorities, and missed opportunities to get to the bottom of an issue. The facilitator intervened three times in the previous example. First, the facilitator assisted the presenter to move from sharing general information about the situation to a reminder about the need for clearly and succinctly framing the question or issue that she is bringing to the team for assistance. Once the presenter put her question forth, however, multiple team members immediately began asking questions and offering assistance. Needed information was still lacking; therefore, the facilitator interrupted to share her observations about the process team members were using to provide support and asked them to reflect on how their behaviors matched the team meeting ground rules. The facilitator reframed the discussion by summarizing what had been learned at this point and asked the presenter to share information about context as outlined on the Individual Family Staffing Report. The team again began to offer random suggestions based on their personal areas of expertise. The third time the facilitator intervened, she asked the presenter to reflect on how the process was helpful. At this point, the presenter's feedback caused the team to realize they had not been sharing information in a useful way to the PSP or consistent with how they want to operate as a team. The facilitator summarized and asked the team members a process-based, action-oriented question to help them coordinate their supports for the presenter, which they then did. The team meeting facilitator must be comfortable with stopping the conversation to help team members ensure they are providing supports in ways that are consistent with effective team meeting practices and the ground rules established by the team. The role of the facilitator is to support both the presenter and the rest of the team with being efficient, effective, accurate, timely, evidence based, and helpful. The facilitator must ensure the presenter's needs are met and that they leave the meeting with a clear plan for next steps.

TEAM MEETING CHALLENGES AND SOLUTIONS

A PSP approach to teaming requires an infrastructure that supports regular (in most situations, weekly) team meetings. Bringing together individuals with diverse experience and expertise can present challenges in terms of access, costs, time, participation, and acculturation. The final points of this chapter include team meeting considerations often presented as challenges that team leaders need to be prepared to address in order to conduct successful team meetings.

Culture of the Team Meeting

Practitioners unfamiliar with working on a team using a PSP approach often lack understanding of the importance of the team meeting or may appear disengaged. In general, meetings can be viewed as extra or a waste of time by busy practitioners. The team meeting in a PSP approach serves as the

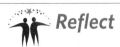

safety net to ensure that no child or family falls through the cracks and, thereby, does not receive necessary supports and services. The team meeting facilitator and program management can assist practitioners by helping them understand that every team member is responsible for every child and family enrolled in the program, not just those families for whom they serve as primary provider. Practitioners indicate their support for the ongoing intervention plan by signing the Individual Family Staffing Report. The undivided attention of every team member is necessary so that all members know when and how to share their discipline-specific as well as person-specific knowledge and expertise.

Compensation for Participation in Team Meetings

The additional costs associated with paying team members to participate in team meetings is an implementation challenge for states and programs that must rely on contract service providers and who have not previously required attendance at team meetings. States and local programs using a PSP approach to teaming must adequately compensate all team members to ensure attendance and participation. For those programs with salaried staff members, adjusting to a team meeting is not as difficult and often involves prioritizing the time and adjusting roles and responsibilities of team members. Developing fiscal policies that establish a special rate for teaming time, providing stipends for contractors that include attendance at team meetings, and paying the contractor's regular hourly rate or a portion thereof are viable solutions for programs that must identify funds to pay contracted members for time spent in team meetings.

Making Time for Team Meetings

Finding the time to schedule the team meeting can be particularly challenging for teams that use contracted or part-time service providers, especially when those individuals have obligations that limit their availability. This time constraint is further complicated because all of the other team members must arrange their schedules to accommodate the limited availability of the contracted therapist. Adding another contracted member to the team with limited availability would further limit options for team meeting time. Using contract providers is a viable and necessary strategy for many early intervention programs; however, careful consideration is required by the program manager or coordinator to ensure some overlap and compatibility of individual schedules to allow for a common team meeting time. The more people on the team, the more complicated scheduling the team meeting becomes.

Using Technology to Support Team Meetings

Sometimes the size of the geographic area to be covered by the team and the distance team members must travel can negatively affect the team's ability to meet regularly. Although face-to-face interaction is the preferred method for conducting team meetings, using technology such as conference calls and web-based meetings may be necessary and most cost effective. Conference calling options include using a telephone conferencing service that allows all team members to dial a toll-free telephone number with an assigned pass code or initiating the conference call from the program office using a speakerphone and enough conference telephone lines to connect team members joining from alternate locations. Many web-based meeting options allowing for audio and/or video conferencing are currently available ranging from no-cost to monthly service fees. These options require an Internet connection, computer, and webcams.

Unavailability of Core Team Members

The lack of access to a core team member either on a short- or long-term basis is a particular challenge for some teams, particularly those in remote areas. A PSP approach is compromised when a required team member is unavailable for the team meeting. A strategy that has been successfully by teams for short periods of time to temporarily bridge missing areas of expertise is to gain access to the needed discipline from another team within the program or to contract with other entities to provide support during team meetings either in person or via technology. In circumstances in which core team members are unavailable on a long-term basis, creative recruitment strategies may be necessary to attract potential employees or contractors. For example, a program might be able to identify a practitioner willing to contract for team meetings only, but the practitioner may be willing to expand available hours once they are involved in the teaming process. When gaining access to an individual only for purposes of providing support within the context of the team meeting, the program must provide training and orientation to ensure this practitioner understands natural learning environment practices, coaching, and a PSP approach to teaming.

Team Member Participation in Meetings

For program leadership and individual practitioners unaccustomed to working on a team, the way in which information and support are provided and received may be different than prior experiences. Individual team members' personalities related to how they share information, learn, and interact directly affects the work of the team. When working alone or using other teaming approaches, if team members disagree, experience personality conflicts, or do not trust and respect one another, then the impact on the families served by that individual is minimal to none. In contrast, individual team members using a PSP approach need one another in terms of knowledge, skills, and resources in order to effectively support the families. The culture of the team and the ways team members interact with one another are magnified at the team meeting when they must all work together toward mutually agreed-on outcomes. Dysfunction among team members prohibits efficient team interaction and directly decreases the quality of services provided to the child and family. Program management and the team meeting facilitator must ensure that individual team members learn how to work together, accepting and building on one another's personality characteristics to enhance rather than inhibit their ability to function as a team.

Colleague-to-Colleague Coaching During Team Meetings

As previously stated, the primary purpose of the team meeting is to provide opportunities for team members to coach and support one another. Colleague-to-colleague coaching, however, can be perceived by many practitioners as more difficult than coaching family members (Rush & Shelden, 2020). Whereas family members are seeking specific supports from the PSP, team members presented with opportunities to build the capacity of another team member through coaching may feel like they will be stepping on the toes of the other person, making assumptions about the other person's knowledge and skills, avoiding answering the other person's questions, or being viewed as lacking the needed expertise when choosing to bring up an issue or seek further understanding rather than remain quiet or tell the person what to do. Opportunities for team members to coach and support one another may also be overshadowed by other important aspects of the team meeting (e.g., updates, logistical issues, scheduling). The team facilitator must ensure that opportunities for coaching are prioritized and continuously be aware of serendipitous moments during which coaching would be the most effective approach for achieving the desired results.

CONCLUSION

Team meetings are a required component of a PSP approach to teaming. Effective team meetings help ensure that family members have timely access to all team members' expertise, knowledge, and resources. Identifying a common planning time and funding that will enable all team members to participate will be an initial challenge to overcome for many programs. Ground rules, facilitation, thoughtfully planned meeting logistics, the use of a meeting facilitator, clearly defined roles of all meeting participants, and adoption of a prepublished agenda can result in team meetings that better meet the needs of team members and maximize efficient use of time.

Guidelines for the Role of the Facilitator in the Team Meeting

- Prepublish the agenda.

- Start and stop the meeting on time.

- Ensure that all items on the agenda are addressed.

- Establish and maintain the structure of the meeting.

- Ensure full participation of all participants.

- Control the air time of participants.

- Ensure that people staffing have an action plan and receive what they need.

- Ensure that staffing time is used only for staffing.

Guidelines for Presenting Information in the Team Meeting

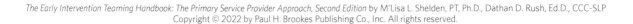

WELCOME TO THE PROGRAM

Welcome to the program ensures that all team members have knowledge of new children and families being served by the team. Welcome to the program should take approximately 5 minutes.

- Prior to the meeting, develop a clear understanding of the families' reason(s) for seeking program supports and any information learned about family priorities.

- During the meeting, share

  - Reason for referral

  - Information gathered about child interests, activity settings, and family priorities

  - Steps in the early intervention process that have been completed

  - Supports needed from other team members

PRIMARY COACHING OPPORTUNITIES

Primary coaching opportunities obtain resources and/or supports (i.e., role assistance) from other team members to ensure that you are effectively addressing the family's priorities. Primary coaching opportunities can last 10–15 minutes.

- Prior to the meeting, identify your need for role assistance from other team members and determine how to present the situation to the rest of the team in a concise manner. The following are questions to consider.

  - What is your question or issue?

  - What type of role assistance are you seeking (e.g., information, resources, strategies, acknowledgment that you are doing the right thing, assistance thinking through a situation, joint visit from a colleague)?

  - What is your or the parent's current knowledge/actions taken regarding this topic/issue?

  - If the issue is child learning, then what are the current interests and activity settings that serve as the context for intervention?

  - What are the current family priorities?

  - What is the minimum amount of information you need to share to ensure team members understand the situation?

- During the meeting, state your need for role assistance in the form of a question or an issue.

- Provide feedback to other team members regarding whether they are giving you the support and assistance you need.

- Restate or clarify your question(s) or issue(s) as needed.

- Ensure that you have a concrete and specific action plan before the facilitator moves to the next item on the agenda.

QUARTERLY UPDATES

Quarterly updates ensure that all children and families are brought to the attention of the full team on at least a quarterly basis. If a family is brought to the team during the primary coaching opportunities section of the agenda, then this may also serve as the quarterly update. Quarterly updates should take no longer than 5 minutes.

- Prior to the meeting, review the staffing report from the previous update. Determine what progress has been made or changes in status have occurred.

- During the meeting, share

  - Current focus of the visits regarding child learning, parenting support, and parent support (see Appendix 7G)

  - The current plan for the family

  - Next steps

Guidelines for How to Provide Coaching in the Team Meeting

- Be certain that you clearly understand the presenter's question or issue.

- Seek clarification of the question or issue, if necessary.

- Be certain that you know what the presenter already knows, has done, or is thinking in relation to the issue or question before providing additional information or ideas.

- Be respectful of other team members' lines of questioning. Allow others to finish their questions, comments, or lines of thinking prior to jumping in with another question or before sharing additional information.

- Listen to what the other team members are asking or sharing. If your thoughts, questions, and ideas are addressed, then you do not need to jump into the conversation.

- Only one person should talk at a time.

- Direct your questions or information to the presenter, rather than another team member.

- Stay on topic. The focus should be on the presenter.

- Share the air time with other team members.

- Asking questions means that you are open to varied possibilities as answers. Having a predetermined answer that you are trying to get the presenter to say is coaxing rather than coaching.

- Information should be shared only after the question or issue has been adequately defined and the presenter has been given the opportunity to reflect on their actions, intentions, ideas, and possible solutions/actions.

- Avoid giving advice (e.g., statements that include the following words: *should, ought to, need to*).

- Ensure that the presenter is getting the type of role assistance they intended.

- Check for the presenter's understanding of any information that is being shared. Listen to the presenter and read their body language as feedback regarding whether they are receiving the type of role assistance they want/need.

- Ensure that the presenter has a concrete and specific plan to implement prior to ending the coaching conversation.

- Ensure that the plan includes a mechanism for sharing the outcomes of plan implementation either with the entire team or key individuals during a follow-up meeting/conversation.

- The team meeting facilitator has ultimate control of the meeting. Their requests to close a conversation should be respected.

The Early Intervention Teaming Handbook: The Primary Service Provider Approach, Second Edition by M'Lisa L. Shelden, PT, Ph.D., Dathan D. Rush, Ed.D., CCC-SLP

Checklist for Selecting a Primary Service Provider Approach to Teaming Meeting Facilitator

Team: _____   Date: _____

Potential facilitator's name: _____

Circle each response that indicates a positive characteristic of the potential facilitator.	Yes	No
Is always on time	Y	N
Has the respect of other team members	Y	N
Is flexible but focused	Y	N
Is diplomatic without compromising	Y	N
Speaks up	Y	N
Is fair	Y	N
Has an awareness of time and can use it effectively	Y	N
Multitasks effortlessly	Y	N
Is good at teamwork	Y	N
Likes and believes in teaming	Y	N
Holds true to the program values and beliefs	Y	N
Seeks consensus among team members	Y	N
Gets others talking	Y	N
Can redirect when someone is talking too much	Y	N
Summarizes, synthesizes, and/or explains others' thoughts or ideas	Y	N
Develops tools, forms, or checklists to help him- or herself and others do his, her, or their work	Y	N
Gives feedback without feelings being hurt	Y	N
Uses a coaching interaction style with families and colleagues with fidelity	Y	N
Recognizes the need to talk about the use of evidence-based practices or the lack thereof	Y	N
Can delegate responsibility to others	Y	N
Moves the agenda forward	Y	N
Ensures that all agenda items are addressed but knows when to allow time for deeper discussion and learning opportunities	Y	N
Has time to address and prepare for team meeting tasks outside the team meeting	Y	N
Builds the capacity of other team members to take responsibility for the team meeting process	Y	N
Enforces the team ground rules	Y	N

At-a-Glance
Primary Service Provider Team Meeting Facilitation

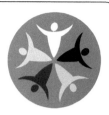

Prior to the Meeting

- Ensure agendas are prepared at least 3 months in advance of meeting date to post quarterly updates from this week's meeting to agenda in 3 months.
- Close the agenda 24 hours prior to the meeting.
- Review the agenda and assign approximate time for each agenda item:
  - Primary coaching opportunities—10 minutes
  - Welcome to the program
    - New referral—15 minutes
    - Follow-up—5 minutes
  - Quarterly update—5 minutes
  - Allow time for unexpected primary coaching opportunities

Beginning the Meeting

- Ensure phones are silenced and off the table, contact notes and other documentation are put away, and all team members are present and focused.
- Provide copies of agenda or display on screen.
- Start the meeting on time.
- Refer to the agenda and ask "Who has a primary coaching opportunity that is not already on the agenda?"
- Do not allow for any other items to be added to the agenda unless time permits at the end of the meeting.

Primary Coaching Opportunities

- Refer to the agenda and ask "(Name of team member), what is the question or issue that you are bringing to the team for support?"
- Ensure team members coach versus tell

Optional questions if not addressed:

- What have you and the caregiver discussed?
- What have you already tried?
- What is the activity setting?
- How do you think your question or issue might best be addressed?

Conclusion:

- What is your plan?
- What feedback do you have for the team about the helpfulness of their support?

Welcome to the Program

New referrals

- Let's all refer to the *Worksheet for Selecting the Most Likely Primary Service Provider.*
- (Team member presenting), beginning with Tier 1, take us through the information you have gathered so far.

Follow-up prior to individualized family service plan (IFSP)

- Based on the bullets on the IFSP, what additional information does the team need at this point?
- What support is needed from the team?

Quarterly Updates

- (Team member presenting), using the bullets on the IFSP as a guide, what information does the team need about (child's name) and their family?
- What additional supports do you need from the team?
- Team members, what questions do you have for (team member presenting)?
- (Team member presenting), what is your plan for moving forward?
- Recorder lists on agenda in 3 months.

Ending the Meeting

- How helpful was our meeting today?
- What could we start doing, stop doing, or do differently to improve our meeting?
- Looking at our agenda for next week, who do we need to add or remove at this point?
- Who still needs to schedule and plan joint visits in the time remaining?

(continued)

Self-Assessment

- What did I and/or the team learn and/or change as a result of the selection of the *most likely* primary service provider (PSP) process, joint visit, and/or team meeting?
- How do team interactions build my/other team member's knowledge and skills for the current and future situations?
- How do selection of the *most likely* PSP, joint visit planning, joint visit implementation, and team meeting interactions compare with the characteristics and implementation conditions for using a PSP approach to teaming?
- What will I and/or my team continue to do? What is working?

Your Plan

- What do I want to continue to improve or do differently as the team meeting facilitator?
- What additional supports do I need?
- How am I preparing the back-up facilitator to lead the meetings when I am not present?
- What is my plan for building the capacity of the back-up facilitator?

Worksheet for Selecting the Most Likely Primary Service Provider

Core team as options for primary service provider (PSP)

Early childhood (EC) _____   Occupational therapist (OT) _____

Physical therapist (PT) _____   Speech-language pathologist (SLP) _____   Other _____

Most likely PSP(s) identified based on

	Parent/family factors	Child factors	Environmental factors	Practitioner factors	Most likely PSP options selected (list)	Secondary service provider (SSP) options selected (list)
Tier 1	List priorities with contexts *"Beginning with box one, Tier I what do we know about this family?"* List parent/physician request	List diagnosis/condition/needs (long-term view) List interests/activity settings	Circle natural learning environments • Home • Community • Preschool • Child care • Other	List knowledge/expertise (personal/professional) *"Based on the information shared so far, what knowledge and expertise would be helpful for the PSP to have?"*	*"Based on the information shared so far, who would be a most likely PSP for this family?"*	Role overlap
Tier 2	Family dynamics Individual parent/caregiver characteristics • Language/culture • Knowledge/expertise • Diagnosis/condition • Other		Safety Distance from program office	Primary service area in geographic region Billability Prior relationship Rapport	*"Based on the information shared so far, who would still be a most likely PSP for this family?"*	Role overlap
Tier 3	Availability			Availability		Role overlap
				Most likely PSP is:	**Role gap? If so, explain:**	**Role assist (SSP):**

Notes:

If more than one most likely PSP is identified, ask: "Based on the information shared, who are our options for most likely PSP for this family and why?" "Considering all factors discussed and long-term view, who should we recommend to the family?"

Guidelines for Agenda Building for the Team Meeting

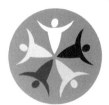

- All primary coaching opportunities, quarterly updates, welcome to the program, transitions, and closures must be posted to the agenda 24 hours prior to the start time of the team meeting. Agendas are located on the shared drive.

- No additional items may be added to the agenda within 24 hours of the staffing meeting unless the situation requires immediate support. If the situation requires immediate support and occurs within 24 hours of the staff meeting, then you may request that the item to be added to the agenda at the beginning of the team meeting.

- Transitions and closures will be posted to the agenda for team members' awareness only and will not be discussed during the meeting unless a team member has a particular question that would involve more team members than the primary service provider.

- Time frames will be assigned to each agenda item by the team meeting facilitator prior to the team meeting.

Team Meeting Agenda

Date: _____

Team members present: _____

_____

_____

_____

_____

_____

Primary coaching opportunities

Primary service provider (PSP)	Family	Question/issue

Quarterly updates

PSP	Family

Welcome to the program	*Transitions*	*Closures*
Family PSP	Family PSP	Family PSP

Individual Family Staffing Report

Family name: _____   Team meeting date: _____

Child's name: _____   Last review in team meeting: _____

Primary service provider: _____

Secondary service provider(s): _____

Type of staffing (check one)	Discussion/outcome
☐ **Welcome to the program** (before the individualized family service plan) Information needed by other team members • Reason for referral • Information gathered about child interests, activity settings, and family priorities • Steps in the early intervention process that have been completed • Supports needed from other team members	**Plan:**
☐ **Primary coaching opportunity** Information needed by other team members • Question/issue you are bringing to the team for support • Your or the parent's current knowledge/actions taken regarding this topic/issue • If child learning, then current interests and activity settings that serve as the context for intervention • Current parent priorities • Video share	**Role assistance** 1. Response to the question/issue discussed during team meeting Plan: *And/or* 2. Joint visit with _____ on _____ at _____ Plan for joint visit: • Conversation to occur with parent: • Context for joint visit and why: • Person taking lead in joint visit and why: • When to debrief joint visit: *(continued)*

☐ **Quarterly update**	**Plan:**
Information needed by other team members	
Child learning	
• Child's current interests and activity settings	
• Ways in which you and parent are promoting child's participation	
• How your actions and/or interactions relate to the parent priorities	
Parenting support (e.g., sleep, behavior, nutrition, toileting)	
• Topics, questions, or issues currently being addressed	
• Ways in which previous supports are being addressed	
Parent support (e.g., housing, transportation, employment, medical)	
• Topics, questions, or issues currently being addressed	
• Ways in which previous supports are being addressed	
• Informal and formal resources to meet identified needs	
☐ **Transition**	**Transition plan:**
Information needed by other team members	
• Transition plan	
☐ **Closure**	**Follow-up:**
Information needed by other team members	
• Reason for closure	

Team members present (signature and discipline):

_____   _____

_____   _____

_____   _____

_____   _____

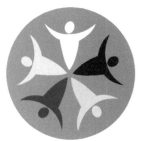

CHAPTER 8

The Future of the Primary Service Provider Approach to Teaming in Early Childhood Intervention

The Early Childhood Technical Assistance Center (2014) surveyed state Part C coordinators and of the 37 respondents, 28 states are using the PSP approach statewide or in some areas. The version being implemented within each state is highly contingent on the consultant(s) and or trainer(s) used to support state and/or program implementation. A challenge related to using a PSP approach to teaming exists because the field of early childhood intervention, national consultants and state technical assistant providers, state early intervention systems, programs providing early intervention services, early intervention practitioners, and families in receipt of early intervention services have not adopted a common definition related to using a PSP under Part C (see Chapter 1).

In the early 2000s, we proposed a new model of team interaction building on the work of Woodruff and McGonigel (1988) that redefined transdisciplinary teaming for purposes of early intervention under Part C (see Chapter 1). This model of team interaction was identified as a PSP approach to teaming. The definition was, and continues to be, based on research and identified characteristics and implementation conditions to assist in operationalizing the teaming practices. Although practitioners and programs talk about using transdisciplinary and PSP approaches, the lack of detail and consensus has created confusion and misunderstanding about what a PSP teaming approach in early intervention looks like and how the practices can be efficiently and effectively implemented.

Additional challenges remain beyond identifying an agreed-on definition of a PSP approach to teaming. The discussion regarding the need for further research is not to invalidate what is currently known about the effectiveness of using a primary provider approach to teaming (see Chapter 2); rather, it is necessary to provide further understanding of the characteristics, expand information about the implementation conditions, and identify new details for how to support teams of practitioners in successfully implementing this approach across family, child, environmental, and practitioner factors. This chapter puts forth issues that have continued to be challenges for moving the field of early childhood intervention and the practices associated with using a PSP approach to teaming forward since the initial publication of this text in 2013.

CHALLENGES

Many challenges exist relative to using a PSP approach to teaming in early intervention. The challenges discussed in this section more broadly affect the field at large and are all long-term issues that have been with early intervention since its inception and are not related solely to using a PSP approach to teaming. Using a PSP approach, however, brings many of the challenging issues to the forefront of program implementation and tests the systems' abilities to acclimate in the presence of new research that requires attention to a host of implications.

Challenge 1: Questions From the Field Related to the
Effectiveness, Cost, and Outcomes for Children and Families

Recognizing the questions about efficacy and use of a PSP approach to teaming is important to support states, programs, practitioners, and families in further understanding and implementing the characteristics and implementation conditions associated with this approach. New questions typically arise as programs and practitioners investigate or initiate implementation. Chapter 2 includes empirically based, foundational information that supports using a PSP approach to teaming. When considered in conjunction with implementing natural learning environment practices and an interaction style (i.e., coaching) that builds the capacity of parents and other care providers to support their children, using a primary provider, team lead, key worker, and so forth becomes an efficient and effective means of organizing supports and services for children and their families. The request that is often voiced is for comparative data relative to a teaming approach that uses a primary provider and multidisciplinary or interdisciplinary models of team interaction. More specifically, programs, practitioners, professional associations, and parents want to know about the differences or similarities in child and family outcomes and costs. We agree that large-scale studies would contribute to the available data supporting the use of a PSP approach to teaming. We also see the need for efficacy, cost, and outcome data on the continued use of multidisciplinary and interdisciplinary teaming approaches and how they are consistent with the implementation of evidence-based early intervention practices (i.e., natural learning environment practices, capacity building, effective helpgiving).

Challenges exist to implementing studies of early intervention teaming models. They include, but are not limited to, obtaining funding necessary to implement a large-scale study of teaming in early intervention; defining the characteristics of multidisciplinary and interdisciplinary teaming approaches; identifying teams that demonstrate fidelity to a particular teaming approach; capturing team-based data, regardless of the approach being used (e.g., meetings, collaboration among team members outside of team meetings); capturing individual practitioner intervention practices; implementing a study large enough to have intervention and control groups that represent a typical early intervention program's population served; and identifying the costs associated with the teaming approaches being studied. The pilot study included in Chapter 2 was our nonfunded attempt at implementing a comparative study of two teaming approaches. Although this study has limitations, it does provide an informative look at the factors to consider when comparing teaming approaches. Now that early intervention programs are required to report on defined child and family outcomes on an annual basis, these data could be used to compare outcomes across teaming approaches if the characteristics of specific models of team interaction could be further identified.

Challenge 2: Research Related to the Necessary
Knowledge and Skills of the Primary Service Provider

The real question is related to who should serve as the PSP (i.e., which discipline). We put forth a core team requirement in which all members, with the exception of the dedicated service coordinator, must be considered as a potential primary provider. Some programs, teams, technical assistance providers, and administrators feel that one discipline, most commonly the role of educator (e.g., early intervention specialist, developmental specialist, special instructor, early interventionist, developmental therapist, early childhood educator, early childhood special educator, teacher), should always serve as the PSP with consultation or coaching from therapists, nurses, psychologists, nutritionists, and so forth. This decision may likely be based on chronic issues that most early intervention programs experience regardless of the teaming approach used. These include, but are not limited to, a perceived or real lack of availability, costs, and knowledge of early intervention and use of family-centered practices by therapists. The notion of the lack of availability of therapists has caused many programs to adopt a scarcity mentality, which promotes using the disciplines that are more prevalent (e.g., educators, nurses) and reserves those disciplines that are not readily accessible for special circumstances or children with the most severe need, thus reinforcing a hierarchical teaming relationship. The cost of therapists is a valid factor based on supply and demand in the marketplace. Programs choose to hire or contract with more educators because of the number of children and families to be seen and because of the availability of people to serve in a sometimes broadly defined educator role costs less than a therapist. The difficulty that programs face in identifying therapists willing

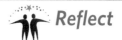

Reflect

If your team has difficulty finding enough members, then how does this affect your decisions for who serves as primary service provider?

to work in early intervention requiring a more nontraditional approach (e.g., home visiting, flexible scheduling, attending team meetings) is a common challenge as well as finding therapists who understand how to work with family members and other care providers instead of having a professionally centered, therapist–child focus.

At the time of the second edition of this text, research does not exist to stipulate that one particular discipline is better or should be used more frequently than another when identifying a PSP. The teaming approach put forth in this book defines the PSP as the best and most qualified individual on the team to mediate the parents' abilities to promote child learning within the context of everyday activities. Part C requires a multidisciplinary perspective. Core teams that are minimally comprised of an educator, OT, PT, SLP, and service coordinator ensures multidisciplinary representation at all times throughout the IFSP process. Professional associations and state early intervention programs have developed competencies or recommendations for practitioners working in early intervention (AOTA, 2010, 2014; APTA Academy of Pediatric Physical Therapy, 2013; APTA Section on Pediatrics, 2010; ASHA, 2008a, b; DEC, 2014; Pilkington, 2006; Vanderhoff, 2004; Workgroup on Principles and Practices in Natural Environments, 2007a, b, c). We have also put

forth the concept of role expectation in early intervention in which all team members are required to have knowledge in early childhood development across all domains, parenting resources, and parent support. Studies that compare teams using a PSP approach to teaming as defined in this text with teams using an approach in which the PSP is always one particular discipline (e.g., educator, nurse) would provide insight into the overall effectiveness of specific disciplines serving in the role of primary provider.

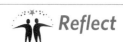

Reflect

How can you ensure that you have an adequate variety of disciplines with enough time available to serve as primary service provider?

Challenge 3: Fiscal Issues

Fiscal issues have long been a challenge for most states and early intervention programs because IDEA 2004 has never been adequately and appropriately funded. As a result, states and programs have been required to pursue third party reimbursement for early intervention services. Taken at face value, what third parties require to justify payment appears to be inconsistent with the implementation of evidence-based practices in early intervention. For example, early intervention research and practice indicates that practitioners should focus on family priorities, strengths and abilities, and parent mediation of child participation in natural contexts and settings (Dunst, 2004). Third party payers require documentation that demonstrates practitioners focus on intervention that remediates the child's skill-based impairments that are medically necessary and related to the disciplinary expertise of the provider. At the time of the publication of the second edition of this text, most third party payers still do not reimburse practitioners for time spent participating in team meetings, joint visits, or parent education, particularly return demonstration by the parent. In essence, third parties will currently pay for non–evidence-based practices as long as they are provided by the approved discipline (e.g., passive sensory stimulation to improve sensory processing, nonspeech oral-motor exercises to address speech sound problems, stretching exercises to decrease spasticity), but refuse to pay for the most effective practices, specifically parent-mediated child learning taught by a billable discipline (Dunst, 2006; Ketelaar et al., 1998; Mahoney, 2009; Mahoney & Perales, 2005; Mahoney et al., 2006; Warren & Brady, 2007; Woods et al., 2004). Curiously, for an adult with dementia or the inability to perform a self-care task, Medicaid, Medicare, and private insurance have typically paid for education activities for family members who will be responsible for caring for the insured adult. For example, consider an 80-year-old female, Mrs. Hernandez, with Alzheimer's disease recovering from a total hip replacement. She is unable to care for herself (i.e., hygiene, self-feed) and cannot remember to comply with the precautions following hip surgery. In this situation, the therapist would focus on teaching the family members how to care for Mrs. Hernandez to ensure the postsurgical precautions were followed as well as supporting them in safely and effectively caring for her. The therapist would be reimbursed for the educational services provided, not just the portion of the visit where the therapist worked with Mrs. Hernandez. In contrast, whenever the insured member is an infant or toddler who cannot speak, move, or provide independent self-care, in many cases, the practitioner can only be paid for the time working directly with the child.

Part C requires practitioners to ensure that family members know how to confidently and competently care for their infant or toddler in order to support the child's learning and development when the practitioner is not present. If Part C practitioners are implementing the required evidence-based interventions, then they seemingly can never receive full payment for the time spent with the child and family. Many practitioners in states in which programs depend on third party reimbursement feel they are faced with choosing between billing for their time or implementing effective practices.

The specific question related to the cost of a PSP approach to teaming has yet to be empirically determined, although several early studies suggested that choosing a primary provider as the liaison from a program to support families and their children may prove to be more cost efficient (Barnett & Escobar, 1990; Barnett et al., 1988; Borrill et al., 2001; Eiserman et al., 1990; Tarr & Barnett, 2001; Warfield, 1995). In the pilot study in Chapter 2, the PSP teaming approach did cost less than the multidisciplinary teaming approach to which it was compared. This included the provision of joint visits and payment to practitioners for time spent in team meetings. The program participating in the study identified alternative payment sources in order to pay the practitioners for these activities during and beyond the study. This can be insurmountable for some programs, particularly those completely reliant on third party reimbursement.

The challenges to the field (and beyond) include advocating for adequate federal and state funding for early intervention under Part C so that programs are not completely dependent on third party reimbursement. Another challenge is to the entities that provide third party payment for early intervention services. Medicaid and private insurers should pay for evidence-based practices in early childhood intervention and not pay for those interventions that lack evidence. This reconsideration could actually result in a financial savings for third party payers and will most certainly enhance child and family outcomes without additional costs. In the meantime, early intervention programs should consider central billing support for both contracted and employed practitioners until additional federal and state funding is available and third party payers reprioritize payment for services. Centralizing billing emphasizes recoupment for all allowable costs while simultaneously supporting practitioners in their decision making and ability to implement evidence-based early intervention practices.

Challenge 4: Use of Evidence-Based Practices

Using a PSP approach to teaming requires that all team members recognize and implement the best and most appropriate evidence-based intervention to support parents and other care providers in mediating child participation and learning. Team members then work collaboratively through a PSP or team liaison to address the identified child and family outcomes. Using a PSP approach to teaming does not in and of itself ensure the implementation of evidence-based practices (see Chapter 1). The team should provide an added safety net or mechanism for increased accountability to implement evidence-based practices rather than only preferred practices by individual team members. For example, without a team in place, each practitioner is solely responsible for the choice of interventions they implement with a child and family. Unfortunately, the interventions chosen may or may not be evidence based. Imagine a PT who chooses to teach a parent how to stretch the heel cords of a toddler with mild diplegic cerebral palsy because the child prefers to walk on their toes. Unfortunately, this PT has either 1) not reviewed current literature and is implementing an intervention that she feels is appropriate but is not supported by the research or 2) is aware of the literature and disagrees because she feels the practice has been beneficial to other children with whom she has previously worked. To the parent, this most likely seems like a direct intervention to support a developing problem, and the parent places her trust in the PT and is willing to do whatever is needed to support her child. Furthermore, this practice is billable to third party payers, which reinforces the therapist's current approach to decision making related to intervention. In contrast, if this PT was working on a team adhering to the characteristics and implementation conditions of a PSP approach, then they would be required to regularly report on current intervention plans, progress on IFSP outcomes, and new plans for supporting parent mediation of child participation. Other team members would have the opportunity to ask and should question how the PT's heel cord stretching instruction matches with the *Mission and Key Principles for Providing Services in Natural Environments* (Principles 1 and 7; Workgroup on Principles and Practices in Natural Environments, 2007b). Specifically, other team members should request that the PT produce available evidence that supports the selected approach to intervention of stretching heel cords for toe walking in a toddler with diplegic cerebral palsy. The PT on this team has the responsibility to provide the requested information to her team members and, in a sense, justify her approach based on current standards. The team should serve as the child's and family's virtual insurance policy for receiving the most state-of-the-art services available at any given time.

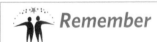

Remember

The team should serve as the child's and family's virtual insurance policy for receiving the most state-of-the-art services available at any given time.

The gap between available evidence and implementing evidence-based practices is well documented. Several studies identified reasons why practitioners do not use evidence-based practices, including lack of time to stay current, inability to gain access to information (cannot access or do not know how), and personal choice regarding preferred interventions (Campbell et al., 2009; Campbell & Halbert, 2002; Gersten, 2001; Schreiber et al., 2008; Zipoli & Kennedy, 2005). Authors representing the primary disciplines that work in early intervention documented the first generation of research related to what we knew at that time to be evidence-based practices within each of the core disciplines associated with early intervention (Guralnick, 1997). The authors also noted the gap in research to practice, with some speculation that the gap between what was known and what was implemented could be as great as 15 years (Fixsen et al., 2013; McLean & Cripe, 1997). A substantial gap still exists between research and practice, even in the presence of recommended practice standards (AOTA, 2010, 2014; APTA Academy of Pediatric Physical Therapy, 2013; APTA Section on Pediatrics, 2010; ASHA, 2008a, b; DEC, 2014; Pilkington, 2006; Vanderhoff, 2004; Workgroup on Principles and Practices in Natural Environments, 2007a, b, c) and guidance for how to obtain and use the most current research available to support intervention with young children and their families (Bennett & Bennett, 2000; Dunst et al., 2002; Johnson, 2006; Law, 2000; Maher et al., 2004; Odom et al., 2005).

One of the challenges to implementing a PSP teaming approach is practitioner belief that no evidence exists to support this method of teaming (see Chapter 3). We provided the research foundations supporting the use of a PSP approach to teaming (see Chapter 2). Interestingly, some of the very practitioners who question or refuse to participate on a team using a PSP approach are using teaming and intervention practices that are either outdated or lack evidence to prove their effectiveness. Practitioner implementation of evidence-based practices under Part C is now required by law. As a result, programs must consider how to ensure compliance with this provision. Using a PSP approach to teaming provides a structure for supporting implementation of evidence-based practices.

Challenge 5: Professional Development

The field of early childhood intervention is faced with the major challenge of ongoing professional development (Bruder, 2010; Bruder et al., 2009, 2019; Campbell et al., 2009; Clark et al., 2004; Dunst, 2009; Stayton et al., 2009; Winton & McCollum, 2008; Woods & Snyder, 2009). Many issues exist in the preservice and in-service venues related to supporting evidence-based teaming practices in early intervention. A PSP approach to teaming involves interaction among members from various disciplines. This is a particular challenge related to preservice preparation, which is discipline specific and often lacks opportunities for interaction and access to students from other fields who would likely be working together on an early intervention team. A common rationale for the lack of interdisciplinary training is an absence of space/time within the curriculum for teaming content and cross-disciplinary learning opportunities. Confounding this concern related to curricular content is the role expectation of practitioners serving in early intervention, particularly on a team using a PSP approach (e.g., general knowledge of typical child development across all domains, family systems, parenting, effective helpgiving). Many Leadership Education in Neurodevelopmental Disabilities programs and University Centers for Excellence in Developmental Disabilities provide meaningful interdisciplinary experiences for the students involved that often include a focus on teaming. The number of students able to participate, however, is often limited to a select number of graduate students with a focus on life span issues and with only a brief amount of time available to address early intervention. The lack of opportunity for students to participate in fieldwork experiences with programs using a PSP approach to teaming is another limitation for preservice education. Student knowledge and experiences can also be restricted by the preferences, beliefs, expertise, and understanding of their faculty. The federally funded Early Childhood Personnel Center is a comprehensive initiative to develop early childhood competencies shared across disciplines to be used at the preservice and in-service level.

Professional development activities that offer evidence-based information for practitioners currently in the work force can be difficult to gain access to due to availability or fiscal issues. In-service opportunities that focus on teaming are almost nonexistent. Many of the same challenges for preservice education exist in the in-service arena, including time, acquisition of knowledge beyond one's own discipline (i.e., role expectation), and access to interdisciplinary learning experiences. Availability of training topics for practitioners who work in early intervention is often limited to non–evidence-based content and/or focuses on practitioner-implemented techniques that promote dependency of the practitioner and decrease the willingness to teach others. This type of training shifts the focus from parent-implemented interventions that promote child participation in everyday activities when the practitioner is and is not present. Practitioners should have filters in place when selecting in-service training events to assist them in determining if the information being provided is based on sound, current research. McWilliam's (1999) characteristics of controversial practices (listed in Chapter 5) still stands the test of time and can serve as a set of red flags or cautions (filters) related to continuing education and professional development opportunities for practitioners to consider. His recommendations can serve as filters or a vetting process to determine whether a particular training is a worthy investment of a practitioner's time and money. In conjunction with considering evidence-based interventions, practitioners should also follow the guidance of Part C, the DEC Recommended Practices (2014), and the *Mission and Key Principles for Providing Services in Natural Environments* (Workgroup on Principles and Practices in Natural Environments, 2007b) for how early intervention services should be provided.

Understanding how to use a team-based approach in early childhood intervention should begin at the preservice level and continue as a part of ongoing professional development. Preservice and in-service faculty should teach practices based on current research to ensure that learners are good at what works. Faculty must also implement evidence-based teaching practices and provide conceptual and theoretical frameworks when teaching promising or controversial practices. Critically important, all learners (preservice and in-service) should have interdisciplinary experiences (rather than being trained in silos) in which they become familiar with other disciplines and how to work together to ensure positive outcomes for children with disabilities and their families.

Challenge 6: Medical Community Understanding

Physicians traditionally served as a primary referral source for children needing specialized services (e.g., nursing, occupational therapy, physical therapy, speech-language pathology) and determined the type and amount of service provided. Part C has always promoted the involvement of physicians in referral, IFSP development, and intervention. The role of the physician, however, is as an equal team member, assisting in developing a plan to meet the prioritized outcomes of the child and family. Due to changes in Part C since the late 1990s, related to payment for services via third party reimbursement, early intervention providers have become increasingly dependent on physician referrals for approval of payment for therapy services that are deemed medically necessary. Many physicians continue to prescribe specialized services based on the child's diagnosis or severity of impairments, delay, or disability, which is most often based on physician preference rather than evidence. The mission of early intervention is to "build upon and provide supports and resources to assist family members and other caregivers to enhance children's learning and development through everyday learning opportunities" (Workgroup on Principles and Practices in Natural Environments, 2007b, p. 2). When physicians refer children for traditional multidisciplinary services provided by discipline-specific therapists, a mismatch exists between the physician's understanding and the mission of early intervention and current evidence-based practices for working with infants and toddlers with disabilities and their families. A conundrum is created for early intervention programs and practitioners because the physician is the conduit for obtaining payment for services from third party payers. Teams using a PSP approach can be placed in an even more vulnerable position when a physician refers for and expects the delivery of multiple services. An example of this is when a parent is referred to early intervention by the physician and has prescriptions for occupational therapy, physical therapy, and speech-language therapy. The early intervention program describes the teaming approach used in their area to the parent, which, in turn, causes the parent to question why the program would not comply with the physician's orders for therapy. The early intervention program is placed in the position of having to defend the teaming approach and point out the physician's lack of knowledge related to evidence-based practices in early intervention under Part C. The relationship between the parent and program is potentially off to a contentious beginning due to a circumstance that could have been avoided.

The most helpful referral from the medical community to an early intervention program happens as soon as any question of delay or diagnosis of a condition resulting in developmental delay occurs on the part of the parent and/or physician. The referral should request evaluation and treatment. Once the early intervention program has interviewed the family, evaluated the child, and assessed prioritized outcomes, one of the practitioners involved should contact the referring physician to extend an invitation to the IFSP meeting, but minimally to obtain input for developing the IFSP. Service delivery decisions occur at the IFSP meeting, following the development of the child and family outcome statements. A designated team member should contact the physician regarding the final decision about outcomes and service delivery as well as provide a copy of the IFSP, with parental permission. The PSP and/or service coordinator should maintain ongoing contact with the physician to update them on the child's progress. This process builds trust between the early intervention program and physician over time by keeping the physician informed and involved.

If a physician questions using a PSP approach, then a designated team member should contact the physician to answer any questions and provide additional information regarding the approach. The American Academy of Pediatrics Council on Children with Disabilities Report (Adams et al., 2013) on the needed collaboration between IDEA Part C and the medical home specifically references the use of coaching, natural learning environment practices, and a PSP approach to teaming (see https://pediatrics.aappublications.org/content/132/4/e1073). This report can serve as a useful resource for early intervention programs to share with referring physicians to promote their understanding of the reason for structuring the delivery of services using a primary provider to promote optimal outcomes for the child and family with the fewest number of people involved. See Chapter 5 for bullet points explaining a PSP approach to teaming to physicians.

CONCLUSION

Many early intervention practitioners have questions initially and ongoing about how to work as a member of a team using a PSP. The DEC Recommended Practices (2014), the *Mission and Key Principles for Providing Early Intervention Services in Natural Environments* (Workgroup on Principles and Practices in Natural Environments, 2007b), and the Part C federal regulations (IDEA 2004) clearly delineate the involvement of teams comprised of individuals from multiple disciplines in the design and delivery of early childhood supports and services. Discipline-specific professional organizations have followed suit in providing information relative to functioning as a PSP in early intervention. Although questions and challenges remain, the research that exists related to teaming, coaching, and using natural learning environment practices indicates that the benefits to children, families, and other team members are worth the struggles (perceived and real).

This text has focused on using a PSP approach to teaming to support young children with disabilities and their families in early intervention. The team (as defined by this text) is responsible for implementing natural learning environment practices using a coaching style of interaction for enhancing the knowledge and skills of the family and other care provider(s) in order to promote positive family functioning, maximize opportunities for child learning, and facilitate expansion of existing development-enhancing experiences within the context of everyday life. Early intervention programs must use practices that are effective and efficient for children with disabilities and their families as well as consistent with how young children learn. The team is responsible for holding its members accountable for the providing the most current evidence-based practices.

Although the SLP in the opening story of this text was initially skeptical of the PT's explanation of evidence-based teaming practices, he was open to further investigating the merit and possibilities of the practice, even though the information was incongruent with his current knowledge, skills, and experience. Reflecting back over the past 30 years, he realizes that his decision was life changing—not only for his own, but also for all of the children and families we both have had the privilege to serve.

Primary Service Provider Teaming Scenario Matrix Index

Page	Chapter	Type	Topic	Child characteristics	Coach	Coachee
64	3	Script	Need to increase contract hours of occupational therapist (OT)	No specific child	Early intervention coordinator (EIC)	OT contractor
72	3	Script	Perceived need of primary service provider (PSP) to refer a child to outside services	Child with severe disabilities	EIC	Early intervention team
76	3	Script	Recommend team member to serve as PSP based on discipline and diagnosis	Children with diagnosis of torticollis	EIC	Physical therapist (PT)
94	4	Narrative	Develop participation-based individualized family service plan (IFSP) outcomes	Child with suspected diagnosis of autism	Early intervention service coordinator (EISC)	Parents
133	5	Narrative	Use the three components of a visit to the park	Infant with a diagnosis of lissencephaly	PT	Mother
136	5	Script	Request a PSP be replaced by another discipline	Child with global delays	Early intervention team	OT/EISC (blended role)
152 159	5	Script 1 Script 2	Use the Worksheet for Selecting the Most Likely PSP with different team configurations	Child with a diagnosis of cerebral palsy	EIC	Early intervention team
173	6	Script	Develop the joint visit plan	Child with a diagnosis of Down syndrome	Speech-language pathologist (SLP) (Secondary service provider)	Early childhood special educator (PSP)
177	6	Script	Implement the joint visit plan	Child with a diagnosis of Down syndrome	SLP (Secondary service provider)	Early childhood special educator (PSP)
182	6	Script	Debrief the joint visit plan	Child with a diagnosis of Down syndrome	SLP (Secondary service provider)	Early childhood special educator (PSP)
194	7	Script	Present a primary coaching opportunity related to family support	No specific child	Early intervention team	OT
199	7	Script	Team meeting facilitates a challenging situation	Child with challenging behaviors	Team meeting facilitator	Early intervention team

Commonly Asked Questions

Topic	Question	Chapter	Page number(s)
Research	What is the research behind this teaming model?	2	25
Research	Why can't we use other teaming models?	2	25
Research	What studies compare primary service provider (PSP) with the way we have always provided services?	2	25
Explanation	How do you explain using a PSP approach to teaming to a parent, physician, or other community member?	5	113
Explanation	What is the role of the service coordinator when using a PSP?	5	113
Explanation	Can the service coordinator ever be the PSP?	3	63
Explanation	What is the difference between transdisciplinary and PSP models?	1	1
Explanation	What if a practitioner is not comfortable with another member of the team serving as the PSP?	3	63
Explanation	How do you address those children with severe disabilities who need more than one provider on a regular basis?	3	63
Explanation	How does this work with children with autism, cerebral palsy, apraxia, and so forth?	5, 8	113, 215
Explanation	What if we need specialized equipment that is only found in our center/clinic?	5, 8	113, 215
Explanation	When do we refer out for services?	3, 5	63, 113
Liability	What are the liability issues for a team member from one discipline to do what another team member would typically do?	3	63
Liability	Isn't it unethical, illegal, or against my practice act to do PSP?	3	63
Logistics	How do you transition families to this approach?	3, 5	63, 113
Logistics	What is the average caseload?	3, 5	63, 113
Logistics	How many people are on a team?	3	63
Logistics	How do vision, hearing, and behavior specialists fit into this approach?	3	63
Logistics	What do you do when a PSP goes on maternity leave, vacation, or has an extended illness?	3, 5, 7	63, 113, 189
Individualized family service plan (IFSP)	How do you document this on the IFSP?	4	87
IFSP	How do you determine frequency/intensity?	3, 5	63, 113
IFSP	What if the practitioner needs to go more frequently?	5	113
IFSP	Is the entire team listed on the IFSP?	4, 5	87, 113
Selection of PSP	How and when do you choose the PSP?	5	113
Selection of PSP	How do you address a physician's prescription for multiple services?	5	113
Selection of PSP	What if we do not have the necessary expertise on our team?	1, 6	1, 169
Selection of PSP	What do we do if the best practitioner for a family is full or cannot provide the frequency/intensity needed?	5	113
Selection of PSP	How do we ensure families have access to all of the expertise they need?	3, 5	63, 113
Scheduling	How do you schedule this way?	5	113

Topic	Question	Chapter	Page number(s)
Team meetings	How often does the team meet?	7	189
Team meetings	How long do team meetings last?	7	189
Team meetings	Is every child discussed at every team meeting?	7	189
Team meetings	How do you schedule team meetings when everyone on the team works different hours or works for early intervention a few hours a week?	7	189
Joint visits	How do you support the PSP on a joint visit?	5, 6	113, 169
Joint visits	How do both practitioners on a joint visit complete both of their sessions?	6	169
Changing the PSP	How often do you need to change the PSP?	5	113
Billing	How do you bill for this?	5	113
Billing	How can you bill for two therapists in the home at the same time?	5, 6	113, 169
Costs	What are the costs associated with using this approach?	2, 5	25, 113

References

Adams, R. C., & Snyder, P. (1998). Treatments for cerebral palsy: Making choices of intervention from an expanding menu of options. *Infants & Young Children, 10*(4), 1–22.

Adams, R. C., Tapia, C., & The Council on Children with Disabilities. (2013). Early intervention, IDEA part C services, and the medical home: Collaboration for best practice and best outcomes. *Pediatrics, 132*(4), e1073–e1088; https://doi.org/10.1542/peds.2013-2305

American Occupational Therapy Association. (2010). *AOTA practice advisory on occupational therapy in early intervention.* Retrieved from http://www.aota.org/~/media/Corporate/Files/Practice/Children/AOTA-Advisory-on Primary-Provider-in-EI.pdf

American Occupational Therapy Association. (2014). *AOTA practice advisory: Occupational therapy practitioners in early intervention.* https://www.aota.org/~/media/Corporate/Files/Practice/Children/Practice-Advisory-Early-Intervention.pdf

American Occupational Therapy Association (2019). *AOTA practice advisory: Occupational therapy practitioners in early intervention.* https://www.aota.org/-/media/Corporate/Files/Practice/Children/Practice-Advisory-Early-Intervention.pdf

American Physical Therapy Association Academy of Pediatric Physical Therapy (2013). *Using a primary service provider approach to teaming.* https://pediatricapta.org/includes/factsheets/pdfs/13%20Primary%20Service%20Provider.pdf?v=1

American Physical Therapy Association Academy of Pediatric Physical Therapy. (2019). *Using a primary service provider approach to teaming.* https://pediatricapta.org/includes/factsheets/pdfs/13%20Primary%20Service%20Provider.pdf?v=1

American Physical Therapy Association Section on Pediatrics. (2010). *Team-based service delivery approaches in pediatric practice.* https://pediatricapta.org/includes/fact-sheets/pdfs/Service%20Delivery.pdf?v=1.1

American Speech-Language-Hearing Association. (2008a). *Roles and responsibilities of speech-language pathologists in early intervention* [Technical Report]. Rockville, MD: Author.

American Speech-Language-Hearing Association. (2008b). *Roles and responsibilities of speech-language pathologists in early intervention: Guidelines* [Technical Report]. Rockville, MD: Author.

Antoniadis, A., & Videlock, J. L. (1991). In search of teamwork: A transactional approach to team functioning. *Infant-Toddler Intervention, 1*, 157–167.

Atwater, S. W., McEwen, I. R., & McMillan, J. (1982). Assessment of the reliability of pediatric screening: A tool for occupational and physical therapists. *Physical Therapy, 62*(9), 1265–1268.

Bagnato, S. J., Suen, H. K., & Fevola, A. V. (2011). "Dosage" effects on developmental progress during early childhood intervention. *Infants & Young Children, 24*(2), 117–132.

Barnett, W. S., & Escobar, C. M. (1990). Economic costs and benefits of early intervention. In S. J. Meisels & J. P. Shonkoff (Eds.), *Handbook of early childhood intervention* (pp. 560–582). Cambridge University Press.

Barnett, W. S., Escobar, C. M., & Ravsten, M. T. (1988). Parent and clinic early intervention for children with language handicaps: A cost-effectiveness analysis. *Journal of the Division for Early Childhood, 12*, 290–298.

Bell, A., Corfield, M., Davies, J., & Richardson, N. (2009). Collaborative transdisciplinary intervention in early years: Putting theory into practice. *Child: Care, Health and Development, 36*, 142–148.

Bell, S. T. (2004). *Setting the stage for effective teams: A meta-analysis of team design variables and team effectiveness.* Unpublished doctoral dissertation, Texas A & M University, College Station, Texas.

Bell, S. T. (2007). Deep-level composition variables as predictors of team performance: A meta-analysis. *Journal of Applied Psychology, 92*, 595–615.

Bennett, S., & Bennett, J. W. (2000). The process of evidence-based practice in occupational therapy: Informing clinical decisions. *Australian Occupational Therapy Journal, 47*, 171–180.

Borkowski, M. A., & Wessman, H. C. (1994). Determination of eligibility for physical therapy in the public school setting. *Pediatric Physical Therapy, 6*(2), 61–67.

Borrill, C. S., Carletta, A. J., Dawson, J. F., Garrod, S., Rees, A., & West, M. A. (2001). *The effectiveness of health care teams in the National Health Service.* Aston Centre for Health Service Organisation Research, Aston Business School, Aston University.

Bowman, C. L., & McCormick, S. (2000). Comparison of peer coaching versus traditional supervision effects. *Journal of Educational Research, 93*(4), 256–261.

Boyer, V. E., & Thompson, S. D. (2014). Transdisciplinary model and early intervention: Building collaborative relationships. *Young Exceptional Children, 17*(19), 19–32. doi:10.1177/1096250613493446

Briggs, M. H. (1997). *Building early intervention teams: Working together for children and families.* Aspen.

Brito, A. T., & Lindsay, G. (2016). Understanding the initial impact of early support and key working training through the voices of trainers, training participants, and families. *Infants & Young Children, 29*(1), 71–88.

Bruce, C. D., & Ross, J. A. (2008). A model for increasing reform implementation and teacher efficacy: Teacher peer coaching in grades 3 and 6 mathematics. *Canadian Journal of Education, 31*(2), 346–370.

Bruder, M. B. (2010). Early childhood intervention: A promise to children and families for their future. *Exceptional Children, 76,* 339–355.

Bruder, M. B., Catalino, T., Chiarello, L. A., Mitchell, M. C., Deppe, J., Gundler, D., Kemp, P., LeMoine, S., Long, T., Muhlenhaupt, M., Prelock, P., Schefkind, S., Stayton, V., & Ziegler, D. (2019). Finding a common lens: Competencies across professional disciplines providing early childhood intervention. *Infants & Young Children, 32*(4), 280–293. doi:10.1097/IYC.0000000000000153

Bruder, M. B., & Dunst, C. J. (2005). Personnel preparation in recommended early intervention practices: Degree of emphasis across disciplines. *Topics in Early Childhood Special Education, 25*(1), 25–33.

Bruder, M. B., Mogro-Wilson, C. M., Stayton, V. D., & Dietrich, S. L. (2009). The national status of in-service professional development systems for early intervention and early childhood special education practitioners. *Infants & Young Children, 22*(1), 13–20.

Campbell, P. H., Chiarello, L., Wilcox, M. J., & Milbourne, S. (2009). Preparing therapists as effective practitioners in early intervention. *Infants & Young Children, 22*(1), 21–31.

Campbell, P. H., & Halbert, J. (2002). Between research and practice: Provider perspectives on early intervention. *Topics in Early Childhood Special Education, 22,* 213–226.

Campbell, P. H., & Sawyer, L. B. (2007). Supporting learning opportunities in natural settings through participation-based services. *Journal of Early Intervention, 29,* 287–305. doi:10.1177/105381510702900402

Caracci, H., Reynolds, S., & Ivey, C. (2018, October). Made to measure: Determining pediatric therapy dosages. *OT Practice,* 10–13.

Carr, S. H. (1989). Louisiana's criteria of eligibility for occupational therapy services in the public school system. *American Journal of Occupational Therapy, 43*(8), 503.

Chiarello, L. A. (2017). Excellence in prompting participation: Striving for the 10 Cs-client-centered care, consideration of complexity, collaboration, coaching, capacity building, contextualization, creativity, community, curricular changes, and curiosity. *Pediatric Physical Therapy, 29*(3), S16–S22. doi:10.1097/PEP.0000000000000382

Clark, G., Polichino, J., Jackson, L., & The Commission on Practice. (2004). Occupational therapy services in early intervention and school-based programs. *American Journal of Occupational Therapy, 58*(6), 681–685.

Clow, P., Dunst, C. J., Trivette, C. M., & Hamby, D. W. (2005). Educational outreach (academic detailing) and physician prescribing practices. *Cornerstones, 1*(1), 1–19.

Cole, K. N., Dale, P. S., & Mills, P. E. (1990). Defining language delay in young children by cognitive referencing: Are we saying more than we know? *Applied Psycholinguistics, 11,* 291–302.

Cole, K. N., & Mills, P. E. (1997). Agreement of language intervention triage profiles. *Topics in Early Childhood Special Education, 17,* 119–130.

Cole, K. N., Mills, P. E., & Harris, S. R. (1991). Retrospective analysis of physical and occupational therapy progress in young children: An examination of cognitive referencing. *Pediatric Physical Therapy, 3,* 185–189.

Cripe, J. W., Hanline, M. F., & Daley, S. E. (1997). Preparing practitioners for planning intervention for natural environments. In P. J. Winton, J. A. McCollum, & C. Catlett (Eds.), *Reforming personnel preparation in early intervention: Issues, models, and practical strategies* (pp. 337–350). Paul H. Brookes Publishing Co.

Daniels, W. R. (1993). *Orchestrating powerful regular meetings: A manager's complete guide.* Pfeiffer and Company.

De Drue, C. K. W., & West, M. A. (2001). Minority dissent and team innovation: The importance of participation in decision-making. *Journal of Applied Psychology, 86,* 1191–1201.

DeGangi, G. A., Wietlisbach, S., Poisson, S., Stein, E., & Royeen, C. (1994). The impact of culture and socioeconomic status on family-professional collaboration: Challenges and solutions. *Topics in Early Childhood Special Education, 14,* 503–520.

Dinnebeil, L. A., Hale, L. M., & Rule, S. (1996). A qualitative analysis of parents' and service coordinators' descriptions of variables that influence collaborative relationships. *Topics in Early Childhood Education, 16,* 322–347.

Dinnebeil, L. A., Hale, L. M., & Rule, S. (1999). Early intervention program practices that support collaboration. *Topics in Early Childhood Education, 19,* 225–235.

Division for Early Childhood. (2014). DEC recommended practices in early intervention/early childhood special education 2014. Retrieved from http://www.dec-sped.org/recommendedpractices

Donovan, M. S., Bransford, J. D., & Pellegrino, J. W. (Eds.). (1999). *How people learn: Bridging research and practice*. National Academies Press.

Doyle, M., & Straus, D. (1993). *How to make meetings work: The new interaction method*. Berkley.

Dunn, W., Cox, J., Foster, L., Mische-Lawson, L., & Tanquary, J. (2012). Impact of a contextual intervention on child participation and parent competence among children with autism spectrum disorders: A pretest–posttest repeated-measures design. *American Journal of Occupational Therapy, 66*, 520–528. doi:10.5014/ajot.2012.004119

Dunst, C. J. (2004). An integrated framework for practicing early childhood intervention and family support. *Perspectives in Education, 22*(2), 1–16.

Dunst, C. J. (2005). Framework for practicing evidence-based early childhood intervention and family support. *CASEinPoint, 1*(1), 1–11. Retrieved from https://fipp.ncdhhs.gov/wp-content/uploads/caseinpoint_vol1_no1.pdf

Dunst, C. J. (2006). Parent-mediated everyday child learning opportunities: I. Foundations and operationalization. *CASEinPoint, 2*(2), 1–10. Retrieved from https://fipp.ncdhhs.gov/wp-content/uploads/caseinpoint_vol2_no2.pdf

Dunst, C. J. (2009). Implications of evidence-based practices for personnel preparation development in early childhood intervention. *Infants & Young Children, 22*(1), 44–53.

Dunst, C. J., & Bruder, M. B. (2006). Early intervention service coordination models and service coordinator practices. *Journal of Early Intervention, 28*(3), 155–165.

Dunst, C. J., Bruder, M. B., & Espe-Sherwindt, M. (2014). Family capacity-building in early childhood intervention: Do context and setting matter? *School Community Journal, 24*(1), 37–48.

Dunst, C. J., Bruder, M. B., Trivette, C. M., & Hamby, D. W. (2006). Everyday activity settings, natural learning environments, and early intervention practices. *Journal of Policy and Practice in Intellectual Disabilities, 3*, 3–10.

Dunst, C. J., Bruder, M. B., Trivette, C. M., Raab, M., & McLean, M. (2001). Natural learning opportunities for infants, toddlers, and preschoolers. *Young Exceptional Children, 4*(3), 18–25 (Erratum in *4*(4), 25).

Dunst, C. J., & Deal, A. G. (1994). A family-centered approach to developing individualized family support plans. In C. J. Dunst, C. M. Trivette, & A. G. Deal (Eds.), *Supporting and strengthening families: Methods, strategies and practices* (pp. 73–88). Brookline Books.

Dunst, C., Hamby, D., & Brookfield, J. (2007). Modeling the effects of early childhood intervention variables on parent and family well-being. *Journal of Applied Quantitative Methods, 2*(3), 268–288.

Dunst, C. J., Hamby, D., Trivette, C. M., Raab, M., & Bruder, M. B. (2000). Everyday family and community life and children's naturally occurring learning opportunities. *Journal of Early Intervention, 23*, 151–164. doi: 10.1177/10538151000230030501

Dunst, C. J., Herter, S., & Shields, H. (2000). Interest-based natural learning opportunities. In S. Sandall & M. Ostrosky (Eds.), *Natural environments and inclusion* (Young Exceptional Children Monograph Series No. 2) (pp. 37–48). Sopris West Educational Services.

Dunst, C.J., & Trivette, C.M. (2009). Capacity-building family-systems intervention practices. *Journal of Family Social Work, 12*, 119–143.

Dunst, C. J., Trivette, C. M., & Cutspec, P. A. (2002). Toward an operational definition of evidence-based practices. *Centerscope, 1*(1), 1–10.

Dunst, C. J., Trivette, C. M., & Hamby, D. W. (2010). Meta-analysis of the effectiveness of four adult learning methods and strategies. *International Journal of Continuing Education & Lifelong Learning, 3*(1), 91–112.

Dunst, C. J., Trivette, C. M., Humphries, T., Raab, M., & Roper, N. (2001). Contrasting approaches to natural learning environment interventions. *Infants & Young Children, 14*(2), 48–63.

Dunst, C. J., Trivette, C. M., & Johanson, C. (1994). Parent–professional collaboration and partnerships. In C. J. Dunst, C. M., Trivette, & A. G. Deal (Eds.), *Supporting and strengthening families: Methods, strategies, and practices* (Vol. 1, pp. 197–211). Brookline Books.

Early Childhood Technical Assistance Center. (2014). *Service delivery approaches and models*. Retrieved from https://ectacenter.org/topics/eiservices/approaches-models.asp

Education of the Handicapped Act Amendments of 1986, PL 99-457, 20 U.S.C. §§ 1401 *et seq.*

Eiserman, W. D., McCoun, M., & Escobar, C. M. (1990). A cost-effectiveness analysis of two alternative program models for serving speech-disordered preschoolers. *Journal of Early Intervention, 14*, 297–317.

Erez, A., LePine, J. A., & Elms, H. (2002). Effects of rotated leadership and peer evaluation on the functioning and effectiveness of self-managed teams: A quasi-experiment. *Personnel Psychology, 55*, 929–948.

Farley, S. K., Sarracino, T., & Howard, P. M. (1991). Development of a treatment rating in school systems: Service through objective measurement. *American Journal of Occupational Therapy, 45*(10), 898–906.

Fewell, R. R. (1983). The team approach to infant education. In S. G. Garwood & R. R. Fewell (Eds.), *Educating handicapped infants: Issues in development and intervention* (pp. 299–322). Aspen.

Fixsen, D., Blasé, K., Metz, A., & Van Dyke, M. (2013). Statewide implementation of evidence-based programs. *Exceptional Children, 79*, 213–230. doi:10.1177/001440291307900206

García-Grau, P., McWilliam, R. A., Martínez-Rico, G., Morales-Murillo, C. P. (2019) Child, family, and early intervention characteristics related to family quality of life in Spain. *Journal of Early Intervention, 41*, 44–61.

Garland, C., McGonigel, M., Frank, A., & Buck, D. (1989). *The transdisciplinary model of service delivery.* Child Development Resources.

Gee, B. M., Lloyd, K., Devine, N., Tyrrell, E., Evans, T., Hill, R., Dineen, S., & Magalogo, K. (2016). Dosage parameters in pediatric outcome studies reported in 9 peer-reviewed occupational therapy journals from 2008 to 2014: A content analysis. *Rehabilitation Research and Practice*, 1–14.

Gersten, R. (2001). Sorting our roles of research in the improvement of practice. *Learning Disabilities Research and Practice, 16*, 45–50.

Giangreco, M. F. (1986). Delivery of therapeutic services in special education programs for learners with severe handicaps. *Physical and Occupational Therapy in Pediatrics, 6*(2), 5–15.

Golden, G. S. (1980). Nonstandard therapies in developmental disabilities. *American Journal of Diseases in Children, 134*, 487–491.

Gomm, A. (2006). Service coordination models: Implications for effective state Part C early intervention systems. *Journal of Early Intervention, 28*(3), 172–174.

Graham, F., Rodger, S., & Ziviani, J. (2009). Coaching parents to enable children's participation: An approach for working with parents and their children. *Australian Occupational Therapy Journal, 56*(1), 16–23. doi:10.1111/j.1440-1630.2008.00736.x10.1111/j.1440-1630.2008.00736.x

Greco, V., & Sloper, P. (2004). Care coordination and key worker schemes for disabled children: Results of a UK-wide survey. *Child: Care, Health and Development, 30*, 13–20.

Guralnick, M. J. (1997). *The effectiveness of early intervention.* Paul H. Brookes Publishing Co.

Hackman, J. R. (1987). The design of work teams. In J. W. Lorsch (Ed.), *Handbook of organizational behavior* (pp. 315–342). Prentice Hall.

Hallam, R. A., Rous, B., Grove, J., & LoBianco, T. (2009). Level and intensity of early intervention services for infants and toddlers with disabilities: The impact of child, family, system, and community-level factors on service provision. *Journal of Early Intervention, 31*, 179–196.

Hanft, B. E., Rush, D. D., & Shelden, M. L. (2004). *Coaching families and colleagues in early childhood.* Paul H. Brookes Publishing Co.

Harris, S. (1996). How should treatments be critiqued for scientific merit? *Physical Therapy, 76*(2), 175–181.

Harrison, P. J., Lynch, E. W., Rosander, K., & Borton, W. (1990). Determining success in interagency collaboration: An evaluation of processes and behaviors. *Infants & Young Children, 3*, 69–78.

Haynes, U. (1976). The UCP National Collaborative Infant Project. In T. D. Tjossem (Ed.), *Intervention strategies for high risk infants and young children* (pp. 509–534). University Park Press.

Holpp, L. (1999). *Managing teams.* McGraw-Hill.

Homa, K., Regan-Smith, M., Foster, T., Nelson, E. C., Liu, S., Kirkland, K. B., Heimarck, J., & Batalden, P. B. (2008). Coaching physicians in training to lead improvement in clinical microsystems: A qualitative study on the role of the clinical coach. *International Journal of Clinical Leadership, 16*, 37–48.

Hong, S. B., & Reynolds-Keefer, L. (2013). Transdisciplinary team building: Strategies in creating early childhood educator and health care teams. *International Journal of Early Childhood Special Education, 5*(1), 30–44.

Houtrow, A., Murphy, N., & The Council on Children with Disabilities. (2019). Prescribing physical, occupational, and speech therapy for children with disabilities. *Pediatrics, 143*, 1–14.

Hughes-Scholes, C. H., Gatt, S. L., Davis, K., Mahar, N., & Gavidia-Payne, S. (2015). Preliminary evaluation of the implementation of a routines-based early childhood intervention model in Australia: Practitioners' perspectives. *Topics in Early Childhood Special Education, 36*(1), 30–42.

Humphrey, R., & Wakeford, L. (2008). Development of everyday activities: A model for occupation-centered therapy. *Infants & Young Children, 21*(3), 230–240. doi:10.1097/01.IYC.0000324552.77564.9810.1097/01.IYC.0000324552.77564.98

Hwang, A. W., Chao, M. Y., & Liu, S. W. (2013). A randomized controlled trial of routines-based early intervention for children with or at risk for developmental delays. *Research in Developmental Disabilities, 34*(10), 3112–3123. doi:10.1016/j.ridd.2013.06.037

Individuals with Disabilities Education Act Amendments (IDEA) of 1997, PL 105-17, 20 U.S.C. §§ 1400 *et seq.*

Individuals with Disabilities Education Act (IDEA) of 1990, PL 101-476, 20 U.S.C. §§ 1400 *et seq.*

Individuals with Disabilities Education Improvement Act (IDEA) of 2004, PL 108-446, 20 U.S.C. §§ 1400 *et seq.*

Johnson, C. J. (2006). Getting started in evidence-based practice for childhood speech-language disorders. *American Journal of Speech-Language Pathology, 15*, 20–35.

Justice, T., & Jamieson, D. (1998). *The complete guide to facilitation: Enabling groups to succeed.* HRD Press.

Kayser, T. A. (2011). *Building team power: How to unleash the collaborative genius of work teams for increased engagement, productivity, and results* (2nd ed.). McGraw-Hill.

Keilty, B., & Galvin, K. M. (2006). Physical and social adaptations of families to promote learning in everyday experiences. *Topics in Early Childhood Special Education, 26*, 219–233. doi:10.1177/02711214060260040301

Kellegrew, D. H. (2000). Constructing daily routines: A qualitative examination of mothers with young children with disabilities. *American Journal of Occupational Therapy, 54*, 252–259. doi:10.5014/ajot.54.3.252

Ketelaar, M., Vermeer, A., Helders, P. J. M., & Hart, H. (1998). Parental participation in intervention programs for children with cerebral palsy: A review of research. *Topics in Early Childhood Special Education, 18*(2), 108–117.

King, G., Strachan, D., Tucker, M., Duwyn, B., Desserud, S., & Shillington, M. (2009). The application of a transdisciplinary model for early intervention services. *Infants & Young Children, 22*, 211–223.

Kingsley, K., & Mailloux, Z. (2013). Evidence for the effectiveness of different service delivery models in early intervention services. *American Journal of Occupational Therapy, 67*, 431–436. http//dx.doi.org/10.5014/ajot.2013.006171

Kramer, J. M., Hwang, I. T., Levin, M., Acevedo-Garcia, D., & Rosenfeld, L. (2018). Identifying environmental barriers to participation: Usability of a health-literacy informed problem-identification approach for parents of young children with developmental disabilities. *Child Care Health and Development, 44*(2), 249–259. doi:10.1111/cch.12542

Krassowski, E., & Plante, E. (1997). IQ variability in children with SLI: Implications for use of cognitive referencing in determining SLI. *Journal of Communication Disorders, 30*, 1–9.

Kuhn, M., & Marvin, C. A. (2016). "Dosage" decisions for early intervention services. *Young Exceptional Children, 19*(4), 20–34.

Kurtts, S. A., & Levin, B. B. (2000). Using peer coaching with preservice teachers to develop reflective practice and collegial support. *Teaching Education, 11*, 297–310.

Larsson, M. (2000). Organising habilitation services: Team structures and family participation. *Child: Care, Health and Development, 26*, 501–514.

Law, M. (2000). Strategies for implementing evidence-based practice in early intervention. *Infants & Young Children, 13*(2), 32–40.

Law, M., Darrah, J., Pollack, N., King, G., Rosenbaum, P., Russell, D., Palisano, R., Harris, S., Armstrong, R., & Watt, J. (1998). Family-centered functional therapy for children with cerebral palsy. *Physical and Occupational Therapy in Pediatrics, 18*(1), 83–102.

Lee, S., & Kahn, J. V. (2000). A survival analysis of parent-child interaction in early intervention. *Infant-Toddler Intervention, 10*, 137–156.

Lim, C. Y., Law, M., Khetani, M., Pollock, N., & Rosenbaum, P. (2016). Participation in out-of-home environments for young children with and without developmental disabilities. *OTJR: Occupation, Participation and Health, 36*(3), 112–125. doi:10.1177/1539449216659859doi: 10.1177/1539449216659859

Limbrick, P. (2004). *Early support for children with complex needs: Team around the child and the multi-agency keyworker.* Interconnections.

Limbrick, P. (2005). Integrated programmes and the primary interventionist in early childhood intervention. *PMLD Link, (18)2, Issue 54*, 9–12.

Limbrick-Spencer, G. (2001). *The keyworker: A practical guide.* WordWorks.

Lowenthal, B. (1992). Interagency collaboration in early intervention: Rationale, barriers, and implementation. *Transdisciplinary Journal, 2*, 103–111.

Maher, C. G., Sherrington, C., Elkins, M., Herbert, R. D., & Moseley, A. M. (2004). Challenges for evidence-based physical therapy: Accessing and interpreting high-quality evidence on therapy. *Physical Therapy, 84*, 644–654.

Mahoney, G. (2009). Relationship-focused intervention (RFI): Enhancing the role of parents in children's developmental intervention. *International Journal of Early Childhood Special Education, 1*(1), 79–94.

Mahoney, G., & Perales, F. (2005). Relationship-focused intervention with children with pervasive developmental disorders and other disabilities: A comparative study. *Journal of Developmental and Behavioral Pediatrics, 26*(2), 77–85.

Mahoney, G., Perales, F., Wiggers, B., & Herman, B. (2006). Responsive teaching: Early intervention for children with Down syndrome and other disabilities. *Down Syndrome: Research and Practice, 11*, 18–28.

Malone, D. M., & Gallagher, P. A. (2010). Special education teachers' attitudes and perceptions of teamwork. *Remedial and Special Education, 31*(5), 330–342.

Mangin, M. M. (2014). Capacity building and districts' decision to implement coaching initiatives. *Education Policy Analysis Archives, 22*(56), 1–25. doi:10.14507/epaa.v22n56.2014

McGonigel, M. J., Woodruff, G., & Roszmann-Millican, M. (1994). The transdisciplinary team: A model for family-centered early intervention. In L. J. Johnson, R. J. Gallagher, M. J. LaMontagne, J. B. Jordan, J. J. Gallagher, P. L. Huntinger, & M. B. Karnes (Eds.), *Meeting early intervention challenges: Issues from birth to three* (2nd ed., pp. 95–131). Paul H. Brookes Publishing Co.

McLean, L. K., & Cripe, J. W. (1997). The effectiveness of early intervention for children with communication disorders. In M. J. Guralnick (Ed.), *The effectiveness of early intervention* (pp. 349–428). Paul H. Brookes Publishing Co.

McWilliam, R. A. (1999). Controversial practices: The need for reacculturation of early intervention fields. *Topics in Early Childhood Special Education, 19*(3), 177–188.

McWilliam, R. A. (2000). It's only natural to have early intervention in the environments where it's needed. *Young Exceptional Children Monograph Series No. 2: Natural Environments and Inclusion,* 17–26.

McWilliam, R. A., & Stevenson, C. M. (2019). *Routines-Based Interview Checklist (with Ecomap).* Retrieved from http://eieio.ua.edu/uploads/1/1/0/1/110192129/rbi_checklist_with_ecomap_with_edits_12.23.19.pdf

Moeller, M. P., Carr, G., Seaver, L., Stredler-Brown, A., & Holzinger, D. (2013). Best practices in family-centered early intervention for children who are deaf or hard of hearing: An international consensus statement. *Journal of Deaf Studies and Deaf Education, 18*(4), 429–45. doi:10.1093/deafed/ent034

Nandiwada, D. R., & Dang-Vu, C. (2010). Transdisciplinary health care education: Training team players. *Journal of Health Care for the Poor and Underserved, 21*(1), 26–34.

Nash, J. K. (1990). Public Law 99-457: Facilitating family participation on the multidisciplinary team. *Journal of Early Intervention, 14,* 318–326.

Nash, J. M. (2008). Transdisciplinary training: Key components and prerequisites for success. *American Journal of Preventive Medicine, 35,* S133–S140.

Nickel, R. E. (1996). Controversial therapies for young children with developmental disabilities. *Infants &Young Children, 8*(4), 29–40.

Notari, A. R., Cole, K. N., & Mills, P. E. (1992). Cognitive referencing: The (non)relationship between theory and application. *Topics in Early Childhood Education, 11*(4), 22–38.

O'Connor, B. (1995). Challenges of interagency collaboration: Serving a young child with severe disabilities. *Physical and Occupational Therapy in Pediatrics, 15,* 89–109.

Odom, S. L., Brantlinger, E., Gersten, R., Horner, R. H., Thompson, B., & Harris, K. R. (2005). Research in special education: Scientific methods and evidence-based practices. *Exceptional Children, 71,* 137–148.

Orelove, F. P., & Sobsey, R. (1996). *Educating children with multiple disabilities: A transdisciplinary approach.* Paul H. Brookes Publishing Co.

Palisano, R. J., & Murr, S. (2009). Intensity of therapy services: What are the considerations? *Physical and Occupational Therapy in Pediatrics, 29*(2), 107–112.

Park, J., & Turnbull, A. P. (2003). Service integration in early intervention: Determining interpersonal and structural factors for success. *Infants & Young Children, 16*(1), 48–58.

Pell, A. R. (1999). *The complete idiot's guide to team building.* Alpha Books.

Peterson, C. A., Luze, G. J., Eshbaugh, E. M., Jeon, H., & Kantz, K. R. (2007). Enhancing parent–child interaction through home visiting: Promising practice or unfulfilled promise. *Journal of Early Intervention, 29,* 119–140.

Peterson, N. (1987). *Early intervention for handicapped and at-risk children: An introduction to early childhood special education.* Love Publishing.

Pilkington, K. O. (2006). Side by side: Transdisciplinary early intervention in natural environments [Electronic Version]. *OT Practice, 11*(6), 12–17.

Raab, M. (2005). Interest-based child participation in everyday learning activities. *CASEinPoint, 1*(2), 1–5.

Rogelberg, S. G., Shanock, L. R., & Scott, C. W. (2012). Wasted time and money in meetings: Increasing return on investment. *Small Group Research, 43*(2), 236–245.

Rosenbaum, P., & Stewart, D. (2002). Alternative and complementary therapies for children and youth with disabilities. *Infants & Young Children, 15*(1), 51–59.

Rosenthal, R. (1994). Parametric measures of effect size. In H. Cooper & L.V. Hedges (Eds.), *The handbook of research synthesis* (pp. 231–244). Russell Sage Foundation.

Rosin, P., Whitehead, A. D., Tuchman, L. I., Jesien, G. S., Begun, A. L., Tuchman, L. I., & Irwin, L. (1996). *Partnerships in family-centered care: A guide to collaborative early intervention.* Paul H. Brookes Publishing Co.

Rush, D., Everhart, K., Sexton, S., & Shelden, M. (2020). The roadmap for assessing meaningful participation: Gathering information, participation-based assessment, and IFSP development. In M. McLean, R. Banerjee, J. Squires, & K. Hebbeler (Eds.), *DEC recommended practices monograph series No. 7: Assessment* (pp. 81–94). Division for Early Childhood of the Council for Exceptional Children.

Rush, D. D., & Shelden, M. L. (1996). On becoming a team: A view from the field. *Seminars in Speech and Language, 17*(2), 131–142.

Rush, D. D., & Shelden, M. L. (2005). Evidence-based definition of coaching practices. *CASEinPoint, 1*(6), 1–6.

Rush, D. D., & Shelden, M. L. (2020). *The early childhood coaching handbook* (2nd ed.). Paul H. Brookes Publishing Co.

Schreiber, J., Stern, P., Marchetti, G., Provident, I., & Turocy, P. S. (2008). School-based pediatric physical therapists' perspectives on evidence-based practice. *Pediatric Physical Therapy, 20*(4), 292–302.

Section on Pediatrics of the American Physical Therapy Association. (2010). *Team-based service delivery approaches in pediatric practice.* Retrieved from https://pediatricapta.org/includes/fact-sheets/pdfs/Service%20Delivery.pdf

Shelden, M. L., & Rush, D. D. (2007). Characteristics of a primary coach approach to teaming in early childhood programs. *CASEinPoint, 3*(1), 1–8.

Shelden, M. L., & Rush, D. D. (2010). A primary coach approach to teaming and supporting families in early childhood intervention. In R. A. McWilliam (Ed.), *Working with families of young children with special needs* (pp. 175–202). Guilford Press.

Shonkoff, J. P., Hauser-Cram, P., Krauss, M. W., & Upshur, C. C. (1992). Development of infants with disabilities and their families: Implications for theory and service delivery. *Monographs of the Society for Research and Child Development, 57*(6), 1–153.

Silver, L. B. (1995). Controversial therapies. *Journal of Child Neurology, 10*(1), S96–S100.

Silverman, K., Hong, S., & Trepanier-Street, M. (2010). Collaboration of teacher education and child disability health care: Transdisciplinary approach to inclusive practice for early childhood pre-service teachers. *Early Childhood Education Journal, 37*, 461–468.

Sloper, P. (2004). Facilitators and barriers for coordinated multi-agency services. *Child: Care, Health and Development, 30*(6), 571–580.

Sloper, P., Greco, V., Beecham, J., & Webb, R. (2006). Key worker services for disabled children: What characteristics of services lead to better outcomes for children and families? *Child: Care, Health and Development, 32*(2), 147–157.

Sloper, P., & Turner, S. (1992). Service needs of families of children with severe physical disability. *Child: Care, Health and Development, 18*(5), 259–282.

Soodak, L. C., & Erwin, E. J. (2000). Valued member or tolerated participant: Parents' experiences in inclusive early childhood settings. *Journal of The Association for Persons with Severe Handicaps, 25*, 29–41.

Spagnola, M., & Fiese, B. H. (2007). Family routines and rituals: A context for development in the lives of young children. *Infants & Young Children, 20*(4), 284–299. doi:10.1097/01.IYC.0000290352.32170.5a

Starfield, B., & Shi, L. (2004). The medical home, access to care, and insurance: A review of the evidence. *Pediatrics, 113*(Supplement 4), 1493–1498.

Stayton, V. D., Dietrich, S. L., Smith, B. J., Bruder, M. B., Mogro-Wilson, C., & Swigart, A. (2009). State certification requirements for early childhood special educators. *Infants & Young Children, 22*(1), 4–12.

Stormont, M., & Reinke, W. M. (2012). Using coaching to support classroom-level adoption and use of interventions within school-wide positive behavioral interventions and support systems. *Beyond Behavior, 21*(2), 11–19. Retrieved from https://files.eric.ed.gov/fulltext/ED540776.pdf

Swanson, J., Raab, M. R., Roper, N., & Dunst, C. J. (2006). Promoting young children's participation in interest-based everyday learning activities. *CASEtools, 2*(5), 1–22.

Tarr, J. E., & Barnett, W. S. (2001). A cost analysis of Part C early intervention services in New Jersey. *Journal of Early Intervention, 24*(1), 45–54.

Trivette, C. M., & Dunst, C. J. (2007). *Capacity-building family-centered help-giving practices.* Winterberry Press.

Trivette, C. M., Dunst, C. J., Hamby, D. W., & O'Herin, C. E. (2009). Characteristics and consequences of adult learning methods and strategies. *Practical Evaluation Reports, 2*(1), 1–32.

Tschantz, J. M., & Vail, C. O. (2000). Effects of peer coaching on the rate of responsive teacher statements during a child-directed period in an inclusive preschool setting. *Teacher Education and Special Education, 23*, 189–201.

Vanderhoff, M. (2004). Maximizing your role in early intervention. *PT: Magazine of Physical Therapy, 12*(12), 48–54.

Warfield, M. E. (1995). The cost-effectiveness of home visiting versus group services in early intervention. *Journal of Early Intervention, 19*, 130–148.

Warren, S. F., & Brady, N. C. (2007). The role of maternal responsivity in the development of children with intellectual disabilities. *Mental Retardation and Developmental Disabilities Research, 13*, 330–338.

Weaver, R. G., & Farrell, J. D. (1997). *Managers as facilitators: A practical guide to getting work done in a changing workplace.* Berret-Koehler.

Weller, J., Boyd, M., & Cumin, D. (2014). Teams, tribes and patient safety: Overcoming barriers to effective teamwork in healthcare. *Postgraduate Medical Journal, 90*, 149–154.

West, M. A. (2012). *Effective teamwork: Practical lessons from organizational research* (3rd ed.). Blackwell.

West, M. A., Brodbeck, F. C., & Richter, A. W. (2004). Does the 'romance of teams' exist? The effectiveness of teams in experimental and field settings. *Journal of Occupational and Organization Psychology, 77*, 467–473.

Winton, P. J., & McCollum, J. A. (2008). Preparing and supporting high-quality early childhood practitioners: Issues and evidence. In P. J. Winton, J. A. McCollum, & C. Catlett (Eds.), *Practical approaches to early childhood professional development: Evidence, strategies, and resources* (pp. 1–12). Zero to Three Press.

Wolery, M. (1983). Proportional change index: An alternative for comparing child change data. *Exceptional Children, 50*, 167–170.

Woodruff, G., & McGonigel, M. (1988). Early intervention team approaches: The transdisciplinary model. In L. J. Johnson, R. J. Gallagher, M. J. LaMontagne, J. B. Jordan, J. J. Gallagher, P. L. Huntinger, & M. B. Karnes (Eds.), *Early childhood special education: Birth to three* (pp. 163–181). Council for Exceptional Children.

Woods, J. (2008). Providing early intervention services in natural environments. *ASHA Leader, 13*(4), 14–17, 23.

Woods, J., Kashinath, S., & Goldstein, H. (2004). Effects of embedding caregiver-implemented teaching strategies in daily routines on children's communication outcomes. *Journal of Early Intervention, 26*(3), 175–193.

Woods, J. J., & Snyder, P. (2009). Interdisciplinary doctoral leadership training in early intervention: Considerations for research and practice in the 21st century. *Infants & Young Children, 22*(1), 32–43.

Workgroup on Principles and Practices in Natural Environments. (2007a, November). *Agreed upon practices for providing early intervention services in natural environments.* Retrieved from https://ectacenter.org/~pdfs/topics /families/AgreedUponPractices_FinalDraft2_01_08.pdf

Workgroup on Principles and Practices in Natural Environments. (2007b, November). *Mission and key principles for providing services in natural environments.* Retrieved from https://ectacenter.org/~pdfs/topics/families /Finalmissionandprinciples3_11_08.pdf

Workgroup on Principles and Practices in Natural Environments. (2007c, November). *Seven key principles: Looks like/doesn't look like.* Retrieved from https://ectacenter.org/~pdfs/topics/families/Principles_LooksLike_ DoesntLookLike3_11_08.pdf

York, J., Rainforth, B., & Giangreco, M. F. (1990). Transdisciplinary teamwork and integrated therapy: Clarifying the misconceptions. *Pediatric Physical Therapy, 2,* 73–79.

Zeng, B., Law, J., & Lindsay, G. (2012). Characterizing optimal intervention intensity: The relationship between dosage and effect size in interventions for children with developmental speech and language difficulties. *International Journal of Speech-Language Pathology, 14*(5), 471–477.

Zipoli, R. P., Jr., & Kennedy, M. (2005). Evidence-based practice among speech-language pathologists: Attitudes, utilization, and barriers. *American Journal of Speech-Language Pathology, 14,* 208–220.

Index

Note: Page numbers followed by *f* indicate figures and those followed by *t* indicate tables.